TSUBO

TSUBO

Vital Points for Oriental Therapy

by Katsusuke Serizawa, M. D.

Japan Publications, Inc.

© 1976 by Katsusuke Serizawa

Published by JAPAN PUBLICATIONS, INC., Tokyo and New York

Distributors:
UNITED STATES: *Kodansha International/USA, Ltd., through Harper & Row, Publishers, Inc., 10 East 53rd Street, New York, New York 10022.* SOUTH AMERICA: *Harper & Row, Publishers, Inc., International Department.* CANADA: *Fitzhenry & Whiteside Ltd., 195 Allstate Parkway, Markham, Ontario, L3R 4T8.* MEXICO AND CENTRAL AMERICA: *HARLA S. A. de C. V., Apartado 30–546, Mexico 4, D. F.* BRITISH ISLES: *International Book Distributors Ltd., 66 Wood Lane End, Hemel Hempstead, Herts HP2 4RG.* EUROPEAN CONTINENT: *Fleetbooks, S. A., c/o Feffer and Simons (Nederland) B. V., 61 Strijkviertel, 3454 PK De Meern, The Netherlands.* AUSTRALIA AND NEW ZEALAND: *Bookwise International, 1 Jeanes Street, Beverley, South Australia 5007.* THE FAR EAST AND JAPAN: *Japan Publications Trading Co., Ltd., 1–2–1, Sarugaku-cho, Chiyoda-ku, Tokyo 101.*

First edition: January 1976
Tenth printing: November 1987

ISBN 0–87040–350–8

Printed in Japan

Preface

Many people in the world today persist in believing that there is something inexplicably mystical about oriental medicine. It is true that oriental therapy can effect cures in cases of certain ailments for which Western medical science lacks explanations. But this success does not rest on miracles. Oriental medical science is a rational system organized around the theory of meridians and tsubo —the basic matter of this book—and substantiated by three thousand years of practical experience. In spite of—or perhaps because of—the differences in their philosophies, in recent years, oriental and occidental therapies have been approaching each other in many instances.

In the face of the stresses and frustrations of modern living, many people are afflicted with sicknesses that are psychological in origin. To a large extent, these sicknesses, which may take the forms of headaches, ringing in the ears, dizziness, palpitations, shortness of breath, and chills in the hands and feet, remain unexplained by Western medicine. Nor is this surprising, because the Western system, whereby the name of the sickness is first ascertained and then treatment is instituted, is balked by diseases for which there seem to be no namable physiological causes. Oriental therapy—particularly tsubo therapy— is able to solve problems that seem unsolvable by occidental methods because of the nature of its general approach. Oriental medicine acts on the belief that organic disorders reflect themselves at certain places on the body surface (these places are the tsubo) and conversely that pressure or other treatment on these places can not only relieve pathological symptoms, but also put the entire physical organism in good working condition. It is because oriental therapy can be used for both chronic symptoms and for psychologically caused sickness that it offers hope for further, more complete agreement with the medical science of the West.

This book presents a broad and detailed account of oriental medical philosophy, the theories of the meridians, and tsubo systems, and various kinds of treatments—massage, shiatsu massage, acupuncture, and moxa combustion— that can be used by the reader in the home to relieve conditions that may have been causes of extended suffering. The tsubo themselves are categorized in the text according to the twelve meridian systems governing body functions. The effects of treatment on the tsubo are carefully explained, the methods of treatment are set forth in detail, and the locations of the tsubo are shown on clear charts. The plan and content of the volume make it suitable for use by amateur and medical specialist alike.

In concluding these remarks, I should like to offer my warmest thanks to Iwao Yoshizaki, president of the Japan Publications, Inc; to Miss Yotsuko Watanabe and to Richard L. Gage, who translated the text into English.

December, 1975

KATSUSUKE SERIZAWA

CONTENTS

Tsubo by Energy Systems

Lung Meridian (肺経, *Fei-ching*)

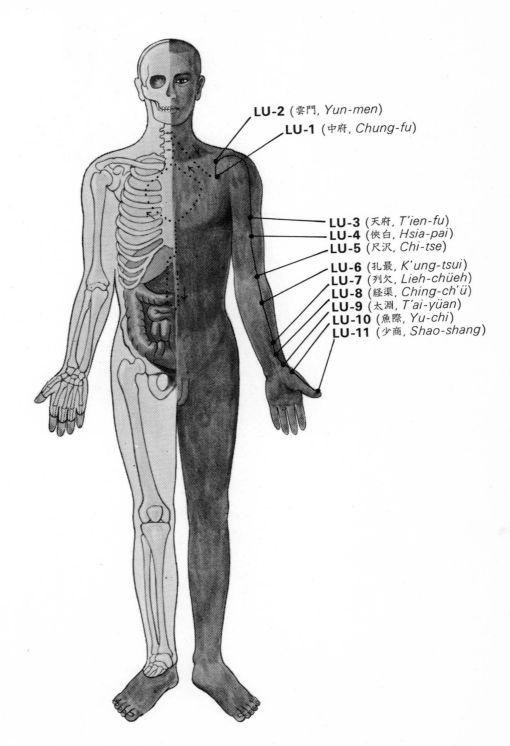

LU-2 (雲門, *Yun-men*)
LU-1 (中府, *Chung-fu*)

LU-3 (天府, *T'ien-fu*)
LU-4 (俠白, *Hsia-pai*)
LU-5 (尺沢, *Chi-tse*)

LU-6 (孔最, *K'ung-tsui*)
LU-7 (列欠, *Lieh-chüeh*)
LU-8 (経渠, *Ching-ch'ü*)
LU-9 (太淵, *T'ai-yüan*)
LU-10 (魚際, *Yu-chi*)
LU-11 (少商, *Shao-shang*)

Large Intestine Meridian (大腸経, *Ta-ch'ang-ching*)

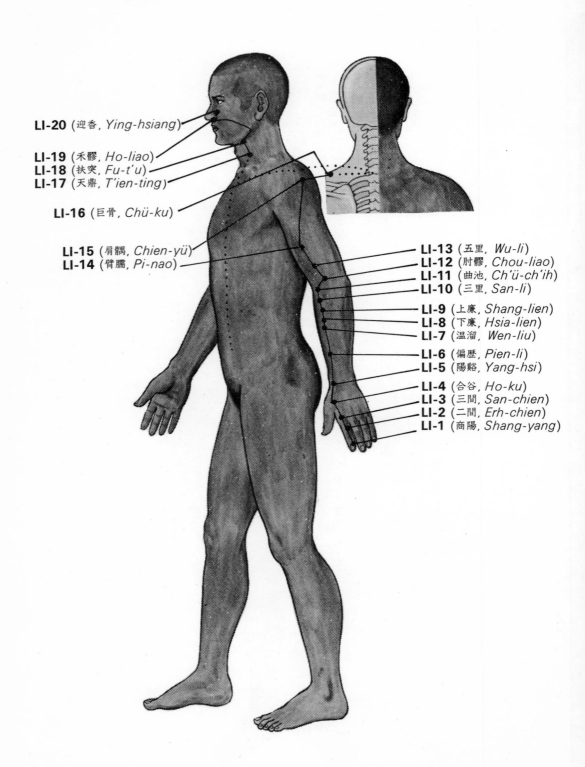

LI-20 (迎香, *Ying-hsiang*)

LI-19 (禾髎, *Ho-liao*)
LI-18 (扶突, *Fu-t'u*)
LI-17 (天鼎, *T'ien-ting*)

LI-16 (巨骨, *Chü-ku*)

LI-15 (肩髃, *Chien-yü*)
LI-14 (臂臑, *Pi-nao*)

LI-13 (五里, *Wu-li*)
LI-12 (肘髎, *Chou-liao*)
LI-11 (曲池, *Ch'ü-ch'ih*)
LI-10 (三里, *San-li*)

LI-9 (上廉, *Shang-lien*)
LI-8 (下廉, *Hsia-lien*)
LI-7 (温溜, *Wen-liu*)

LI-6 (偏歴, *Pien-li*)
LI-5 (陽谿, *Yang-hsi*)

LI-4 (合谷, *Ho-ku*)
LI-3 (三間, *San-chien*)
LI-2 (二間, *Erh-chien*)
LI-1 (商陽, *Shang-yang*)

Stomach Meridian (胃経, *Wei-ching*)

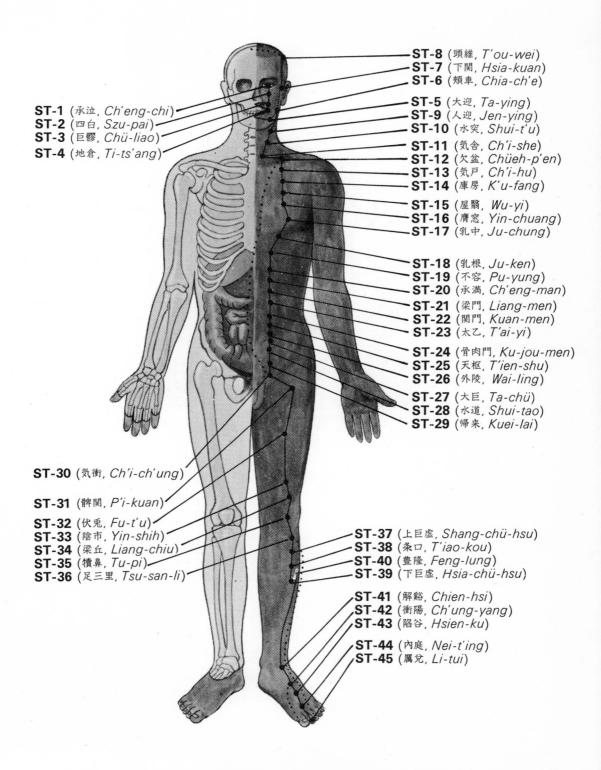

ST-8 (頭維, *T'ou-wei*)
ST-7 (下関, *Hsia-kuan*)
ST-6 (頬車, *Chia-ch'e*)

ST-1 (承泣, *Ch'eng-chi*)
ST-2 (四白, *Szu-pai*)
ST-3 (巨髎, *Chü-liao*)
ST-4 (地倉, *Ti-ts'ang*)

ST-5 (大迎, *Ta-ying*)
ST-9 (人迎, *Jen-ying*)
ST-10 (水突, *Shui-t'u*)

ST-11 (気舎, *Ch'i-she*)
ST-12 (欠盆, *Chüeh-p'en*)
ST-13 (気戸, *Ch'i-hu*)
ST-14 (庫房, *K'u-fang*)

ST-15 (屋翳, *Wu-yi*)
ST-16 (膺窓, *Yin-chuang*)
ST-17 (乳中, *Ju-chung*)

ST-18 (乳根, *Ju-ken*)
ST-19 (不容, *Pu-yung*)
ST-20 (承満, *Ch'eng-man*)
ST-21 (梁門, *Liang-men*)
ST-22 (関門, *Kuan-men*)
ST-23 (太乙, *T'ai-yi*)

ST-24 (骨肉門, *Ku-jou-men*)
ST-25 (天枢, *T'ien-shu*)
ST-26 (外陵, *Wai-ling*)

ST-27 (大巨, *Ta-chü*)
ST-28 (水道, *Shui-tao*)
ST-29 (帰来, *Kuei-lai*)

ST-30 (気衝, *Ch'i-ch'ung*)

ST-31 (髀関, *P'i-kuan*)

ST-32 (伏兎, *Fu-t'u*)
ST-33 (陰市, *Yin-shih*)
ST-34 (梁丘, *Liang-chiu*)
ST-35 (犢鼻, *Tu-pi*)
ST-36 (足三里, *Tsu-san-li*)

ST-37 (上巨虚, *Shang-chü-hsu*)
ST-38 (条口, *T'iao-kou*)
ST-40 (豊隆, *Feng-lung*)
ST-39 (下巨虚, *Hsia-chü-hsu*)

ST-41 (解谿, *Chien-hsi*)
ST-42 (衝陽, *Ch'ung-yang*)
ST-43 (陥谷, *Hsien-ku*)

ST-44 (内庭, *Nei-t'ing*)
ST-45 (厲兌, *Li-tui*)

Spleen Pancreas Meridian (脾経, *P'i-ching*)

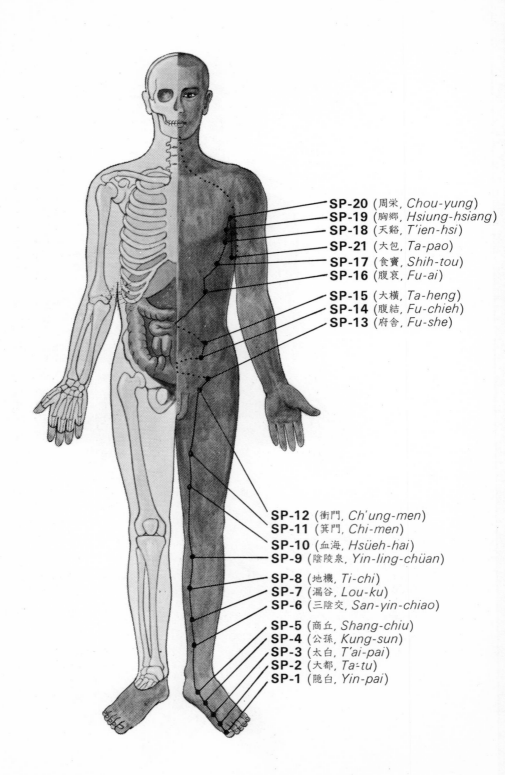

SP-20 (周栄, *Chou-yung*)
SP-19 (胸郷, *Hsiung-hsiang*)
SP-18 (天谿, *T'ien-hsi*)
SP-21 (大包, *Ta-pao*)
SP-17 (食竇, *Shih-tou*)
SP-16 (腹哀, *Fu-ai*)
SP-15 (大横, *Ta-heng*)
SP-14 (腹結, *Fu-chieh*)
SP-13 (府舎, *Fu-she*)

SP-12 (衝門, *Ch'ung-men*)
SP-11 (箕門, *Chi-men*)
SP-10 (血海, *Hsüeh-hai*)
SP-9 (陰陵泉, *Yin-ling-chüan*)
SP-8 (地機, *Ti-chi*)
SP-7 (漏谷, *Lou-ku*)
SP-6 (三陰交, *San-yin-chiao*)
SP-5 (商丘, *Shang-chiu*)
SP-4 (公孫, *Kung-sun*)
SP-3 (太白, *T'ai-pai*)
SP-2 (大都, *Ta-tu*)
SP-1 (隠白, *Yin-pai*)

Heart Meridian (心経, *Hsin-ching*)

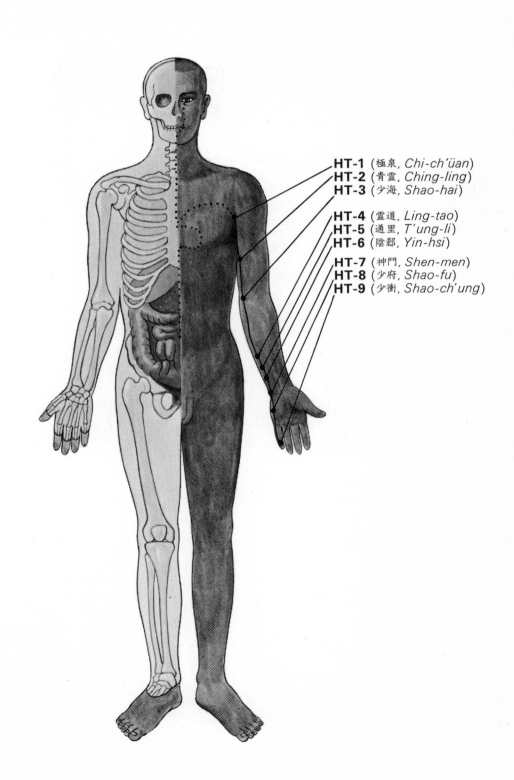

HT-1 (極泉, *Chi-ch'üan*)
HT-2 (青霊, *Ching-ling*)
HT-3 (少海, *Shao-hai*)

HT-4 (霊道, *Ling-tao*)
HT-5 (通里, *T'ung-li*)
HT-6 (陰郄, *Yin-hsi*)

HT-7 (神門, *Shen-men*)
HT-8 (少府, *Shao-fu*)
HT-9 (少衝, *Shao-ch'ung*)

Small Intestine Meridian (小腸経, *Hsiao-ch'ang-ching*)

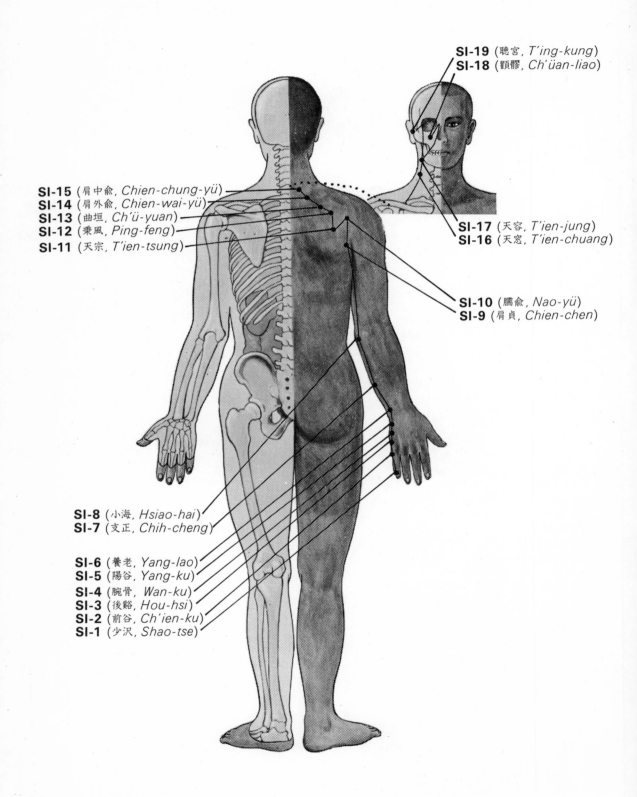

SI-19 (聴宮, *T'ing-kung*)
SI-18 (顴髎, *Ch'üan-liao*)

SI-15 (肩中兪, *Chien-chung-yü*)
SI-14 (肩外兪, *Chien-wai-yü*)
SI-13 (曲垣, *Ch'ü-yuan*)
SI-12 (秉風, *Ping-feng*)
SI-11 (天宗, *T'ien-tsung*)

SI-17 (天容, *T'ien-jung*)
SI-16 (天窓, *T'ien-chuang*)

SI-10 (臑兪, *Nao-yü*)
SI-9 (肩貞, *Chien-chen*)

SI-8 (小海, *Hsiao-hai*)
SI-7 (支正, *Chih-cheng*)

SI-6 (養老, *Yang-lao*)
SI-5 (陽谷, *Yang-ku*)
SI-4 (腕骨, *Wan-ku*)
SI-3 (後谿, *Hou-hsi*)
SI-2 (前谷, *Ch'ien-ku*)
SI-1 (少沢, *Shao-tse*)

Bladder Meridian (膀胱経, *P'an-kung-ching*)

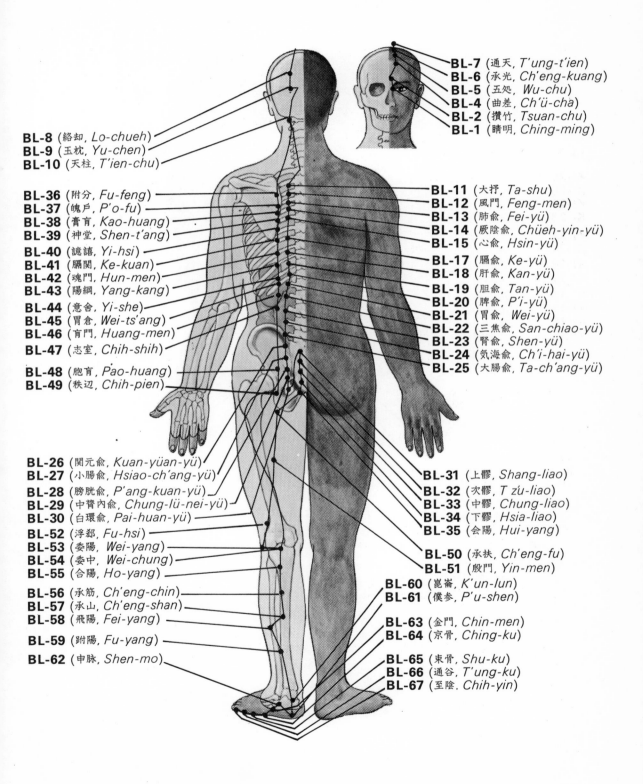

BL-7 (通天, *T'ung-t'ien*)
BL-6 (承光, *Ch'eng-kuang*)
BL-5 (五処, *Wu-chu*)
BL-4 (曲差, *Ch'ü-cha*)
BL-2 (攢竹, *Tsuan-chu*)
BL-1 (睛明, *Ching-ming*)

BL-8 (絡却, *Lo-chueh*)
BL-9 (玉枕, *Yu-chen*)
BL-10 (天柱, *T'ien-chu*)

BL-36 (附分, *Fu-feng*)
BL-37 (魄戸, *P'o-fu*)
BL-38 (膏肓, *Kao-huang*)
BL-39 (神堂, *Shen-t'ang*)
BL-40 (譩譆, *Yi-hsi*)
BL-41 (膈関, *Ke-kuan*)
BL-42 (魂門, *Hun-men*)
BL-43 (陽綱, *Yang-kang*)
BL-44 (意舎, *Yi-she*)
BL-45 (胃倉, *Wei-ts'ang*)
BL-46 (肓門, *Huang-men*)
BL-47 (志室, *Chih-shih*)
BL-48 (胞肓, *Pao-huang*)
BL-49 (秩辺, *Chih-pien*)

BL-11 (大抒, *Ta-shu*)
BL-12 (風門, *Feng-men*)
BL-13 (肺兪, *Fei-yü*)
BL-14 (厥陰兪, *Chüeh-yin-yü*)
BL-15 (心兪, *Hsin-yü*)
BL-17 (膈兪, *Ke-yü*)
BL-18 (肝兪, *Kan-yü*)
BL-19 (胆兪, *Tan-yü*)
BL-20 (脾兪, *P'i-yü*)
BL-21 (胃兪, *Wei-yü*)
BL-22 (三焦兪, *San-chiao-yü*)
BL-23 (腎兪, *Shen-yü*)
BL-24 (気海兪, *Ch'i-hai-yü*)
BL-25 (大腸兪, *Ta-ch'ang-yü*)

BL-26 (関元兪, *Kuan-yüan-yü*)
BL-27 (小腸兪, *Hsiao-ch'ang-yü*)
BL-28 (膀胱兪, *P'ang-kuan-yü*)
BL-29 (中膂内兪, *Chung-lü-nei-yü*)
BL-30 (白環兪, *Pai-huan-yü*)
BL-52 (浮郄, *Fu-hsi*)
BL-53 (委陽, *Wei-yang*)
BL-54 (委中, *Wei-chung*)
BL-55 (合陽, *Ho-yang*)
BL-56 (承筋, *Ch'eng-chin*)
BL-57 (承山, *Ch'eng-shan*)
BL-58 (飛陽, *Fei-yang*)
BL-59 (跗陽, *Fu-yang*)
BL-62 (申脉, *Shen-mo*)

BL-31 (上髎, *Shang-liao*)
BL-32 (次髎, *Tzú-liao*)
BL-33 (中髎, *Chung-liao*)
BL-34 (下髎, *Hsia-liao*)
BL-35 (会陽, *Hui-yang*)
BL-50 (承扶, *Ch'eng-fu*)
BL-51 (殷門, *Yin-men*)
BL-60 (崑崙, *K'un-lun*)
BL-61 (僕参, *P'u-shen*)
BL-63 (金門, *Chin-men*)
BL-64 (京骨, *Ching-ku*)
BL-65 (束骨, *Shu-ku*)
BL-66 (通谷, *T'ung-ku*)
BL-67 (至陰, *Chih-yin*)

Kidney Meridian (腎経, *Shen-ching*)

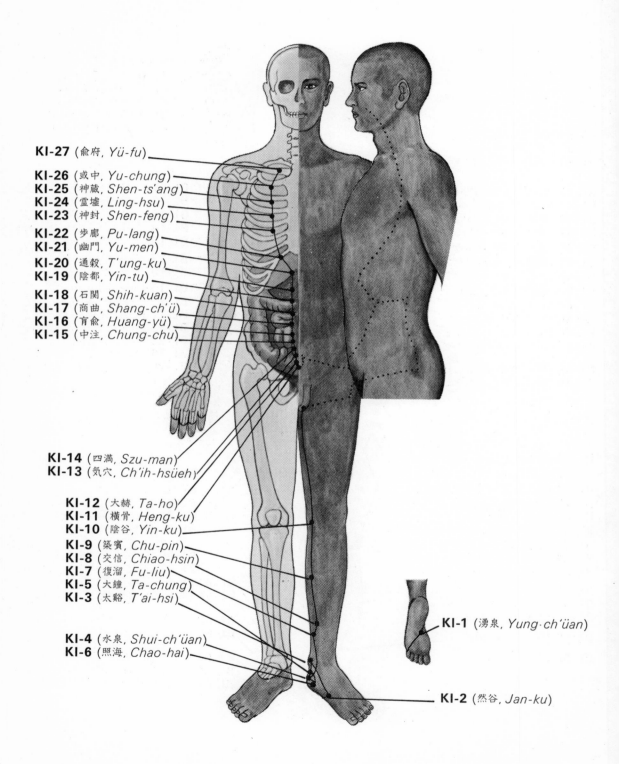

KI-27 (俞府, *Yü-fu*)

KI-26 (或中, *Yu-chung*)
KI-25 (神蔵, *Shen-ts'ang*)
KI-24 (霊墟, *Ling-hsu*)
KI-23 (神封, *Shen-feng*)

KI-22 (歩廊, *Pu-lang*)
KI-21 (幽門, *Yu-men*)
KI-20 (通穀, *T'ung-ku*)
KI-19 (陰都, *Yin-tu*)

KI-18 (石関, *Shih-kuan*)
KI-17 (商曲, *Shang-ch'ü*)
KI-16 (肓俞, *Huang-yü*)
KI-15 (中注, *Chung-chu*)

KI-14 (四満, *Szu-man*)
KI-13 (気穴, *Ch'ih-hsüeh*)

KI-12 (大赫, *Ta-ho*)
KI-11 (横骨, *Heng-ku*)
KI-10 (陰谷, *Yin-ku*)

KI-9 (築賓, *Chu-pin*)
KI-8 (交信, *Chiao-hsin*)
KI-7 (復溜, *Fu-liu*)
KI-5 (大鐘, *Ta-chung*)
KI-3 (太谿, *T'ai-hsi*)

KI-4 (水泉, *Shui-ch'üan*)
KI-6 (照海, *Chao-hai*)

KI-1 (湧泉, *Yung·ch'üan*)

KI-2 (然谷, *Jan-ku*)

Pericardium (Heart Constrictor) Meridian (心包経, *Hsin-pao-ching*)

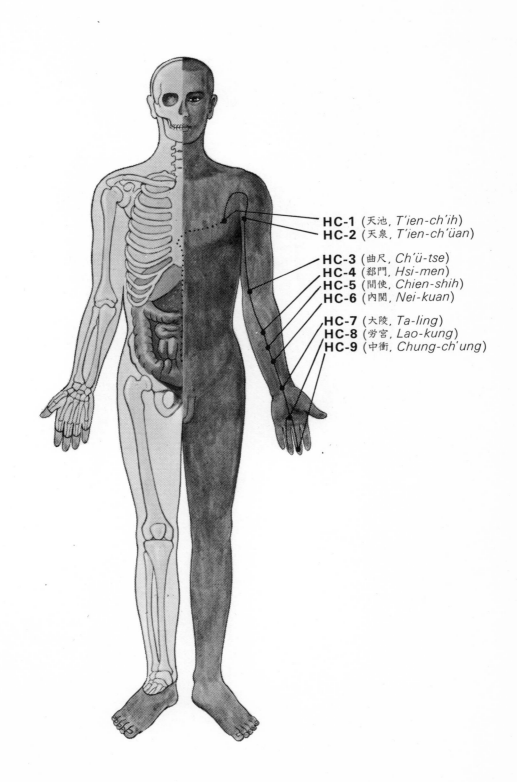

HC-1 (天池, *T'ien-ch'ih*)
HC-2 (天泉, *T'ien-ch'üan*)

HC-3 (曲尺, *Ch'ü-tse*)
HC-4 (郄門, *Hsi-men*)
HC-5 (間使, *Chien-shih*)
HC-6 (内関, *Nei-kuan*)

HC-7 (大陵, *Ta-ling*)
HC-8 (労宮, *Lao-kung*)
HC-9 (中衝, *Chung-ch'ung*)

Triple Heater Meridian (三焦経, *San-chiao-ching*)

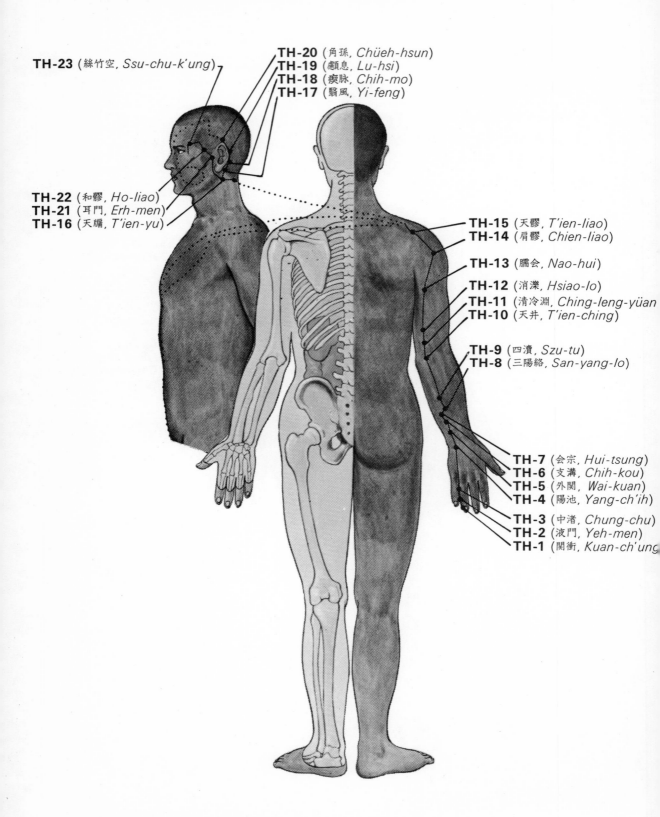

TH-23 (絲竹空, *Ssu-chu-k'ung*)

TH-20 (角孫, *Chüeh-hsun*)
TH-19 (顱息, *Lu-hsi*)
TH-18 (瘛脉, *Chih-mo*)
TH-17 (翳風, *Yi-feng*)

TH-22 (和髎, *Ho-liao*)
TH-21 (耳門, *Erh-men*)
TH-16 (天牖, *T'ien-yu*)

TH-15 (天髎, *T'ien-liao*)
TH-14 (肩髎, *Chien-liao*)

TH-13 (臑会, *Nao-hui*)
TH-12 (消濼, *Hsiao-lo*)
TH-11 (清冷淵, *Ching-leng-yüan*)
TH-10 (天井, *T'ien-ching*)

TH-9 (四瀆, *Szu-tu*)
TH-8 (三陽絡, *San-yang-lo*)

TH-7 (会宗, *Hui-tsung*)
TH-6 (支溝, *Chih-kou*)
TH-5 (外関, *Wai-kuan*)
TH-4 (陽池, *Yang-ch'ih*)

TH-3 (中渚, *Chung-chu*)
TH-2 (液門, *Yeh-men*)
TH-1 (関衝, *Kuan-ch'ung*)

Gall-Bladder Meridian (胆経, *Tan-ching*)

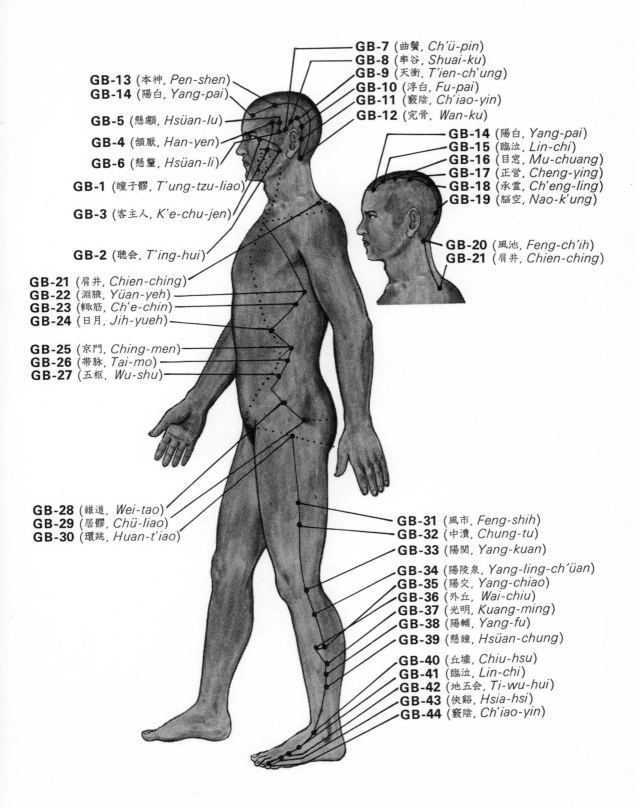

GB-7 (曲鬢, *Ch'ü-pin*)
GB-8 (率谷, *Shuai-ku*)
GB-9 (天衝, *T'ien-ch'ung*)
GB-10 (浮白, *Fu-pai*)
GB-11 (竅陰, *Ch'iao-yin*)
GB-12 (完骨, *Wan-ku*)

GB-13 (本神, *Pen-shen*)
GB-14 (陽白, *Yang-pai*)

GB-5 (懸顱, *Hsüan-lu*)
GB-4 (頷厭, *Han-yen*)
GB-6 (懸釐, *Hsüan-li*)

GB-1 (瞳子髎, *T'ung-tzu-liao*)

GB-3 (客主人, *K'e-chu-jen*)

GB-2 (聴会, *T'ing-hui*)

GB-14 (陽白, *Yang-pai*)
GB-15 (臨泣, *Lin-chi*)
GB-16 (目窓, *Mu-chuang*)
GB-17 (正営, *Cheng-ying*)
GB-18 (承靈, *Ch'eng-ling*)
GB-19 (脳空, *Nao-k'ung*)

GB-20 (風池, *Feng-ch'ih*)
GB-21 (肩井, *Chien-ching*)

GB-21 (肩井, *Chien-ching*)
GB-22 (淵腋, *Yüan-yeh*)
GB-23 (輒筋, *Ch'e-chin*)
GB-24 (日月, *Jih-yueh*)

GB-25 (京門, *Ching-men*)
GB-26 (帯脉, *Tai-mo*)
GB-27 (五枢, *Wu-shu*)

GB-28 (維道, *Wei-tao*)
GB-29 (居髎, *Chü-liao*)
GB-30 (環跳, *Huan-t'iao*)

GB-31 (風市, *Feng-shih*)
GB-32 (中瀆, *Chung-tu*)
GB-33 (陽関, *Yang-kuan*)

GB-34 (陽陵泉, *Yang-ling-ch'üan*)
GB-35 (陽交, *Yang-chiao*)
GB-36 (外丘, *Wai-chiu*)
GB-37 (光明, *Kuang-ming*)
GB-38 (陽輔, *Yang-fu*)
GB-39 (懸鐘, *Hsüan-chung*)

GB-40 (丘墟, *Chiu-hsu*)
GB-41 (臨泣, *Lin-chi*)
GB-42 (地五会, *Ti-wu-hui*)
GB-43 (俠谿, *Hsia-hsi*)
GB-44 (竅陰, *Ch'iao-yin*)

Liver Meridian (肝経, *Kan-ching*)

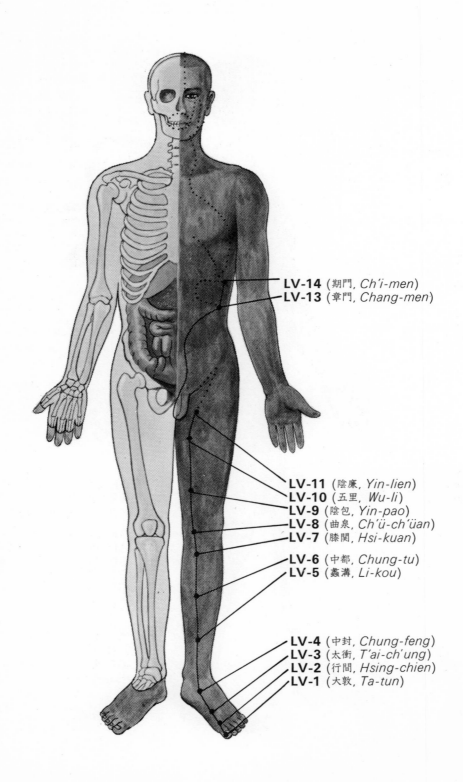

LV-14 (期門, *Ch'i-men*)
LV-13 (章門, *Chang-men*)

LV-11 (陰廉, *Yin-lien*)
LV-10 (五里, *Wu-li*)
LV-9 (陰包, *Yin-pao*)
LV-8 (曲泉, *Ch'ü-ch'üan*)
LV-7 (膝関, *Hsi-kuan*)

LV-6 (中都, *Chung-tu*)
LV-5 (蠡溝, *Li-kou*)

LV-4 (中封, *Chung-feng*)
LV-3 (太衝, *T'ai-ch'ung*)
LV-2 (行間, *Hsing-chien*)
LV-1 (大敦, *Ta-tun*)

Governing Vessel (督脈, *To-mo*)

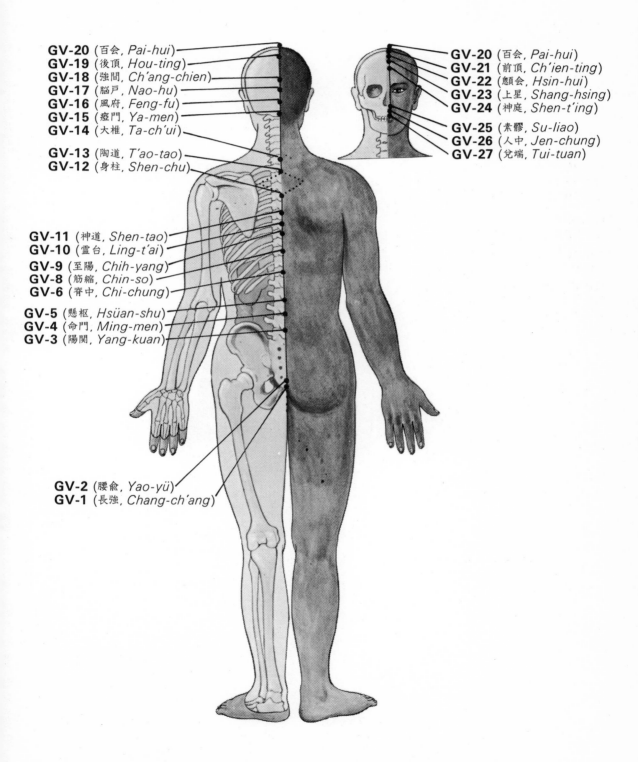

GV-20 (百会, *Pai-hui*)
GV-19 (後頂, *Hou-ting*)
GV-18 (強間, *Ch'ang-chien*)
GV-17 (脳戸, *Nao-hu*)
GV-16 (風府, *Feng-fu*)
GV-15 (瘂門, *Ya-men*)
GV-14 (大椎, *Ta-ch'ui*)

GV-13 (陶道, *T'ao-tao*)
GV-12 (身柱, *Shen-chu*)

GV-11 (神道, *Shen-tao*)
GV-10 (靈台, *Ling-t'ai*)
GV-9 (至陽, *Chih-yang*)
GV-8 (筋縮, *Chin-so*)
GV-6 (脊中, *Chi-chung*)

GV-5 (懸枢, *Hsüan-shu*)
GV-4 (命門, *Ming-men*)
GV-3 (陽関, *Yang-kuan*)

GV-2 (腰俞, *Yao-yü*)
GV-1 (長強, *Chang-ch'ang*)

GV-20 (百会, *Pai-hui*)
GV-21 (前頂, *Ch'ien-ting*)
GV-22 (顖会, *Hsin-hui*)
GV-23 (上星, *Shang-hsing*)
GV-24 (神庭, *Shen-t'ing*)

GV-25 (素髎, *Su-liao*)
GV-26 (人中, *Jen-chung*)
GV-27 (兌端, *Tui-tuan*)

Conception Vessel (任脈, *Ren-mo*)

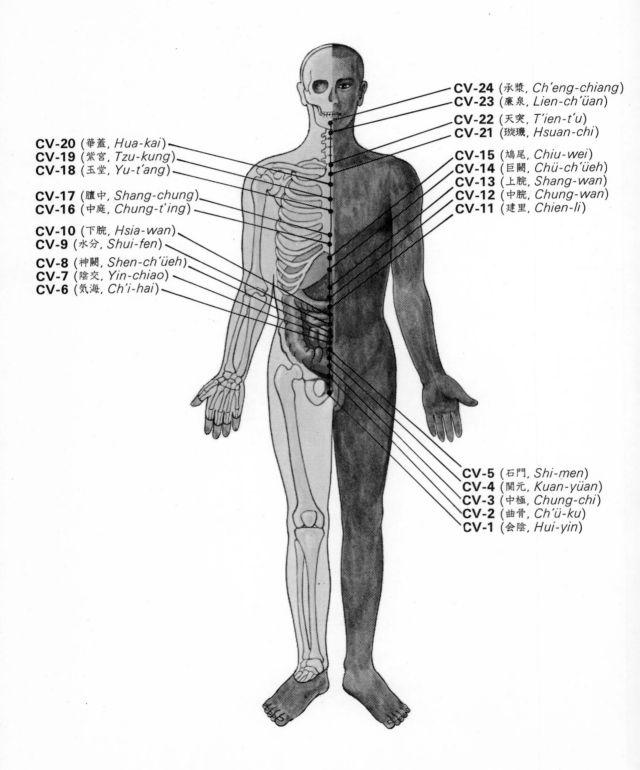

CV-24 (承漿, *Ch'eng-chiang*)
CV-23 (廉泉, *Lien-ch'üan*)
CV-22 (天突, *T'ien-t'u*)
CV-21 (璇璣, *Hsuan-chi*)

CV-20 (華蓋, *Hua-kai*)
CV-19 (紫宮, *Tzu-kung*)
CV-18 (玉堂, *Yu-t'ang*)

CV-15 (鳩尾, *Chiu-wei*)
CV-14 (巨闕, *Chü-ch'üeh*)
CV-13 (上脘, *Shang-wan*)
CV-12 (中脘, *Chung-wan*)
CV-11 (建里, *Chien-li*)

CV-17 (膻中, *Shang-chung*)
CV-16 (中庭, *Chung-t'ing*)

CV-10 (下脘, *Hsia-wan*)
CV-9 (水分, *Shui-fen*)
CV-8 (神闕, *Shen-ch'üeh*)
CV-7 (陰交, *Yin-chiao*)
CV-6 (気海, *Ch'i-hai*)

CV-5 (石門, *Shi-men*)
CV-4 (関元, *Kuan-yüan*)
CV-3 (中極, *Chung-chi*)
CV-2 (曲骨, *Ch'ü-ku*)
CV-1 (会陰, *Hui-yin*)

Bones and Muscles Important in Tsubo Therapy

The following charts show the locations of the major bones and muscles mentioned in the explanations of how to find the tsubo.

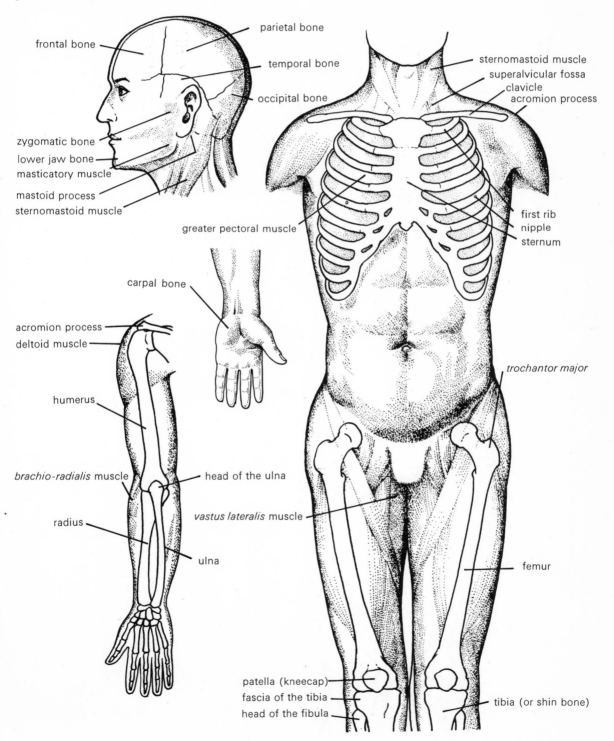

frontal bone

parietal bone

temporal bone

occipital bone

zygomatic bone

lower jaw bone

masticatory muscle

mastoid process

sternomastoid muscle

sternomastoid muscle

superalvicular fossa

clavicle

acromion process

greater pectoral muscle

first rib

nipple

sternum

carpal bone

acromion process

deltoid muscle

humerus

brachio-radialis muscle

radius

head of the ulna

vastus lateralis muscle

ulna

trochantor major

femur

patella (kneecap)

fascia of the tibia

head of the fibula

tibia (or shin bone)

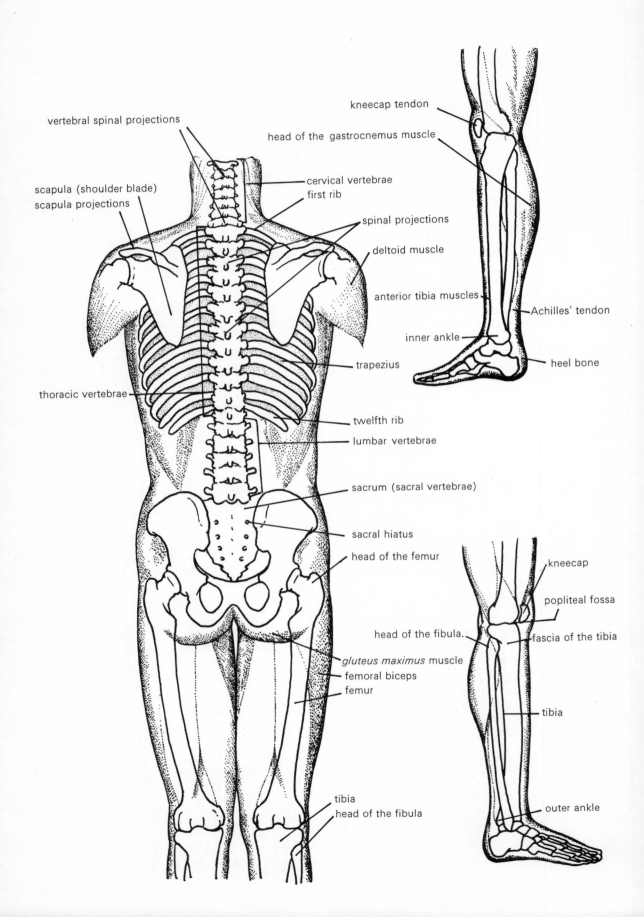

vertebral spinal projections

scapula (shoulder blade)
scapula projections

thoracic vertebrae

kneecap tendon

head of the gastrocnemus muscle

cervical vertebrae
first rib

spinal projections

deltoid muscle

anterior tibia muscles

Achilles' tendon

inner ankle

heel bone

trapezius

twelfth rib

lumbar vertebrae

sacrum (sacral vertebrae)

sacral hiatus

head of the femur

kneecap

popliteal fossa

head of the fibula.

fascia of the tibia

gluteus maximus muscle
femoral biceps
femur

tibia

tibia
head of the fibula

outer ankle

Chapter 1:
TSUBO THERAPY FOR TODAY

1. The Current of Development in Oriental Medicine

We have all experienced occasions in which confusion and vagueness made it necessary to "get to the point" in order to solve a problem. In Japan getting to the "point" is described as pressing the *tsubo*, a word meaning points on the human body, as shall be explained later. In matters of health and physical well-being too, the tsubo are of the greatest importance, for pressing, rubbing, or massaging them or applying acupuncture or moxa to them can relieve many symptoms of illness. The study and treatment of tsubo is a highly significant branch of oriental medicine. Although they are located on the surface of the body, the tsubo are not apparent like the eyes or the nose. It is not possible for the uninitiated person to locate them at once. When the method for finding them is understood, however, the tsubo can be used in treatments that bring about amazing results.

Some people argue that tsubo therapy to cure chronic sicknesses that are unresponsive to modern medical treatment is miraculous or accidental. In fact, however, both interpretations are wrong. Tsubo treatment is based on science and is a therapy of proved validity. A system evolved from three thousand years of medical experience, tsubo treatment can be put to excellent use in daily life in the home. But before explaining how this can be done, I shall discuss the background of oriental medicine and some of the ways in which it differs from occidental medicine.

Western medicine, today considered synonymous with modern medicine, has made great strides and is extremely important in fields in which new medicine's therapy, and application of physical energy can be used in treating certain kinds of sicknesses, in prescribing health regimens, in preventing diseases, and in devising rehabilitation plans. Oriental medicine, long the major medical philosophy in the East and the primary current of therapy in Japan until the late nineteenth century, is very different in approach and practice from the medicine of the West. The reason for the separation of oriental and occidental medicine in Japan is explained as the outcome of oriental medicine's failure to provide protection against contagious illnesses and to give relief from sudden acute inflammations and distress from such things as swelling, fevers, pain, and organic malfunctions. In addition, because it is devoted primarily to the treatment of the individual human being, the oriental medical system is lacking in mass applicability. Undeniably, oriental medicine has faults; but, in terms of promoting well-being and health and in the gradual development of power to resist illness and ability to relieve pain from the symptoms of sickness, it is no way inferior to the medical science of the West. Indeed, in these connections it has some deicided advantages over Western medical science. For this reason, medical scientists in other countries are reconsidering their own systems and the system of the Orient.

According to modern Western medical science, the doctor first diagnoses the sickness of the patient and gives it a name. He then proceeds to prescribe medicines, injections, and other treatment designed to cure that sickness. If he says the patient has a cold, the treatment is the general one given for colds; it is unlikely to take special consideration of the strength and physical characteristics of the specific patient. But if a man and his wife both catch colds, it cannot be the identical sickness since the two people are of different physical makeups and one is probably stronger, or weaker, than the other. An example of something similar is medication for the masses. Since such medication is designed for a broad segment of the population, it must have few harmful side effects. But its efficacy is greatly reduced because of the need to make it serve many different kinds of people. Though it is widely applicable and good for public uses, Western medical treatment fails to take into consideration the characteristics of the individual case. In order to assist the reader in understanding the tsubo-therapy system better and in grasping the differences between it and occidental medical science, I shall devote some space to a discussion of the historical background and the philosophy of oriental medicine.

In spite of the trend to reevaluate it, there are still people who regard oriental therapy as old-fashioned. Though it is not old-fashioned, it is undeniably old, for the Chinese medical system (*Kampo* as it is known in Japanese) has a tradition of three thousand years of development and use. In the past, it was clearly divided into the northern and the southern branch. The southern branch, which developed in the fertile lands south of the Yangtze River, employs herbs and barks, which are brewed or otherwise processed to produce medicines. The northern branch, however, grew up in the barren lands north of the Yellow River, where only low grasses dot the rocky ground. People living in this zone could not rely on herbal concoctions in time of sickness. From experience, however, they learned that stimulation on certain points on the body brings relief from pain. From this knowledge, they gradually evolved the systems of acupuncture, moxa, and massage (*amma*). These three constitute northern Chinese medicine. The massage system prescribes digital pressure or rubbing on the parts of the body that are in pain. Applications of such pressure cure numbness, stiffness, and chills in the affected parts. Over many years of practice and experience with massage, acupuncture, and moxa, the Chinese people came to understand the points on the body where such therapy produces maximum effects. These points are called the tsubo.

Although in its earliest stages Chinese medicine was divided into northern and southern branches, when the nation was unified under the Han dynasty (202 B.C. to A.D. 220), Chinese medicine too was unified into a single system. It was introduced into Japan in the sixth century, roughly a decade after the introduction of Buddhism (traditionally said to have come into Japan in 552). The physical therapies of acupuncture and moxa preceeded the use of medicines, because, it is said, the herbs and other materials needed for the preparation of medicines were likely to spoil during the many days then required to make the sea voyage from China to Japan. Chinese medicine reached a peak of popularity in Japan during the Edo period (1603–1867); but in the late part of this period, Western medical science as known in Germany and Holland began to influence Japanese thought, especially because of its surgical methods and its effectiveness against epidemics. Before long, Western methods had become the main topic of investigation and interest in Japanese medical fields. In recent years, however, as the number of illnesses that do not respond to Western medicine increases and as the limitations of Western medicine cause many people to reflect on its faults, reevaluations of oriental medicine are being made. The fact that oriental medicine has a long tradition of learned systematization reinforced by practical therapeutical application that has been scientifically verified speaks loudly in favor of such reevaluations. In China today Western medical science and traditional Chinese medicine are studied and used in parallel.

2. Oriental Medical Philosophy

When a patient suffers from a headache, stiff shoulders, congestion of the chest, overall sluggishness, numb feet and legs, or any other of a large number of ailments, the modern medical way to diagnose is first to give the sickness a name —cold, high blood pressure, asthma, and so on—and then to treat it. According to the oriental system, however, the physician first diagnoses the symptoms. After he discovers the subjective and objective manifestations of sickness in the patient and applies the distinctive Chinese approach to determine the patient's condition, the physician proceeds to prescribe therapy. Since the symptoms are interpreted on the basis of the patient's total condition, even such apparently localized complaints as inflammation of the ear or the nasal passages require total treatment. While devoted to the same general aim—the relief of suffering—medical practices in the East and in the West pursue different methodologies. In terms of both practical application and theory, Western medicine is based on a clinical approach. In contrast, oriental medicine is based on a system of thought explaining the human body as being composed of organs divided into two major categories: the five *Zo* organs (actually six) and the six *Fu* organs. If these organs work as they ought, the human being is in good health; but malfunctions in them cause illness.

Still more basic to oriental medicine and general thought than the five Zo and six Fu organs, however, is the concept of the two opposing forces, Yang and Yin, which control all nature. The sun and the moon, spring and autumn, north and south, day and night, and all other natural phenomena in the universe represent Yang, the active male element, and Yin, the passive female element. While representing these forces, everything in the natural world is controlled by five elements: wood, fire, earth, gold, and water. This is tantamount to saying that everything in the universe is composed of vegetable matter, heat, earth, minerals, and liquids. Though this system may seem simple to people accustomed to modern scientific and experimental explanations of the universe, the people of the distant past first pondered the nature of their own bodies and become more or less masters of their conditions as an outcome of this philosophy.

Since the human body is part of the world of nature—indeed, is a natural microcosm in itself—it is subject to the same laws that govern the universe. The male is the Yang force; the female is the Yin force, though each sex includes both Yin and Yang elements. The five Zo organs and the six Fu organs occur in Yang-Yin related pairs; and they are all composed of the five elements, wood, fire, earth, gold, and water. Furthermore, just as all things go through cyclical changes, so human beings, as parts of the universe, are borne, live active lives, die, and return to the earth. The weather is not always fair, nor is human life always the same. Sometimes, human beings work with vigor and force; sometimes they experience periods of inactivity and regression. Though we all feel good some of the time, we all experience days of poor physical condition. As the seasons of the year change in orderly cycle, so human beings undergo cyclical patterns of well-being and illness. The basis of oriental medicine is to consider the symptoms of illness as natural phenomena.

The five Zo and six Fu organs are the parts of the human body that enable us to fulfill our roles in the Yang-Yin, male-female, duality. It is necessary to offer a word of caution here, however, about the nature of these organs as interpreted in oriental medicine. Although the names of the organs in the Eastern system correspond to the names of organs as classified in Western medical science, the organs themselves are not always the same in the two systems. In oriental medicine, the five Zo organs are the following: liver, corresponding to the wood element; heart, corresponding to the fire element; spleen, corresponding to the earth element; lungs, corresponding to the gold element; and kidneys, corresponding to the water element. The Zo organs are the active (Yang) elements supporting life in the human body. As might be expected, they are assisted in their functions by passive (Yin) elements, which are the following Fu organs: gall bladder, small intestine, stomach, large intestine, urinary bladder, and *sansho*. The pairing of the Zo and Fu organs is as follows: liver with gall bladder, heart with small intestine, spleen with stomach, (in this case, the organ called spleen is what modern Western medical science calls the pancreas), lungs with large intestine, and kidneys with urinary bladder. In addition to these five pairs, there is one other traditionally held to work together for the well-being of the human body. The heart, as the most important of the organs, is thought to require and to have special protection, provided in the form of an enclosing sac called the *shinpo* (心包, *Hsin-pao*). This is the organ that works together with the sansho (三焦 *San-chiao*), the three sources of heat believed to supply the warmth that is characteristic of the human body throughout life.

People brought up on modern medical science may find this system entirely unconvincing, especially since it does not correspond with what dissection and the study of anatomy teach about the structure of the body. I can only ask that such people remember that oriental and occidental medical systems have grown and developed under the influences of very different religious and philosophical traditions. The important question is not which is right and which is wrong. From the standpoint of Western medical thought, the oriental system includes much that is difficult to accept. Attempting to find the points on which the two agree and performing research experiments in these areas can produce startling results. In fact, processes of this kind are now clarifying the shortcomings and merits of the two, but it seems that a union of them is unfortunately still a long way in the future. I therefore ask that my readers not equate the names of the Zo and Fu organs with those bearing the same names in modern medicine. Instead, the reader should think of them as the functions enabling the human body to live and work within the larger world of nature. This is not necessarily an unreasonable request, since most of us are not absolutely scientifically accurate in referring to our bodies when we have what is called a stomachache or a bodily upset.

The aim of oriental medicine is to take advantage of the miraculous flow of life as it exists, to ensure its well-being, to prevent sickness, and to improve physical appearance. Because the people of the West believe that human beings can alter nature with their own hands, they have evolved surgical methods to amputate bodily organs and even to replace them with artificial ones. Oriental medical philosophy, on the other hand, holds that the human being is only a part of nature. When man is out of line with the rules governing nature, his physical health fails. It follows, then, that to cure illness, the person must be restored to harmony with the rules of nature. The Zo and Fu organs are entrusted with the control of the human body in harmony with these natural rules.

3. Energy Systems: (経絡 *Ching-lo*)

In summary of the preceding material, I can say that the human body is controlled by five (actually six) Zo and six Fu organs. When these organs function normally, the body is in good health. When they malfunction, illness results. In order to explain how these organs are related to the tsubo of the body surface and why pressure, moxa, and acupuncture on the tsubo have therapeutic effects, I must explain the oriental concept of the energy that courses throughout the body from the top of the head to the tips of the toes. The energy for the proper operation of the Zo and Fu organs is provided by a total system divided into one system for each of the organs. The systems are called meridians. In other words, there are the following twelve meridians in the body: the lung meridian (肺経, *Fei-ching*), the large-intestine meridian (大腸経, *Ta-ch'ang-ching*), the stomach meridian (胃経, *Wei-ching*), the spleen-pancreas meridian (脾経, *P'i-ching*), the heart meridian (心経, *Hsin-ching*), the small-intestine meridian (小腸経, *Hsiao-ch'ang-ching*), the bladder meridian (膀胱経, *P'ang-kuang-ching*), the kidney meridian (腎経, *Shen-ching*), the pericardium meridian (心包経, *Hsin-pao-ching*), the triple heater meridian (三焦経, *San-chiao-ching*), the gall-bladder meridian (胆経, *Tan-ching*), and the liver meridian (肝経, *Kan-ching*). Energy travels through the body, beginning at the lung meridian, proceeding through the other meridians in the order listed here, and returning to the lung meridian after having passed through the liver meridian.

Deficiencies and excesses in energy in the systems determine whether the person is healthy or ill. To make possible adjustments of the intensities of energy in the twelve basic systems, there are eight subsystems in the body. These subsystems are called *keimyaku* (経脈, *ching-me*, or vessels.). Of the eight subsystems, the most important are these: the *jinmyaku* (仁脈, *ren-me*, conception vessel), which runs through the center of the front surface of the body from the center of the face through the chest and the abdomen; and the *tokumyaku* (督脈, *tu-me*, governing vessel), which runs down the center of the back of the body from the buttocks, along the spine, and up the neck. In Chinese medicine, these two subsystems are considered paramount in the control of the energy coursing through the body.

The systems and subsystems transport blood and energy (*ki* in Japanese and *ch'i* in Chinese) through the body. According to oriental medical theory, the human being receives a certain amount of energy from his mother at birth and takes in additional energy through the mouth and nose during life. This additional supply reinforces and amplifies the energy received at birth and ensures that circulation through the body is smooth and strong enough to support the functioning of the organs on whose operation life depends. The meridian systems are the paths along which blood and energy are transported to the organs. A slight reduction in the flow causes sickness; cessation of the flow causes death.

In keeping with the oriental belief that everything depends on the opposing forces of Yin and Yang, the energy transportation systems and subsystems of the body are divided into Yin and Yang categories: those associated with the six Zo organs are Yang, and those associated with the six Fu organs are Yin. Symptoms too are divided into Yang and Yin classes. Yang symptoms occurring on the front of the body are called *Yomei* (*Yang-ming*); Yin symptoms occurring on the front of the body are called *Tai'in* (*T'ai-yin*). Yang symptoms occurring on the side of the body are called *Shoyo* (*Shao-yang*); Yin symptoms on the side of the body are called *Ketsuin* (*Chüeh-yin*). Yang symptoms occurring on the back of the body are called *Taiyo* (*T'ai-yang*); and Yin symptoms there are called *Shoin* (*Shao-yin*). Since the stomach energy system belongs to the Fu category, symptoms for it should be described as Yomei, because they are Yang symptoms on the front of the body, and *Ikei*, because they affect the stomach system.

4. Causes of Sickness

Oriental medicine defines two major categories of causes of sickness: external and internal. Both kinds of causes have harmful effects on the body since they retard the energy flow in the meridian systems. The bodies of all human beings are constantly being affected by climate, external temperatures, winds, and the changes of the seasons. Cold may make us uneasy; hot, humid weather makes us sluggish. A bright spring day, on the other hand, makes most people feel fresh and alert. On windy or stormy days, many of us are restless and uneasy. But the natural environment does more than affect the emotions of the human being; acting through the skin, it strongly influences the nerves, the motor system, and the internal organs. Indeed, it is because of the influence of the natural environment on our nerves and motor systems that we have emotional responses to cold, warmth, and so on. As long as the internal bodily functions are able to respond smoothly and efficiently to external influences, the body remains in good health. Unpleasantness arises when responses to these influences are no longer satisfactory. The functioning of the Zo and Fu organs becomes upset with such disagreeable consequences as stomach disturbance, numbness in the hands and feet, and loss of luster in the skin.

Though we are all parts of the natural environment, we must live in human society as well and must therefore maintain many different human relations, some of which are very demanding. The affairs of school, work, family life, and parental duties create emotional and mental situations that are sometimes upsetting. The happiness, anger, anxiety, concern, sadness, shocks, and fears of daily life might be considered as unrelated directly to bodily well-being. But the relationship is undeniable. Oriental medical thought regards these seven emotions —the seven emotional disturbances—as highly important internal causes of sickness. Because they upset the mind, these disturbances immediately affect the functioning of the five Zo and six Fu organs. In addition, excess worry about family matters, mental suffering resulting from the desire for worldly success, gluttony, too much alcohol, and obsessions with sex produce imbalances that generate illnesses. Causes of this kind are neither exclusively internal nor exclusively external. Stagnation of the flow of energy in the meridian systems and malfunctioning of the organs and bodily tissues produce various pathological symptoms.

5. Tsubo

The points called tsubo lie along the fourteen meridian systems—twelve basic systems and two control systems—that extend over the entire body and to the internal organs. Though invisible to the eye, these points, or tsubo, are the locations at which it is easy for the flow of energy in the meridian systems to become sluggish and to stagnate. When the energy flow slows down in the systems associated with organs, malfunctions occur. What happens in the meridian systems might be compared to the way water acts in a hose. Flowing freely from the main, water passes easily along the full length of the hose as long as there is no obstruction. But if something constricts the hose at some point, the flow of water will alter. The point of constriction corresponds to a tsubo in the meridian systems. When there is a malfunction in the Zo or Fu organs, it is manifested in the tsubo in many different ways: pain, numbness, a sense of pressure, stiffness, chills, flushing, spots, small discolorations, depositions of pigment (freckles and so on), and peculiarities in the electrical charges of the skin.

To know which tsubo to employ in therapeutic treatment, it is necessary to know which meridian system is affected. For instance, the tsubo that must be treated to cure a stomachache are different depending on whether the trouble arises as a result of abnormality in the lungs or in the liver. For this reason, oriental medicine insists that each patient be treated as an individual case. It is less important pain and learning what the body wants done to bring about a cure. The complaint may not be cured by a single treatment, for the body may replace one kind of pain signal with another. But if all of the complaint-reactions are treated systematically, one by one, the body will return to the rhythm that is in keeping with the laws of nature. The tsubo are determining factors in reestablishing this rhythm.

There are 365 tsubo on the human body. They occur in places that are physically weak; for example, the depressions at the junctures of muscles, places under the skin where nerves emerge from muscles, the trunks of muscles and nerves, and the spaces between wrinkles in the skin. Sometimes compound alterations in the body make it impossible to observe all of the tsubo, but in technical terms, it is possible to say that, from the standpoint of the physical mechanism of the structure of the human body, the tsubo are weak spots where organic disturbances produce powerful reflex actions.

Throughout my long experience with diagnosis according to tsubo, I have devoted much thought to determining whether this system is rational. In one instance, I conducted clinical comparisons between fifty healthy controls and fifty people suffering from various sicknesses. I examined their pulse rates, the electrical resistance of their skin, and their electromyograms. Allowing for some individual differences, I proved conclusively that skin and muscular alterations in sick people are concentrated in the regions of the tsubo.

6. Effectiveness of Tsubo Therapy

The tsubo treatment for hemorrhoids is to apply pressure, moxa, or acupuncture to tsubo located on the head. Since the treatment works in spite of the apparent lack of relation between the ailing part of the body and the part treated, some people might regard it as miraculous. But it is not. As I have stressed in earlier sections of this book, oriental medical philosophy is basically practical. In extreme terms, its approach is that the cause of the sickness is less important than the symptoms. If the symptoms are accurately understood, the efficacy of treatment is virtually guaranteed.

Although experience has provided oriental medicine with a rich store of undoubtedly effective treatments, experimental research into the reasons for their effectiveness did not begin until this century and is still inadequate. At present, there are many explanations of the operations of the meridian systems and the tsubo. Some modern medical scientists argue that the phenomenon is related to nervous reflexes and especially to the reflex system connecting the internal organs and body walls. Others insist that the working of the Zo and Fu organs and the energy circulation system as explained in the classical Chinese texts is clinically valid and that it represents a flowing fluid different in kind from what modern science explains as nervous functions and blood transportation. Further, Dr. Bonhan Kim of the University of Pyongyang, in Korea, claims to have proved that the meridian systems and the tsubo actually exist in the body tissues. But, on the basis of its usefulness in clinical interpretation and application, I believe that the modern scientific explanation of the meridian systems and the tsubo as nerve reflex action is the most satisfactory. Though it is possible that, in the future, other superior explanations may emerge, I shall use this one as the basis of my discussions.

In brief, the nerve-reflex theory holds that, when an abnormal condition occurs in an internal organ, alterations take place in the skin and muscles related to that organ by means of the nervous system. These alterations occur as reflex actions. The nervous system, extending throughout the internal organs, the skin, the subcutaneous tissues, and the muscles, constantly transmit information about the physical condition to the spinal chord and the brain. These information impulses, which are centripetal in nature, set up a reflex action that causes symptoms of the internal organic disorder to manifest themselves in the surface areas of the body. The reflex symptoms may be classified into the following three major groups: a. sensation reflexes, b. interlocking reflexes, c. autonomic-system reflexes.

a. *Sensation reflexes.* When an abnormal centripetal impulse travels to the spinal chord, reflex action causes the skin at the level of the spinal column affected by the impulse to become hypersensitive. This sensitivity to pain is especially notable in the skin, subcutaneous tissues, and muscles located close to the surface, since these organs are richly supplied with sensory nerves.

b. *Interlocked reflexes.* An abnormality in an internal organ causes a limited contraction, stiffening, or lumping of the muscles in the area near the part of the body that is connected by means of nerves to the afflicted organ. Stiffness in the shoulders, back, arms, and legs are symptoms of this kind. In effect, the interlocked reflex actions amount to a hardening and stiffening of the muscles to protect the ailing internal organ from excess stimulus. When the abnormality in the organ is grave, however, the stiffening of the muscles is not limited to a small area, but extends over large parts of the body. When this stage is reached, the conditions is too serious for home therapy. A specialist must be consulted.

c. *Autonomic-system reflexes.* Abnormalities in the internal organs sometimes set up reflex action in the sweat glands, the sebaceous glands, the pilomotor muscles, and the blood vessels in the skin. The reflex action may cause excess sweat or drying of the skin as the consequence of cessation of sweat secretion. Its effect on the pilomotor muscles may be to cause the condition known as goose flesh. The sebaceous glands may be stimulated to secrete excess sebum, thus causing abnormal oiliness in the skin; or they may stop secreting sebum, thus making the skin abnormally dry. The reflex action may cause chills or flushing because of its effects on the blood vessels in the skin.

I have discussed the ways in which abnormalities in internal organs cause changes in the conditions of the surface organs of the body. But the intimate relation between internal organs and external ones has a reverse effect as well; that is, stimulation to the skin and muscles affects the condition of the internal organs and tissues, since impulses from the outside are transmitted to the inside by means of the spinal chord and the nervous system. For instance, stimulation transmitted to the spinal chord sets up a reflex action in the internal organ that is controlled by the nerves at the level of the spinal column corresponding to the height of the place at which the external stimulus was applied. Stimuli of this kind instigate peristaltic motion or contraction in the organ. The effect of such external stimulation on blood vessels and on the secretion of hormones has been scientifically verified.

Tsubo therapy makes use of the reflex phenomenon by applying massage pressure, shiatsu pressure, moxa, or acupuncture to the skin in order to moderate malfunctions of the internal organs. In other words, to relieve numbness or chilling caused by a distress signal from the nerves to the central nervous system, tsubo therapy employs a different kind of stimulus from a different direction to counter the one causing the distress. Electromyograms and studies of the electrical resistance of the skin reveal that stimulus can remove such symptoms as chilling and stiffness. My own daily research has proved that tsubo therapy can be used against skin and muscle symptoms to cure internal disorders and to return body functions to normality. Recently, it has been learned that injections are more effective if administered in one of the tsubo on the body surface.

7. Limitations of Tsubo Therapy

It is true that tsubo therapy is effective against some of the ailments that modern medicine fails to cure, but it does not work against all of them. Oriental medicine is used to treat the individual in certain cases, but it is powerless to cure victims of such illnesses as cancer, malignant tumors, neoplasms, typhus, dysentery, cholera, severe tuberculosis, syphilis, or contagious skin diseases. Sicknesses clearly caused by bacteria, like acute high fevers and contagious diseases, must be left to modern medical science, which is better equipped to treat them and to offer protection from them. Nor can tsubo therapy do anything to help victims of cerebral hemorrhage, hardening of the blood vessels, in the brain, softening of the brain, or damage to the blood vessels of the brain.

The ailments from which tsubo therapy can offer relief, however, are numerous and include the following: symptoms of chilling; flushing; pain, and numbness; neuralgia; parallelismus; headaches; heaviness in the head; dizziness; ringing in the ears; stiff shoulders arising from disorders of the autonomic nervous system; constipation; sluggishness; chills of the hands and feet; insomnia; malformations of the backbone frequent in middle age and producing pain in the shoulders, arms, and hands; pains in the back; pains in the knees experienced during standing or going up or down stairs. In short, tsubo therapy is more useful in treating ailments in which there is no, or only slight, organic malformation and in which the cause is functional. It is less effective against sicknesses caused by serious irregularities in the organs. It is especially good in cases of people who suffer from no definite illness, but who are sluggish, lack appetite, tire easily, have poor facial color, and are upset in the stomach or intestines. Tsubo treatment can bring relief in such cases because it is not only a specific treatment, but also a regimen designed to promote general health.

Chapter 2:
TREATMENT IN GENERAL

1. Before Treatment

(1) Locations of the tsubo

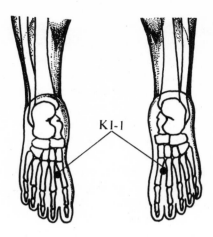

KI-1

The locations of the tsubo are indicated on the charts of the human body in this book. In cases where space permits, the tsubo are shown in pairs, for this is how they usually occur. This presentation is feasible in charts of the shoulders, back, and abdomen. In the cases of the head, neck, hands, and feet, however, the small sizes of the drawings make it difficult to indicate both of each pair of tsubo. Consequently, for the sake of clarity, only one of each is shown. For instance, a tsubo shown on the sole of the right foot has a corresponding partner on the sole of the left foot, though it may not appear on the charts. There are slight differences in the locations of the tsubo depending on the physical makeup of the individual human being. The locations given in the charts of this book are the standard ones. To find the actual ones on the patient's body, rub or press with the fingers in a given diameter around the location given as standard. Even when only one tsubo of a pair is shown on the chart, remember that you must treat both. Arrows are used to indicate the meridian systems.

In describing the locations of the tsubo, I use traditional, relative measurement terms called *sun* and *bu*. One sun is determined as follows. When the person being treated makes a circle by bringing the tip of the middle finger to the tip of the thumb, one sun is the length of the second joint of the middle finger. Or one sun can be the width of the thumb of the person receiving treatment. Five bu are half of one sun.

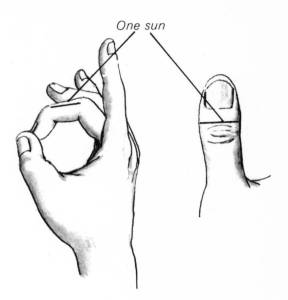

One sun

(2) How to find the tsubo

Rubbing, pinching, and pressing

I have heard complaints that treatment on the tsubo has produced no effect, even when performed according to reliable directions. But in most cases of this kind, the person has been treating what he thought was the correct places without accurately locating the tsubo. Unless treatment is applied directly to the tsubo, effective therapy cannot be expected. In the next few pages, I shall discuss the way to locate the tsubo.

The three methods of finding the tsubo on the patient are these: lightly rubbing the skin, gently pinching the flesh while moving it back and forth, gently pressing the skin with the thumbs or with the four fingers. Once the general location of the tsubo has been determined, check by rubbing the

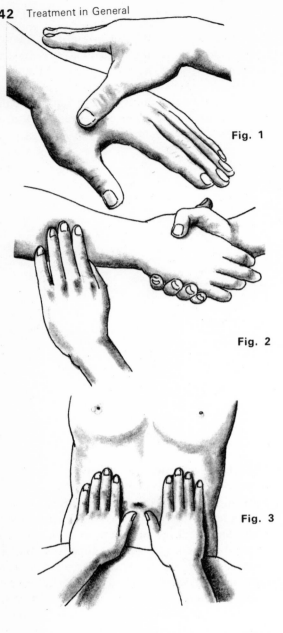

Fig. 1

Fig. 2

Fig. 3

area, then by pinching it, and finally by pressing it. Do not exert great pressure while rubbing and, in pressing, use no more than from three to five kilograms of pressure (bathroom scales are a useful device to gauge the pressure you are exerting).

First lightly touch the tsubo on the right and left sides of the body with both hands. Depending on the part of the body being examined, you must use the hands differently: for the wrists and ankles, touch with the thumbs (Fig. 1); for the arms, legs, and neck, use all four fingers (index, middle, fourth, and little fingers; Fig. 2); for broad areas like the back and the abdominal region, use the palms of the hands (Fig. 3). If the part of the body being investigated is healthy, the skin will feel the same to both hands. If there is an abnormal situation, however, the skin will either be hypersensitive or will feel as if you were touching it through a thin layer of cloth; that is, it will lack sensitivity.

When you have located the site of the abnormal condition, pinch the skin and flesh between your thumb and index finger (Fig. 4) and move it back and forth about four times (Figs. 5 and 6). (People skilled in tsubo therapy can determine the exact location by moving the flesh back and forth only once.) This method is used to determine abnormalities in the subcutaneous tissues. These disorders, as have been explained in the preceding chapter, arise from disorders in the internal organs. If there is something wrong with the patient, you will notice that there is a difference between the way the flesh on the right and left sides of the body feels when pinched. Once again, the difference will be a matter of sensitivity. The flesh will be either hypersensitive or insensitive.

Fig. 4   Fig. 5   Fig. 6

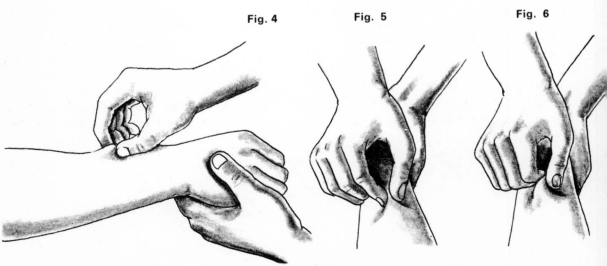

Next use pressure to determine the disorder in the skin, the subcutaneous tissues, the membranes surrounding the muscles, and the muscles themselves. You will be able to tell whether these organs are in pain, are in a state of contraction, or are tense. To find out whether the stiffness is in small spots, lumps, or bands, rotate the balls of your fingers as you apply pressure with them (Figs. 7 and 8).

In looking for the tsubo on the back and abdomen, use the fingers of both hands but be careful to exert equal pressure with them. In this case, pressure of from three to five kilograms should be applied for from three to five seconds. Generally, the patient will lie face-up or face-down or will sit when he has someone examine the tsubo of his body (Figs. 9 and 10). When the tsubo on the back or hips are being examined, the patient must, of course, lie face-down. At this time, the arms of the patient must be at right angles to his spinal column (Fig. 11). During massage or shiatsu treatment, however, the arms may be put in any comfortable position.

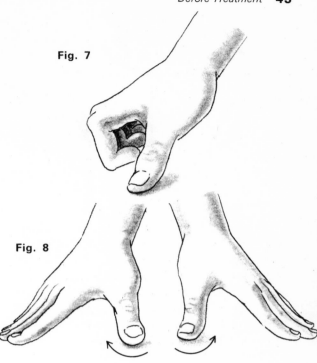

Fig. 7

Fig. 8

Fig. 9

Fig. 10

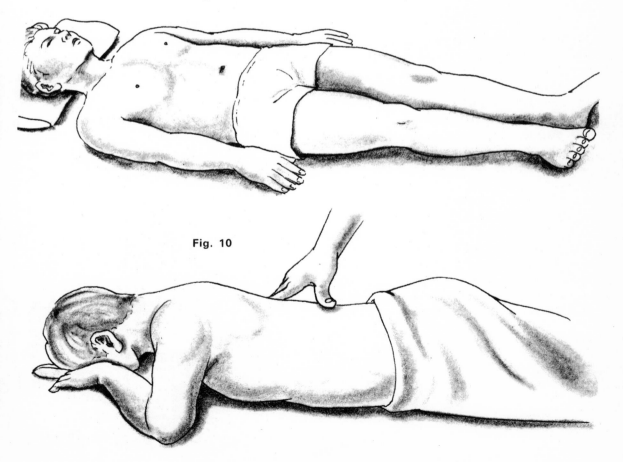

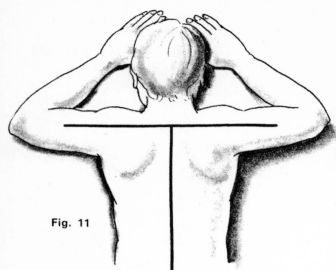

Fig. 11

To summarize the way to look for tsubo then, the process is in three stages. First, rub the skin to test the surface of the body. Next, pinch the flesh to examine the state of the subcutaneous tissues. Finally, press the flesh to examine the condition of the deeper organs. You may feel certain that you have accurately located the tsubo if in the region tested you encounter any of the following symptoms: pain, numbness, stiffness, chills, flushing, small eruptions or rashes, stains or freckless in more than the ordinarily expected quantities, muscular stiffness or tension in band-shaped zones.

When tsubo are hard to find

Sometimes the absence of the symptoms mentioned in the preceding section makes the tsubo hard to locate when it is imperative to find them for treatment designed to contribute to good health or to fulfill some cosmetic purpose. In such instances, the important thing is to understand the locations of the muscles, since, as I have already said, the tsubo are located along the meridian systems, which run in grooves between muscles. The muscles manifest themselves through the skin in different ways in different parts of the body; consequently, to locate a muscle, tense that part of the body. For instance, have the patient bend backward to reveal the muscles of the back. If you are looking for tsubo on the arm, have the patient lie face-down and raise his arms to the side as far as he can. The

muscles of the back of the neck are clearly revealed on the sides of the spinal column. To examine the muscles of the sides of the neck, have the patient turn his face as far to the side as possible. The large muscle in the front of the neck (the sternomastoid muscle) is usually prominent. To make the large muscles of the chest clearly visible, raise both arms to the sides, tense them, and bring them slightly forward. To make the tsubo in the abdominal and side regions easier to locate, have the patient lie face-up and slightly raise his upper body. The muscles in the underside of the forearm become prominent if the elbow is bent and then the wrist is turned in one direction or the other. The muscles on the outer side of the forearm are best seen if the elbow and the wrist are extended. Have the patient spread his legs, extend his knee, and raise his leg to reveal the muscles of the front of the groin and the underside of the thigh.

Finding tsubo with the help of the charts

In explaining the locations of the tsubo it is impossible to avoid such specialized terminology as the *spinal processes of the first cervical vertebra* or the *spinal processes of the third thoracic vertebra*. To help you locate the point you are seeking, I shall give concrete explanations of the procedure to follow. I shall take the tsubo designated GV-14 as my first example.

GV-14 (大椎, *Ta-ch'ui*) is located between the spinal process of the seventh cervical vertebra and the spinal process of the first thoracic vertebra. When you turn your head forward and backward, the bones in the neck that move are the cervical vertebrae. The seventh is the lowest of them.

Fig. 1

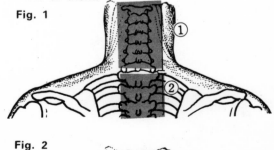

Fig. 2

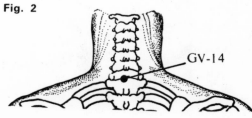

GV-14

First locate the space between the spinal process of the seventh cervical vertebra and the first thoracic vertebra. To do this, look at the chart (Fig. 1). The vertebrae in the section marked with a ① are the cervical vertebrae. At the bottom of each is a small projection; these are the spinal processes. It follows that the small projection at the bottom of the seventh (lowest) cervical vertebra is one of the spinal processes you are seeking. The thoracic vertebrae, which are the section of the spinal column immediately below the cervical vertebrae, are actually twelve in number, though only a few of them—the ones marked with a ② —are shown in this chart. The spinal projection at the bottom of the topmost thoracic vertebra are the one you are looking for, and the tsubo GV-14 is located between it and the spinal process of the seventh cervical vertebra immediately above (Fig. 2). Next, locate the tsubo designated BL-13.

BL-13 (肺兪, *Fei-yü*) is a pair of tsubo located one sun and five bu on either side of the spinal column below the spinal process of the third thoracic vertebra.

Looking at Fig. 3 and recalling what was said in the preceding section on tsubo GV-14, locate the spinal process of the third thoracic vertebra; it is marked No. 3 on the chart. Below this spinal process there is an × on the chart. Move your fingers on a horizontal line on either side of the × for a distance of one sun and five bu in each direction. The places where your fingers are now located (marked with circles on the chart) are the locations of the pair of tsubo designated BL-13. You may use a similar procedure to locate any of the tsubo on the body.

Fig. 3

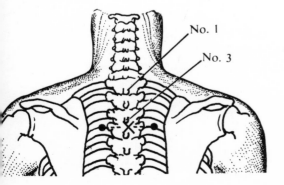

No. 1
No. 3

2. Acupuncture

When the human skin is struck, pricked, or cut, sensory bodies in it feel pain and transmit this sensation along the spinal chord to the brain. Acupuncture makes use of the sensory ability of the skin in amazingly effective therapy. Bringing needles into contact with the skin or inserting them into the skin stimulates sluggish nerves and calms overexcited nerves to cure symptoms of illness. Until only recently, the advocates of exclusive devotion to Western medical science have tended to discount acupuncture as old-fashioned, untrustworthy quackery. Perhaps the employment of the needle, a humble object of daily use, helped discredit acupuncture. Nonetheless, the great achievements made in recent years in China in acupuncture treatment have captured the attention of medical specialists in many parts of the world and have helped remove the onus of quackery from the therapy. Nor is this surprising, for anyone who keeps his mind free of preconceived notions and prejudices can see that oriental medical therapeutical methods are logical and in conformity with modern medicine. This can be said of shiatsu, moxa therapy, and acupuncture as well.

Because of the nature of acupuncture therapy—insertion of a fine needle into the body—it is unsuited to domestic application. Never allow an amateur to practice it on you; instead consult a trained specialist with the required technical skills. Its worldwide interest, however, leads me to give a few words of explanation of acupuncture, even though it is impractical as a home treatment.

The needles used in acupuncture are generally made of gold, silver, iron, platinum, or stainless steel. They are from 0.15 to 0.2 millimeters in diameter and from 3 to 6 centimeters in length. The specialist first disinfects the skin and then applies to it a silver tube containing the needle. The needle is inserted into the skin to a depth of about two centimeters, creating a sensation similar to that produced by contact with a weak electrical current. The needle is then either rhythmically withdrawn and inserted or allowed to remain inserted for from ten to twenty minutes. Sometimes a weak current of electricity is passed through the needle. This stimulus created in this way adjusts the condition of the meridian systems and thus helps relieve symptoms and preserve health. The thin, flexible needle makes use of the resilience of the skin so effectively that the insertions and withdrawals produce practically no pain. Furthermore, when the needle is removed, the skin closes over the opening at once; there is no danger of hemorrhage, bacterial invasion, or infection.

In addition to the standard treatment described above, there are several others. For instance, sometimes very small needles—two millimeters long—are inserted horizontally under the skin, fixed in place with adhesive tape, and allowed to remain for two or three days. The needles cause no discomfort, even when the patient moves; and there is no danger of the needles' breaking. This treatment is effective against pain in joints and against chronic sickness.

A related therapy, which is not exactly acupuncture, works for irritable children subject to nervous hypersensitivity or indigestion. Unlike true acupuncture, this simple treatment is safe enough for use by amateurs in the home. Using the bristle side of a hairbrush, rhythmically and lightly tap the child's skin. The stimulus created by this treatment will improve the child's condition and help him to grow strong.

An interesting recent variation of acupuncture is the use of small magnetized chromium balls (diameter of one millimeter) applied to the skin at a tsubo location and held in place by means of adhesive tape. The small balls stimulate the skin and in this way relieve stiffness in the shoulders and other parts of the body. The effectiveness of this system in combination with other clinical therapy has been recognized by the clinical research laboratory of the Institute of Oriental Medical Physiotherapy of the Tokyo University of Education.

3.   Massage

People all over the world have engaged in massage of one kind or another in all historical periods, for it is the natural reaction to pain or discomfort. Even persons who know nothing of medical science tend to try to find relief by pressing or rubbing a part of the body that hurts or is numb. When a person has walked an unaccustomed amount, upon retirement, he is likely to feel tension and pain in his calves. This is caused by excess action on the part of the nerves in the muscles of the calves and consequent cramps. To soothe the pain, most of us rub or squeeze the muscles.

Traditional oriental massage, or *amma*, is a developed therapeutical system passed from China into Japan, where it underwent much improvement to become a highly popular treatment. Like acupuncture and moxa combustion, amma employs the tsubo areas and the joints. By rubbing and pressing these areas, amma restores organs to proper functioning conditions, creates general bodily harmony, and contributes to health and good looks.

Until the nineteenth century, in Japan, amma massage was considered a major medical treatment. After the introduction of Western medical science and of French-style massage in the late nineteenth century, however, traditional amma lost prestige and became only a pleasant way to recover from fatigue.

In terms of point of origin, development process, and therapeutical principles, amma and Western-style massage are very different. Amma, based on the theory of the tsubo, employs treatment that follows the meridian systems and moves outward from the center of the body to the extremities. Massage, on the other hand, is based on the idea that the heart is the center of the body. Its treatment, therefore, follows the blood vessels (mainly the arteries) and moves inward from the extremities to the heart. The effects of the two treatments differ. Amma relieves weariness, sluggishness, stiff shoulders, heaviness in the head, insomnia, pains in the hips and back, chills of the hands and feet, and swelling. Massage affects the nervous system, joints, muscles, and hormone system. It is effective in treating paralysis caused by apoplexy, infantile paralysis, stiff shoulders caused by age, numbness or pain in the arms, weak stomach, and chronic constipation.

Although the effects vary, the techniques of the two systems closely resemble each other. In fact, today, the distinction between them is rarely maintained. Both are used as ways to relieve fatigue, promote health, and improve appearance. And both are usually called by the one name *massage*. In this book, I too shall include amma under the general name *massage;* but I must make it clear that I am referring to a massage system based on the oriental medical idea of the tsubo.

Before describing the six basic oriental massage techniques, I shall say a few words about massage methods in general. Unless it is specifically stated that massage pressure must be light, each application should consist of a pressure of from three to five kilograms applied for a duration of from three to five seconds. Unless specific directions are given—for instance, "palms of the hands" or "thumbs only"—adjust the use of the hands to the degree and location of the symptom: use the thumbs, index fingers, middle fingers, palms, of four fingers as required by the individual case.

(1)   Light rubbing (*Keisatsu*)

This most widely used massage technique involves stroking and rubbing the body with the hands, which exert a suitable degree of pressure as they massage. The ways in which the hands are used depend on the size of the part of the body being treated. For large areas—the back and shoulders, the abdomen, the arms and forearms, the thighs— the entire palm of the hand is used (Fig. 1). For small zones like the fingers and toes, the areas among the bones of the backs of the hands and the insteps, the upper surfaces of the tendons, and the areas between them, the tip of one or the tips of both thumbs are used (Fig. 2); or the skin and flesh are pinched between the thumbs and the index fingers (Fig. 3). For the head, neck, face, chest, and abdomen, the four fingers (index, middle, fourth, and little fingers) are used (Fig. 4).

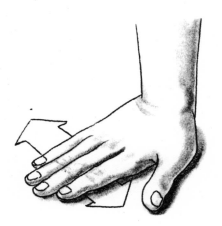

Fig. 1

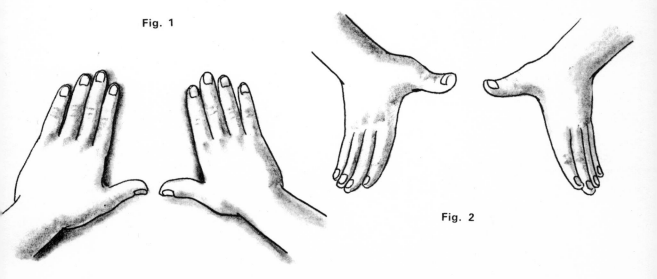

Fig. 2

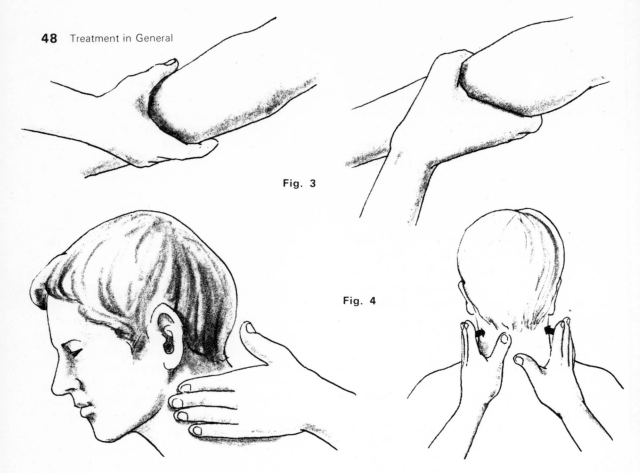

Fig. 3

Fig. 4

For areas of the body where the skin is thick and tough—back, buttocks, thighs, palms, and soles—the base or second knuckles of the four fingers are employed. In rubbing, the fingers must come into firm contact with the skin. The pressure exerted must be completely even throughout the massage; from three to four kilograms is suitable.

This massage method improves blood circulation and the flow of lymph. In addition, it stimulates the nervous system, muscles, and internal organs. Because it improves the sensitivity of the skin, strengthens the flow of blood, improves the functioning of the sweat and sebaceous glands, invigorates respiration in the pores, and provides greater nutrition, the massage system can help develop a lovely, soft skin. In addition, massage of the abdomen regulates the functioning of the stomach and intestines, improves digestion and absorption, and relieves constipation. Light pressing on the affected parts stimulates the circulation of the blood and thereby relieves chilling and numbness caused by paralysis and swelling caused by obstructions in the circulatory system.

Fig. 5

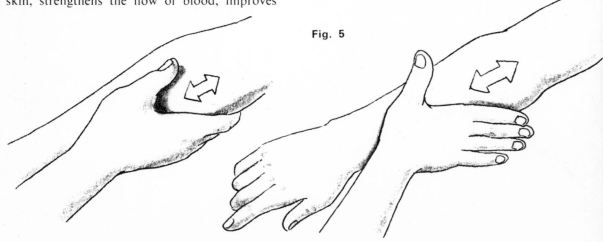

(2) Soft kneading (*Junetsu*)

This is another of the most popular massage techniques; it is used primarily for muscles. Without tensing your fingertips, gently shake your wrists and elbows. As you do this, using either the entire palm or the balls of the fingers, lightly and gently rub the patient's flesh in small, circular motions.

For large muscles in the major parts of the body —back, chest, abdomen, arms, forearms, thighs, lower abdomen—use the palms of both hands to press and knead the flesh (Fig. 5).

For muscles in more restricted zones—head, face, lower back, backs of the hands, legs—press with one or both thumbs as you rotate the flesh in circular motions (Fig. 6).

To rub the long, thick muscles of the neck, shoulders, arms, and legs, you may use the thumbs and index fingers in pinching and kneading actions (Fig. 7).

It is permissible to use both hands together or in alternation to give the kind of massage performed by sports masseurs in treating the larger muscles and muscle groups. It is of the greatest importance to remember not to massage with the fingertips alone, for this mistaken kind of treatment can cause skin abrasions that might make the patient wish he had never submitted to massage therapy at all.

Since this massage method invigorates the circulation in the muscles and stimulates metabolism, it aids in recovery from fatigue and improves muscular contraction powers, resilience, and tone. It is therefore recommended for strengthening the legs and arms of paralytic children, for removing fat from the abdomens of middle-aged people, for relieving weak stomach, and for curing constipation.

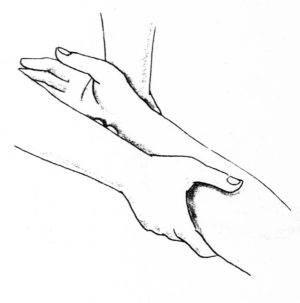

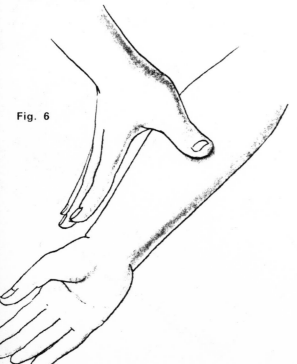

Fig. 6

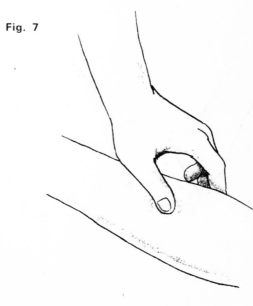

Fig. 7

(3) **Pressure method** (*Appaku*)

Using the palms (Fig. 8), the thumbs (Fig. 9), or the four fingers (Fig. 10), apply pressure to parts of the body, moving inward toward the center.

When using the thumbs or four fingers of one or both hands, apply steady pressure, then slowly release (Fig. 11).

This technique is employed in treating the muscles and joints of the arms and legs and the abdominal region. Since treatment with the thumbs affects the muscles and the nerves, it is used when light pressure causes pain in areas where the nerves emerge from the bone or run close under the skin. Pressure applications should be from three to five kilograms and should last for from three to five seconds. When applying pressure, rest the full weight of your body on your fingertips or hands. It is important to feel as if you were pulling your hands and your fingertips toward you as you apply pressure. Allowing your fingertips to move forward during the pressure application destroys the effect of the treatment.

Since it calms and relaxes hypertense nerves, this treatment is good for neuralgia and cramps. It is especially effective in treating the calves. Light pressure applied to the abdominal region for short periods improves the functioning of the stomach and intestines. Each application of pressure should be on a different part of the abdomen.

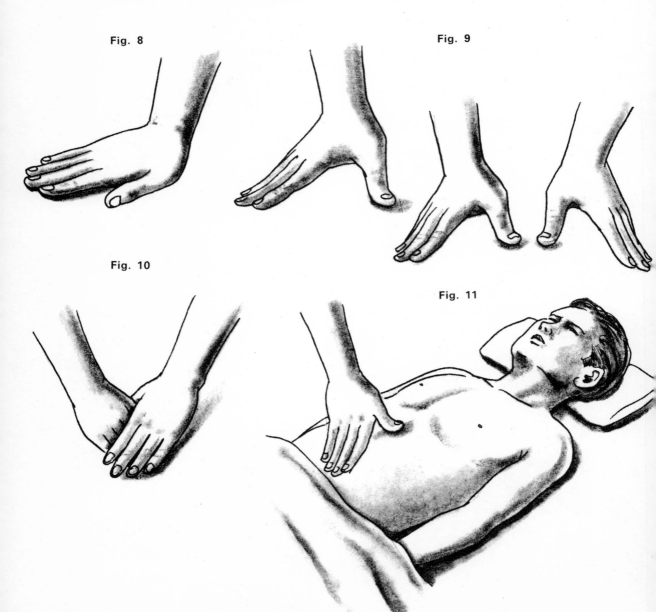

Fig. 8

Fig. 9

Fig. 10

Fig. 11

(4) Vibration (*Shinsen*)

Using the palm and the fingertips, apply light pressure as you vibrate the patient's flesh in short, rhythmical motions (Fig. 12). A skilled masseur can make as many as from ten to forty vibrations each second. The stimulation provided by this treatment improves the functioning of the fine unbranched nerves and the small muscles of the fingers. It is effective against numbness caused by nervous muscular sluggishness and against paralysis.

Fig. 12

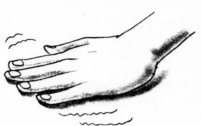

Fig. 13

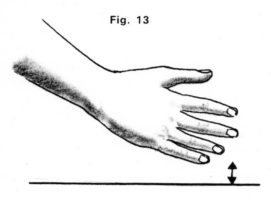

(5) Tapping (*Koda*)

With limber wrists, employ the motions of the entire forearm and hand to tap the patient's body lightly and rapidly. The hands are used in succession, and the tapping must be rhythmical (Fig. 13). For large areas or for parts of the body with hard, big muscles, use your fists (Fig. 14).

For small, tender parts of the body, employ cutting motions of the fingertips or of the four fingers (Figs. 15 and 16). Cup the palm of the hand for tapping soft areas like the abdominal region (Fig. 17).

Fig. 14

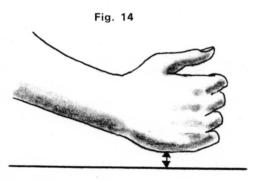

Fig. 15

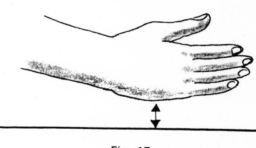

Fig. 16

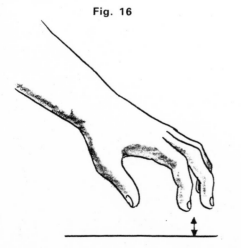

Fig. 17

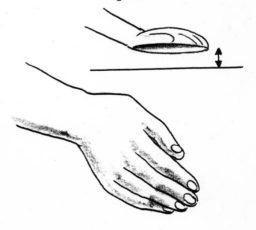

Though, in its rhythmical nature, this method resembles the vibration technique, it is more forceful. A short period of tapping treatment stimulates the nerves and the muscles; a longer period of the same treatment retards their functioning. You must not tense your shoulders, elbows, and wrists as you tap. Furthermore, you must not strike the patient hard. This is especially important in treating a person suffering from high blood pressure. In such instances, light, quiet tapping is essential, for the wrong kind of treatment can have the harmful effect of raising the patient's blood pressure. The pressure of each tapping action should be about one kilogram. A skilled masseur can tap from thirteen to fourteen times a second. Properly executed, tapping treatment can affect the motor nerves of the blood vessels and in this way can stimulate circulation. It helps remove fatigue-causing materials from the system, improves metabolism, and brings relief from muscular fatigue. Light tapping with the fingertips or palms on the chest relieves asthma. Tapping on the abdomen restores vigorous activity to the stomach and intestines and relieves gastroatonia and gastroptosis.

(6)   Squeezing and kneading (*Annetsu*)

For this technique, use the thumbs, the index finger, and the middle finger (Figs. 18 to 20). To massage the areas between bones and at joints, use the tips of the thumbs and the middle fingers. Only the tips of the fingers touch the patient's skin. Gradually increase pressure as you make circular motions with your fingertips. Start at the outer parts of the body and work inward in a spiral. To massage the joints, the wrists, backs of the ankles, and the abdomen, make circular motions with the thumbs and middle fingers. This is a forceful technique that breaks up and contributes to the assimilation of pathological accumulations in the joints. It brings relief to rheumatic joints—which can be treated only after fever, swelling, and pain have ceased—since it relieves stiffness and makes the joints easier to move. It is effective in cases of people who are semiparalyzed as a result of apoplexy and whose joints do not function. It can bring relief to the stiffness, pain, and creaking that sometimes develop in joints of people in their forties and fifties.

These then are the basic massage techniques. They must be used according to the symptoms of the patient and the part of the body affected. After massage, always lightly rub or tap the treated area and have the patient move the joints. This will make him feel much lighter and more supple. The effect of the massage will be increased if the patient lightly and slowly turns his head to right and left and front and back, stretches his arms and legs, raises and lowers his shoulders, and bends his body backward and forward. These actions will further relax muscles from which massage has already reduced tension.

Fig. 18

Fig. 19   **Fig. 20**

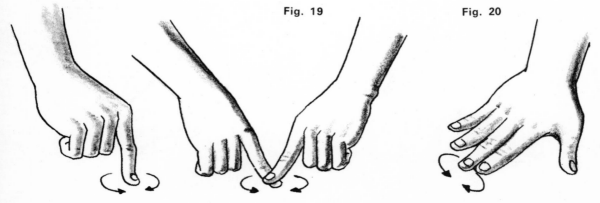

4. Shiatsu Treatment

Although the many different schools and systems of shiatsu therapy in Japan today make it impossible to point to one and to say, "This is the true system," all of them have developed from traditional, ancient amma massage with the addition of certain judo hand techniques (those called *kappo* and *doin*). A characteristic of shiatsu is the application of pressure to the tsubo of the patient's body. These applications are effective because they are regulated to the physique and bodily powers of the patient. Furthermore, the pressure used is varied in accordance with whether the functions of the body must be stimulated, calmed, or reinforced.

According to oriental medical thought, the body functions may be hyperactive (*jissho* condition); in such cases therapy must be applied to calm them. Or the functioning of the organs may be sluggish (*kyosho* condition) and require treatment to stimulate or reinforce them. In the case of shiatsu, practitioners lightly press a tsubo with the fingers. If the patient feels pain, he is exhibiting symptoms of the jissho condition and needs shiatsu treatment to calm his body functioning. If he feels only a pleasant sensation, however, he is exhibiting a kyosho symptom. This means that light rubbing treatment is called for. The theory on which this therapy is based is in accord with modern physical treatment rules.

Pressure is the only thing used in shiatsu, but ways of applying it are varied to suit the needs of the case in hand. Sometimes, pressure is applied to one spot for a short interval and then to another and another in rapid succession. In certain cases, pressure is applied slowly for a long time to a single tsubo. In other cases, it is applied for short intervals on one tsubo but is gradually increased. In other words, the pressure may be light, medium, or strong. The basic methods employed in shiatsu therapy are pressure and motion.

(1) Pressure

The palms, thumbs, or fingers are used in a number of different techniques, which are varied to suit the condition and illness of the patient.
(1) Light pressure that is gradually increased and then slowly decreased.
(2) A quick, light touch with a sudden increase of pressure followed by a sudden release.
(3) Completely natural touch followed by a very slight increase of pressure and a careful, gradual release.

The weight of the practitioner rests on the hands or fingers that are in contact with the patient's body. Using only the strength of the fingers results in sharp pressure that causes pain and reduces the effectiveness of the treatment. It is important that pressure be always directed toward the center of the patient's body. Because of the essential nature of this rule, great stress is put on the position of the body of the shiatsu practitioner. There is no definitely established spatial interval at which pressure should be applied to the patient's body, though from three to five centimeters is generally accepted.

(2) Motion

Like the motion techniques of massage, this part of shiatsu is designed to promote general good condition and to improve the appearance; it has no therapeutic value. In general, it is used in conjunction with shiatsu pressure applications.

The practitioner has the patient sit in a relaxed position and move the joints of the body to the right and left and to the front and back as far as is physiologically possible. This restores limberness and suppleness to the joints and removes stiffness from tendons and connective tissues. Consequently, it helps the patient maintain a youthful body. Shiatsu is too specialized a system for the uninformed person to use. It is always safer to call upon the services of a trained shiatsu practitioner.

5. Moxa Combustion Therapy

Moxa (*mogusa* in Japanese) is a soft material derived from such plants as Chinese wormwood and burned on the skin as is explained below for the therapeutic effects it produces. The theory on which this therapy is based is this. Moxa burned on the skin burns a small amount of the tissue which is dissolved and passed into the blood stream, where it acts as a stimulus to the circulation and to the production of immunizing substances. On the basis of the theory of the relation between the internal organs and the surface of the body, moxa combustion improves the functioning of the organs. Consequently, it is most effective applied to the tsubo. This treatment increases the body's powers of resistance, thus reducing the danger of sickness. In addition, it can be used as a therapeutic system and as an aid in preserving general good condition and preventing illness.

The most widely used method for moxa combustion by specialists and ordinary people as well is direct application. A small amount of moxa is rolled into a cone about the size of a grain of rice—or half that size (Fig. 1). The tsubo related to the disorder of the patient are located, and the moxa is placed directly on the skin at one of the tsubo. Ordinarily, moxa must be ignited and allowed to burn three times on the same place for a single treatment.

In the indirect combustion method (Fig. 2), the moxa cone, of the same size as the one used in the direct method, is not placed on the skin. Instead it is put on a slice of ginger root, garlic, or onion; a piece of flat chives; a dab of bean paste; or a piece of gauze soaked in salt water. The moxa is then ignited and allowed to burn. This method has the advantage of leaving no mark on the skin. Because it produces only moderate heat, it is comfortable and popular.

In addition to these systems, there are two more that are fairly widely used. One involves the use of a container to hold the burning moxa. The other calls for a large amount of moxa—a piece about the size of the end of the thumb—to be placed on the appropriate tsubo. This is ignited. As soon as the skin senses heat, the moxa must be removed with the fingers or with tweezers. Applications of this kind are made from one to three times on the same tsubo. There is no danger of marking the skin with this method.

Fig. 1

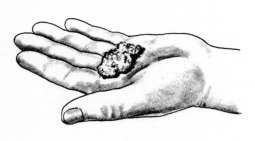

Hold the moxa in both hands.

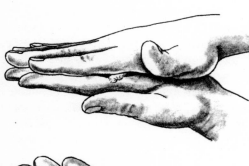

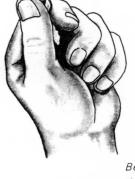

Be careful to shape the moxa into a tight cone before application.

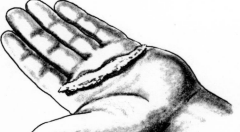

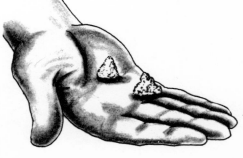

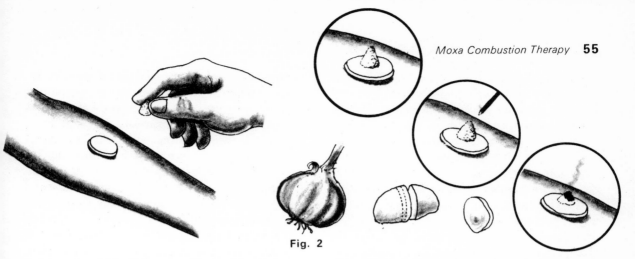

Fig. 2

Moxa is sold in Chinese or oriental pharmacies in coarse, medium, and fine grades. For domestic use, the medium and fine grades are suitable. Good quality moxa, which is fine, pleasant to the touch, and pale yellow, is preferred. It is old and contains no impurities. It therefore burns well and gradually. Coarser, blackish, new moxa contains extraneous material and may burn irregularly or go out during treatment. Use ordinary stick incense to ignite moxa. First light the incense, then, after knocking off whatever ash may have formed on the end of the stick, bring it near the moxa, rotating it all the while. The rotation prevents the moxa from adhering to the incense.

After you have located the tsubo that require treatment, make a cone of moxa, place it on the skin at the location of the tsubo, and ignite it with an incense stick (Fig. 3). Your hands must be dry to prevent the moxa from sticking to your fingers. Rubbing incense ash on the fingertips is a good way to ensure dryness. To keep the moxa in the proper place, wet the skin.

The moment the moxa has ignited, with the index and middle fingers of the left hand, press the skin on either side of the moxa. This will cause that part of the skin to rise slightly thereby reducing the heat it receives from the burning moxa and lessening the danger of marking the skin. Furthermore, raising the skin in this way increases the effectiveness of the treatment. When the moxa has burned completely, remove it from the skin with tweezers or a small brush and make another application.

Fig. 3

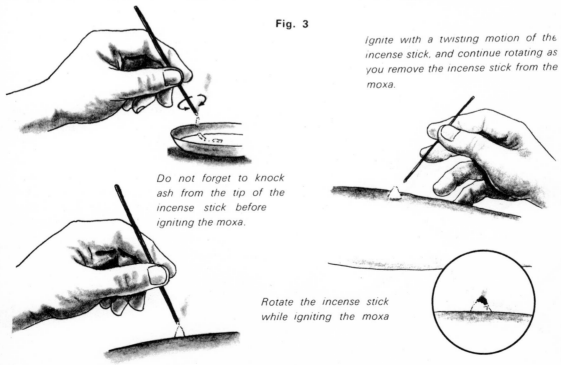

Do not forget to knock ash from the tip of the incense stick before igniting the moxa.

Ignite with a twisting motion of the incense stick, and continue rotating as you remove the incense stick from the moxa.

Rotate the incense stick while igniting the moxa

For adults, make from five to seven applications on the same tsubo; for children, from one to three. The minimum number is preferred. Continue the treatment daily for three weeks. Then rest for one week. If the symptoms that were causing the trouble do not abate as a result of this treatment, after the week's rest, begin again and continue for another three-week period. Follow moxa combustion with light pressure by the fingertips. If the heat has caused a blister, first disinfect the skin with alcohol, then prick the blister with a sterilized needle. Squeeze the water from the blister and reapply moxa. Should infection occur, temporarily stop moxa treatment and coat the infected area with a suitable ointment (for instance, penicillin ointment). Moxa may be applied at any time during the day, but it must not be used on patients who have fever, who are very tired, who are dizzy or have palpitations, who are hungry, or who have just eaten. Moxa may be applied to women who are pregnant or who are in their menstrual periods. If the numbers of applications of moxa or the quantities of the material used in each application are too great, sluggishness, loss of appetite, and listlessness may result. These symptoms will vanish, and the treatment will have its proper effect when adjustments in frequencies and quantities are made. In some instances, it is wise to give moxa treatment no more often than every other day. Always persevere and be consistent in using this therapy. Applying moxa on one day and then resting for two or three will produce no results.

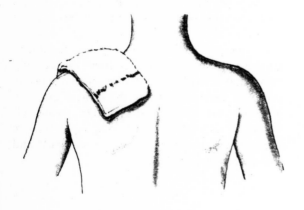

6.   Simple Domestic Treatments

(1)   Hot packs

To relieve stiff shoulders, hypertense muscles, and chills, use a hot pack made by soaking a towel in hot water and wringing it out well. This treatment is effective in all but the most stubborn cases because it stimulates the circulation of the blood. Since the hot towel soon cools, it is more convenient to make use of the many therapeutic heating devices—packs and heating pads—available on the market.

(2)   Paraffin baths

Commercially available paraffin, heated for ten minutes to a temperature that is hot, but not hot enough to burn the skin (about 50 degrees centigrade) makes a good bath for hands or feet that are sore or hypertense. The hand or foot should be lowered into the paraffin, allowed to remain there for about five seconds, raised, then lowered into the paraffin again. Repeat this about ten times. The paraffin will form a coat that fits the hand or foot as closely as a glove or stocking.

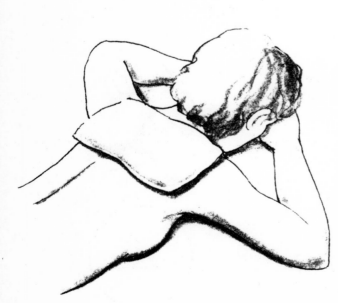

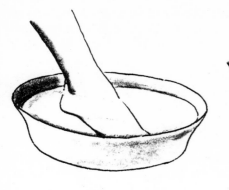

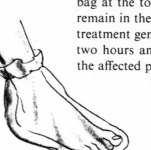

Enclose the hand or foot in a plastic bag, seal the bag at the top, and allow the ailing member to remain in the bag for about thirty minutes. This treatment generates warmth that lasts for one or two hours and that improves the circulation in the affected part of the body.

(3) Hair dryer

The ordinary hair dryer can be used in conjunction with finger massage to bring relief from stiff shoulders, aching arms, aching back, or chills or pains in the joints. The gentle warm air current has an effect very much like that of massage.

(4) Massage devices

There are many massage machines and devices and vibrators of several sorts that can be effectively used for relief from bent back, tension, and discomfort in the chest and back, and from stiffness in the hips and shoulders. Any of the vibrator or roller muscle massage devices is good. You can find relief from sore feet by placing something cylindrical—or roughly cylindrical like a beer bottle—under the arch of the foot and rolling it back and forth.

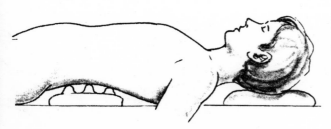

7. Basic Positions for the Patient and the Person Giving Treatment

(1) Treatment of the back

The patient lies in a relaxed position on his stomach. While the person giving the treatment is locating the tsubo, it is imperative for the sake of accuracy that the patient positions his arms so that they form right angles with the spinal column. Once the tsubo have been correctly located, however, the patient may put his arms in any position that he finds comfortable. For massage and shiatsu massage, the person giving the treatment kneels on one knee, leans his upper body forward, and puts the bulk of his weight on his arms. Both elbows must be straight.

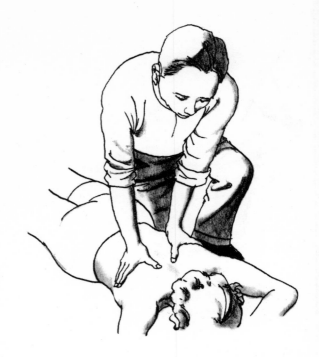

(2) Treatment of the abdominal region

The patient lies comfortably on his back with both knees raised and with mouth slightly open. His arms may be in any comfortable position that does not hinder the activities of the person giving the treatment. The knees are raised to relax the abdominal muscles, which inhibit treatment when they are tense, as they are when the legs are outstretched. The person who gives the treatment is in the position outlined in the section on treating the back.

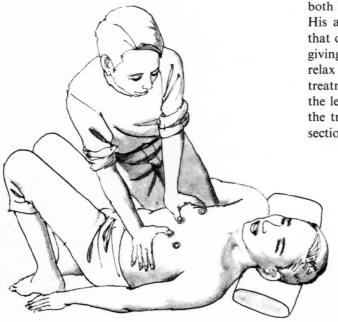

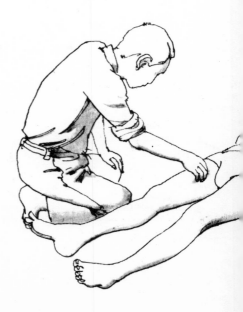

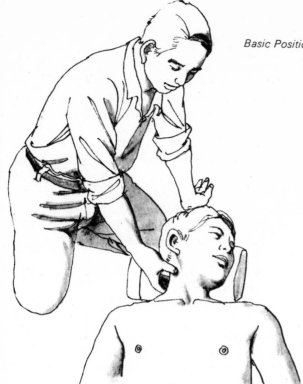

(3) Treating the side of the neck and the throat

The patient lies on his back. The person giving the treatment kneels at his side with his left hand on the floor; the left arm becomes the center of gravity of his body. With his right hand, the person giving the treatment massages the patient's neck and throat. If the patient coughs or becomes red in the face, pressure is too strong, and treatment must be halted.

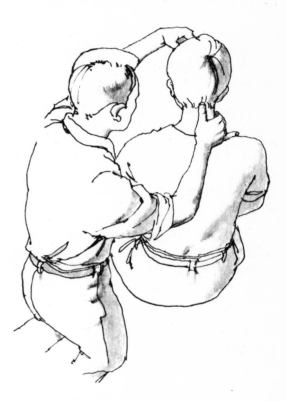

(4) Treating the back of the neck and the hands

The patient sits in a comfortable position with his back straight. The person giving the treatment kneels and supports the head or hand with one of his hands while he applies massage or shiatsu treatment. This kind of therapy may be performed in a standing or kneeling position as well.

(5) Treating the legs and feet

When the fronts of the legs are being treated, the patient lies on his back; he lies on his stomach when the backs of the legs are being treated. The person giving the treatment kneels in a suitable position. When treating the feet, he must support the patient's foot with one hand while massaging or applying shiatsu with the other.

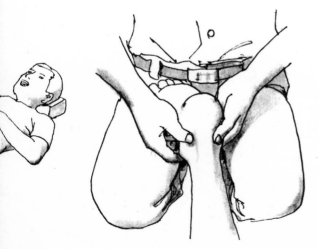

8. General Rules

Anyone who practices the therapies explained in this book at home must keep a number of things in mind.

1) Cut the fingernails short and round

Massage and shiatsu are used against the naked skin of the patient. The person performing such therapy must keep his fingernails trimmed short and round to prevent cutting or otherwise injuring the patient.

2) Clean garments

The person performing treatment must always be clean. This includes well scrubbed hands and face and clean, neat clothing.

3) Patient must relax

Unless the patient is relaxed and comfortable, massage and shiatsu cannot be expected to have full effect. Putting the muscles in the most natural positions possible, the patient must lie as required by the treatment with relaxed shoulders, arms, and legs.

4) Loosen all binding articles of clothing

To prevent obstructions in the blood and lymph circulation, the patient's collar, belt, and any other binding articles of clothing must be loosened before treatment begins.

5) From five to fifteen minutes per area

Although variations to this guideline may be necessary, as a general rule, treat one part of the body for from five to fifteen minutes. A total massage treatment must not last for more than one hour, since excessive treatment can have the reverse effect of tiring the patient. Usually the treatment is repeated daily, though, depending on the case, as often as two or three times a day or as seldom as twice or three times a week may be suitable. In all instances, the frequency and length of treatment and of the pressure used in massage and shiatsu must be gauged to the circumstances and condition of the patient.

6) When to refrain from massage and shiatsu

Do not use these therapeutic systems on patients with fever who must remain quiet. Do not use them in cases of infection or ulceration. Avoid them in cases of phlebothrombosis, vericose veins, aneurysm, or in any instance in which there are poisonous exudations that could spread throughout the body by means of the circulatory system. Further, these treatments must not be used in serious illness involving the lungs, heart, or kidneys; malignant tumors; primary syphilis; or tuberculosis. Massage and shiatsu must not be used on skin that is burned, infected, ulcerous, or subject to any kind of exudation. In the following cases, it may be acceptable to use these methods, but it is wiser to avoid them: advanced arteriosclerosis, high blood pressure resulting from this condition, hemophilia, sicknesses involving fresh hemorrhage, broken bones, or dislocated joints.

Chapter 3:
TREATMENT IN SPECIFIC

1.   Sicknesses That Are Not Strictly Sicknesses

(1)   Impotence

At the age of puberty, as the sexual organs develop, human beings become aware of sexual desires. In the male, this naturally involves erection of the penis. In recent years, however, many men have complained of failure to achieve erection and of impotence. There seems to be no definite illness causing an increase in the numbers of impotent males in our times: the true cause is related to faults in the nature of our civilization. In other words, the kind of impotence most frequent today is largely psychological in origin. For instance, intensification of awareness of sexual matters leads to excessive concern with minor excitements that in more sober times would have been passed over. Furthermore, too much fuss is raised over sex today. This, in combination with the mental stress of living in our complicated social structure, has a bad effect on the sexual abilities of the human male.

In general terms, impotence can result from one of three kinds of causes. First the male can be disinterested in or unexcited by normal sexual intercourse. He may be constitutionally weak. Hormone upsets may have made him ill and may thus have prevented or greatly reduced his sexual desire. Or daily living conditions may exert a debilitating influence on him.

The second major category of causes of impotence involves feelings of sexual inadequacy. This may arise from an actual physical injury to the sexual organs or from feelings of inferiority caused by failure in initial sexual experience.

Finally, serious physical injury or disability can bring about impotence. For instance, damage to the brain or the spinal column, in something like an automobile accident, may produce such an effect. Excess consumption of alcohol, addiction to sleeping pills or stimulants, diabetes, obesity, and other abnormal conditions can reduce or eliminate the male's ability to perform sexually. In cases of these kinds, cure can only be effected on the basis of treatment by a specialist. But psychiatric treatment or a mere change of place in living can do much to relieve impotence caused by psychological factors.

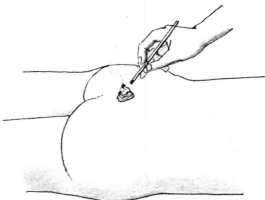

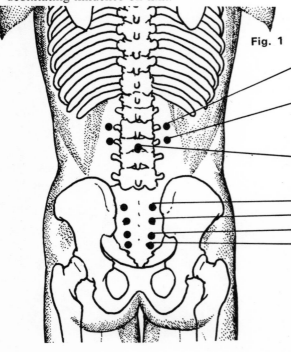

Fig. 1

1. BL-22 (三焦兪, *San-chiao-yu*)
One sun and five bu on either side of the spinal column at points below the first lumbar vertebra.

2. BL-23 (腎兪, *Shen-yü*)
One sun and five bu on either side of the spinal column at points below the spinal projections of the second lumbar vertebra, which is located at the height of the lowest ribs.

3. GV-4 (命門, *Ming-men*)
Below the spinal projections of the second lumbar vertebra; between the tsubo designated BL-23.

4. BL-31 (上髎, *Shang-liao*)
5. BL-32 (次髎, *T'zu-liao*)
6. BL-33 (中髎, *Chung-liao*)
7. BL-34 (下髎, *Hsia-liao*)
Five sacral vertebra fused to form a rear wall for the pelvic cavity. The four tsubo BL-31, BL-32, BL-33, and BL-34 are located beside the openings on either side of the projections of the top four of these vertebrae. The pair of tsubo designated BL-31 is on the level of the topmost of the sacral vertebrae, and the others proceed downward in ascending numerical order.

Acupuncture and moxa combustion have surprising effects in treating impotence for which causes are unclear. They can strengthen the body when it is weakened to the point that sexual powers fail. The first step to take in relieving this condition is to make whatever adjustments are possible in the daily-life environment and in this ‚way to lessen psychological stresses. Then, select six of the following eight tsubo (Fig. 1) for moxa-combustion treatment: BL-22, BL-23, GV-4, BL-31, BL-32, BL-33, and BL-34.

In addition, moxa combustion may be used on the following tsubo related to the kidney meridian: KI-16, CV-4, CV-3, LV-11, LV-9 (Fig. 2), KI-9, and KI-3 (Fig. 3). Treatment is effective if applied from three to five times on each tsubo regularly once a day.

Fig. 2

8. KI-16 (肓兪, *Huang-yü*)
Points located five sun on either side of the navel.

9. CV-4 (関元, *Kuan-yüan*)
Three sun below the navel, or midway between the navel and pubis.

10. CV-3 (中極, *Chung-chi*)
Four sun below the navel, or four-fifths of the length of a line connecting the navel and the pubis.

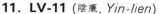

11. LV-11 (陰廉, *Yin-lien*)
About two sun below the crotch on the inner side of the thigh.

12. LV-9 (陰包, *Yin-pao*)
Four sun above the groove formed when the knee bends on the inner side of the thigh. Or four sun above a point directly to the side of the kneecap.

13. KI-9 (築賓, *Chu-pin*)
In the muscle that is the width of the index finger inward of the shin at a point five sun above the inner side of the ankle.

14. KI-3 (太谿, *T'ai-hsi*)
Rear part of the inside of the ankle.

Fig. 3

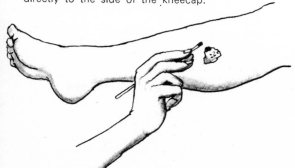

(2) Cramps

After vigorous protracted exercise, chills brought on by swimming, or fatigue arising from any of a number of causes, people often experience extremely painful cramps in the calf muscles when they go to bed at night. Similar conditions arise when a person is recovering, but has not completely recovered, from beriberi or other contagious diseases. Although cramps are more a physiological discomfort than a sickness in the strict sense of the word, they are sometimes unbearable. Consequently, it is a good idea to learn the tsubo where massage and shiatsu therapy can be used to bring relief.

The sciatic nerve, which passes from the lower back to the buttocks and the backs of the thighs before reaching the lower legs, controls the muscles of the calves. Malfunction—especially hyperfunctioning—of the sciatic nerve causes pains and heaviness in the back and calf cramps, which can become chronic.

Sometimes simply squeezing the muscle relieves the condition. When cramps are experienced out of doors—for instance, on the sports field—if the weather is cold, the most important thing is to go indoors at once and raise the body temperature. A hot towel will bring relief from minor cramps.

Since the aim in treatment to relieve cramps is to calm the hyperactive sciatic nerve and limber the muscles, shiatsu therapy is more effective than ordinary massage. The following is the course of treatment I recommend.

First, vigorously squeeze the flesh at BL-27 and BL-28 (Fig. 4). Then apply shiatsu pressure.

When this is finished, repeat the same kind of treatment on BL-54, BL-56, BL-57 (Fig. 5), SP-9, and KI-3 (Fig. 6).

Fig. 4

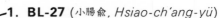

1. BL-27 (小腸俞, *Hsiao-ch'ang-yü*)
The sacral vertebra are fused and formed into the rear wall of the pelvic cavity. These tsubo are located one sun and five bu on either side of the spinal column at points below the spinal projections of the first sacral vertebra.

2. BL-28 (膀胱俞, *P'ang-kuan-yü*)
One sun and five bu on either side of the spinal column at points below the spinal projections of the sacral vertebra.

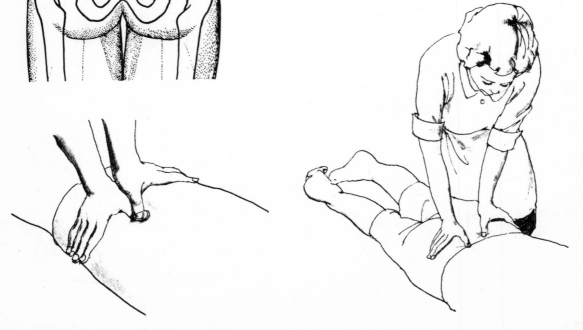

The tsubo BL-54, BL-56, and BL-57 are especially important. Using the thumbs and the four fingers, apply shiatsu pressure to them, first gently and slowly and then more forcefully for from three to seven seconds each. The relief brought by this treatment is amazing.

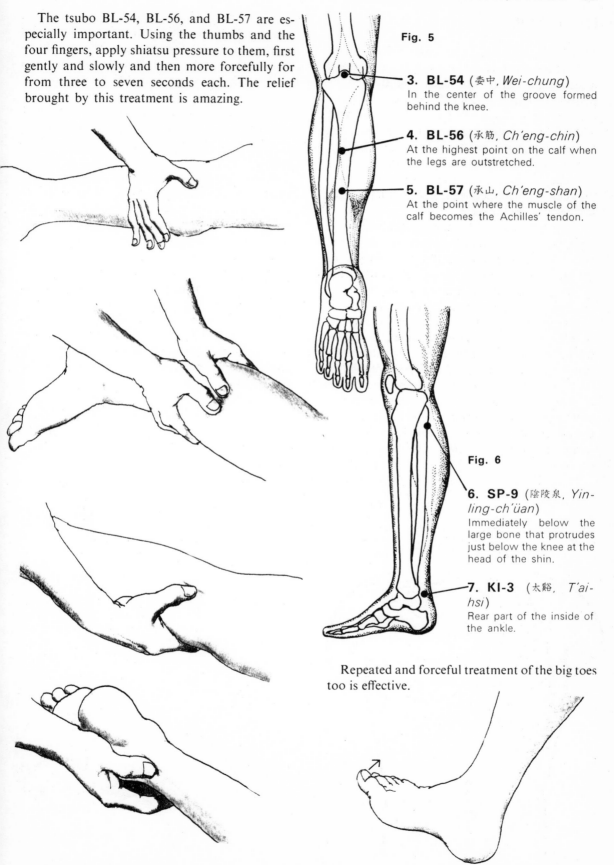

Fig. 5

3. BL-54 (委中, *Wei-chung*)
In the center of the groove formed behind the knee.

4. BL-56 (承筋, *Ch'eng-chin*)
At the highest point on the calf when the legs are outstretched.

5. BL-57 (承山, *Ch'eng-shan*)
At the point where the muscle of the calf becomes the Achilles' tendon.

Fig. 6

6. SP-9 (陰陵泉, *Yin-ling-ch'üan*)
Immediately below the large bone that protrudes just below the knee at the head of the shin.

7. KI-3 (太谿, *T'ai-hsi*)
Rear part of the inside of the ankle.

Repeated and forceful treatment of the big toes too is effective.

(3) **Hiccoughs**

There may ·be some people who accuse me of making too much of a small thing in setting apart a section for the cure of hiccoughs. But for the person who suffers from this unexplained and distressing condition, which can develop suddenly without any warning, hiccoughs are no laughing matter. All that is presently known is that hiccoughs are a kind of irregularity in the breathing brought on by cramps or spasms in the diaphragm. No definitely effecutal internal remedy has been found for them.

The nerves controlling the diaphragm emerge from the third and fourth cervical vertebrae and are called the fourth cervical nerves. They cross the chest and reach the diaphragm, which they contract and relax according to the needs of respiration. Sometimes damage to the cervical vertebrae or the spinal column can cause hiccoughs. Some cases are easily cured, especially when they are caused by eating something violently stimulating or by sickness in the esophagus or the stomach. Others, however, are less tractable, as is likely to be the case when the pathological state causing them is grave. Hiccoughs caused by uremia, alcoholism, infection, peritonitis, and postoperative conditions are of this kind.

Many home remedies claim to cure hiccoughs: repeated deep breaths, tensing the stomach and holding the breath for as long as possible, sneezing, coughing, cold towels or ice on the abdomen, long drinks of water, mustard plasters on the abdomen, sudden shocks, pounding on the back, and so on. But none of these is of completely reliable efficacy. Some people have been known to suffer from hiccoughs for as long as two or three years.

Since the causes are often psychological, treatments of the nerves and of the skin related to the meridians connected to the diaphragm are effective. In my research institute, acupuncture has proved efficacious, even in some of the most stubborn cases. Since acupuncture is not a treatment that the amateur can use with safety, however, I shall explain how to produce the same effects with massage and shiatsu.

The first step is to apply shiatsu pressure to LI-17 and ST-11 (Fig. 7). Do not press too heavily; simply allow the weight of the body to rest on the left hand, which is on the floor, and press with the right hand.

1. LI-17 (天鼎, *T'ien-ting*)
Near the peak of the triangular depression formed by the sternomastoid muscle (the muscle from the base of the neck to the ear; it becomes apparent when the neck is turned full to one side), the trapezius muscle (the large triangular muscle running from the neck to the shoulder tip), and the clavicle. Or three sun to the sides of the Adam's apple and one sun downward, or the outer edge of the sternomastoid.

2. ST-11 (気舎, *Ch'i-she*)
One sun and five bu on either side of the central point in the front of the neck. Inner tip of the clavicles and upper tip of the sternum.

Fig. 7

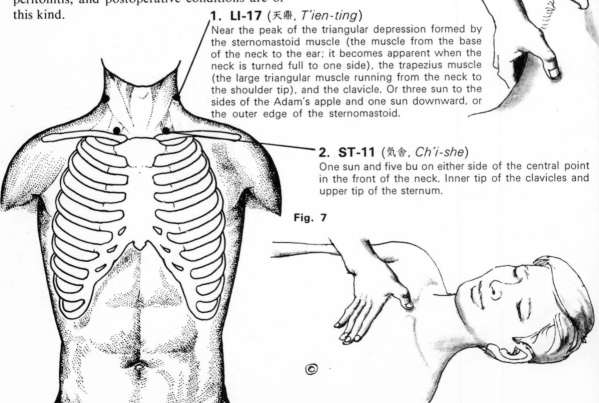

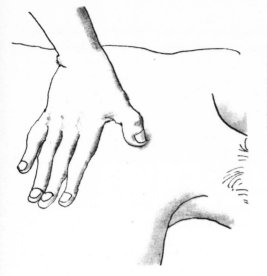

3. BL-17 (膈俞, *Ke-yü*)

one sun and five bu on either side of the spinal column at points below the seventh thoracic vertebra.

Fig. 8

Then apply shiatsu pressure to BL-17 (Fig. 8), CV-15, CV-14, CV-12, ST-19, and LV-14 (Fig. 9).

In this case, make small kneading movements with your hands as you apply pressure.

It is not unusual for the hiccoughs to stop at once with only one acupuncture treatment, and shiatsu massage can produce almost the same effects. Shiatsu is more effective in these cases than moxa combustion.

Fig. 9

4. CV-15 (鳩尾, *Chiu-wei*)
At the diaphragm, or one sun below the lower extremity of the sternum.

5. CV-14 (巨闕, *Chü-ch'üeh*)
Immediately below the diaphragm; two sun below the lower extremity of the sternum.

6. CV-12 (中脘, *Chung-wan*)
Four sun above the navel; midway between the navel and the diaphragm.

7. ST-19 (不容, *Pu-yung*)
On either side of the diaphragm at the front edges of the eighth ribs counted from the top.

8. LV-14 (期門, *Ch'i-men*)
Extremities of the ninth ribs. Or a place located at the boundary between the rib and the abdomen directly below the nipple of the breast.

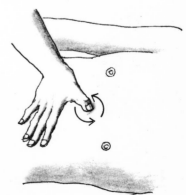

(4) Headaches

Headaches can be caused by definite conditions. They can be the forerunners of such sicknesess as colds, neuralgia, menstrual irregularities, toothache, earache, and internal head pains. On the other hand, they can arise from much vaguer sources that are not specifically illnesses: fatigue, sudden changes in the weather, menstrual upsets, and so on. Causes of headaches may be grouped into three major categories: irregularities in the blood vessels, muscular tension, and psychological upsets.

Headaches caused by irregularities in the blood vessels (migraine) take the form of throbbing on one side of the head and flashes before the eyes. As they grow increasingly severe, they cause nausea. A brief sleep will usually cure them. The pain is said to be caused by the expansion of the blood vessels in the head. People who are totally absorbed in their work often suffer from headaches caused by muscular tension. The muscles of the shoulders stiffen and bring pain in the back of the neck and the back of the head. Difficulties in personal relations with others, minor domestic problems and other psychological matters can make themselves painfully apparent in the form of headaches. In addition, the nerves in the head sometimes cause aching.

To bring relief to this unpleasant condition, one must act according to the nature of the symptoms. Headaches caused by the expansion of the blood vessels can by cured by means of some of the drugs that relax those vessels. Ergotamine, made from the ergot fungus that afflicts the grain rye, has proved especially effective in treating migraine headaches. Exercise, baths, and changes of task and mood relieve the pain caused by tense muscles. Tranquilizers and pain killers are used to combat psychologically produced headaches, but the best cure is to solve the problem bringing about the upsetting condition.

For serious headaches with specific, definite causes, relief can best be found by consulting a physician and having him perform the therapy required by the case in hand. But most people hesitate to make trips to the doctor for ordinary, light headaches. In such instance, the following treatments are effective.

First lightly massage meridians (Nos. ① and ② in Figs. 10 and 11 in the directions indicated by the arrows. Then rub meridian ③ in Fig. 12, making small, circular motions with the palms of both hands. Next, slowly massage meridian ④ (Fig. 13) from BL-10, GB-20 to GB-12 with both thumbs.

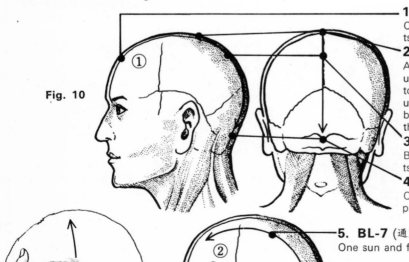

Fig. 10

Fig. 11

1. GV-24 (神庭, *Shen-t'ing*)
One sun and five bu in front of the tsubo designated GV-20.

2. GV-20 (百会, *Pai-hui*)
At the point where a line directly upward from ear to ear crossing the top of the head and a line straight upward from the midpoint of the area between the shoulders to the top of the head intersect.

3. GV-19 (後頂, *Hou-ting*)
Behind and one sun five bu below the tsubo designated GV-20.

4. GV-16 (風府, *Feng-fu*)
One sun below the external occipital protuberance.

5. BL-7 (通天, *T'ung-t'ien*)
One sun and five bu from the very top of the head.

6. BL-4 (曲差, *Ch'ü-ch'a*)
One sun and five bu on either side of a point five above the hairline in the center of the forehead.

7. BL-10 (天柱, *T'ien-chu*)
To the outer side of the two large muscles of the neck where they join the back of the head.

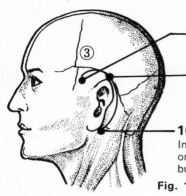

8. GB-7 (曲鬢, *Ch'ü-pin*)
One sun above the highest part of the cheekbone in front of the ear.

9. TH-20 (角孫, *Chüe-hsun*)
Immediately above the ear; or in the depression at the hairline on the occiput at the point of the ear.

10. GB-12 (完骨, *Wan-ku*)
In the depression that is located about the width of one finger above the mastoid process, and about four bu from the hairline.

Fig. 12

For heaviness caused by congestion of the blood in the head, use the thumbs and index fingers of both hands to massage lightly the area from the chest to the clavicles; this involves the area from SI-17 to ST-11. The massage should be done in small, circular motions in the direction of meridian ⑤ (Fig. 13). This will lighten the feeling of the head. After the massage, using either the thumbs or the four fingers, apply shiatsu pressure to each of the tsubo for from three to five seconds each.

The effect of this therapy will be heightened if you combine it with treatment applied to GB-21, BL-13 (Fig. 14), and LI-11 (Fig. 15). Moxa combustion applied to the same tsubo brings equal relief.

11. GB-20 (風池, *Feng-ch'ih*)
Depressions in the lower edge of the occiput two sun on either side of the tsubo designated BL-10.

GB-12

Fig. 13

BL-10

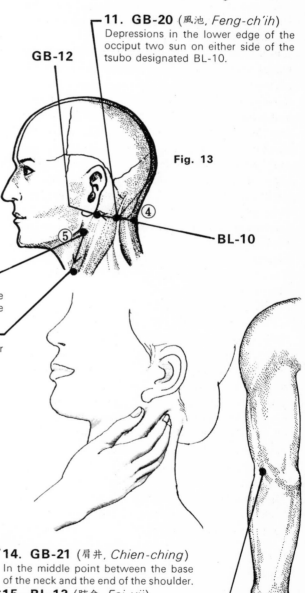

12. SI-17 (天容, *T'ien-yung*)
Below the ear at the corner of the lower jaw. Immediately in front of the sternomastoid muscle.

13. ST-11 (気舎, *Ch'i-she*)
Inner tip of the clavicles and upper tip of the sternum.

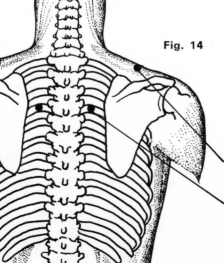

Fig. 14

14. GB-21 (肩井, *Chien-ching*)
In the middle point between the base of the neck and the end of the shoulder.

15. BL-13 (肺俞, *Fei-yü*)
One sun and five bu on either side of the spinal column at points below the spinal projections of the third thoracic vertebra.

16. LI-11 (曲池, *Ch'ü-ch'ih*)
Thumb side of the bend of the elbow. **Fig. 15**

(5) Cricks Caused by Poor Sleeping Positions

Sometimes movement during sleep, when the body is in an unnatural position, causes pain in the neck, the back of the head, or the shoulders when the person awakens the following morning. Sleeping in front of an electric fan, in a cold draft, or in an air-conditioned room can produce the same symptoms, which are especially startling since, generally, the sufferer felt perfectly well the night before. When this happens, it is important first to touch one or all of the following: the trapezius muscles on both sides of the back of the neck (meridian ①, Fig. 16), the sternomastoid muscle running from the sides of the neck forward and diagonally downward (meridian ②, Fig. 17), and the hairline from the nape of the neck to the ears (meridian ③, Fig. 17). These places will probably be stiff and very sensitive to even light digital pressure. The more severe the case, the stiffer the muscles. The neck muscles will not contract normally and may be slightly twisted. For one or two days, the patient is unable to bend his neck; but gradually, in four or five days, he forgets the pain. His neck returns to normal. X-ray photographs usually show no abnormality in instances of the disorder.

The first aim of treatment is to relieve muscular stiffness. To do this, have the patient lie on his back. Apply a heating pad to the back of his neck. If a heating pad is unavailable, use a hot towel covered in a sheet of plastic to prevent rapid cooling. The heat application should last for from fifteen to twenty minutes. In this time, the stiffness in the neck and shoulders should have relaxed. Next massage the two large muscles in meridians ① and ② (Figs. 16 and 17). Use either the thumbs or four fingers in gentle, small, circular motions. Next use fairly strong shiatsu pressure on GB-20, GB-21, SI-17, and ST-11. If the back of the head—the occipital region—is in pain, lightly massage meridians ③ and ④ (Fig. 17).

Fig. 16

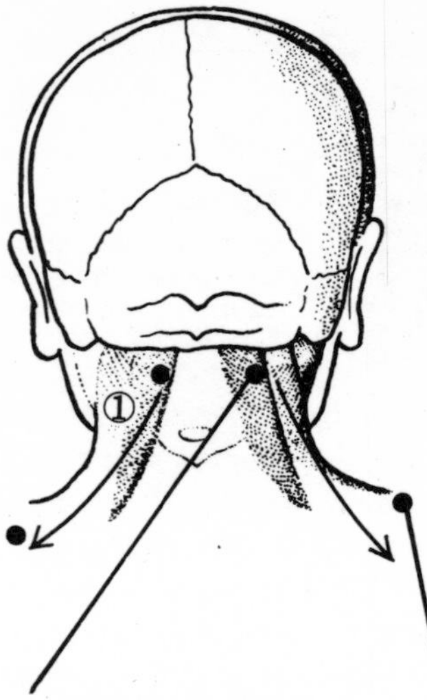

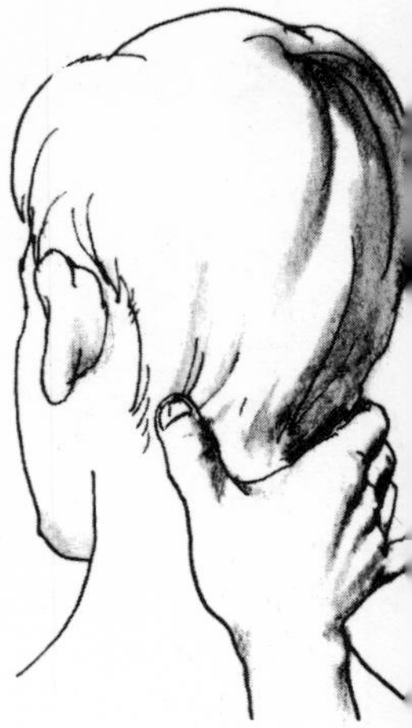

1. BL-10 (天柱, *T'ien-chu*)
To the outer side of the two large muscles of the neck where they join the the back of the head.

2. GB-21 (肩井, *Chien-ching*)
In the middle point between the base of the neck and the end of the shoulder.

Fig. 17

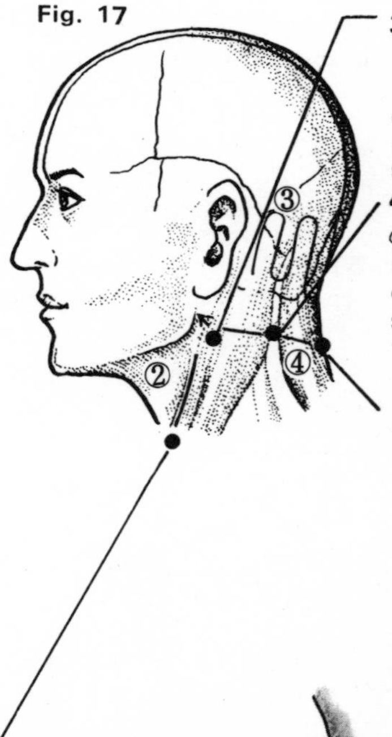

3. SI-17 (天容, *T'ien-yung*)
Below the ear at the corner of the lower jaw. Immediately in front of the sternomastoid muscle.

4. GB-20 (風池, *Feng-ch'ih*)
Depressions in the lower edge of the occiput two sun on either side of the tsubos designated BL-10.

BL-10

5. ST-11 (気舎, *Ch'i-she*)
One sun and five bu on either side of the central point in the front of the neck. Inner tips of the clavicles and upper tip of the sternum.

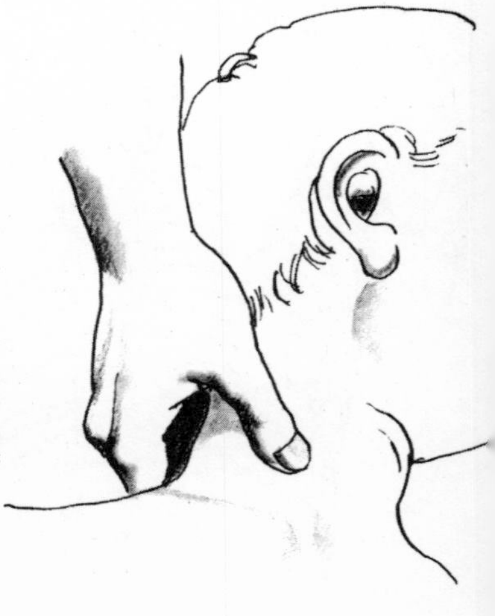

Fig. 18

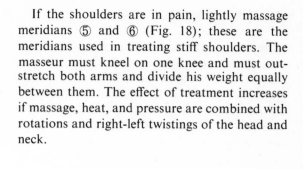

BL-10
GB-21

⑤

⑥

If the shoulders are in pain, lightly massage meridians ⑤ and ⑥ (Fig. 18); these are the meridians used in treating stiff shoulders. The masseur must kneel on one knee and must out-stretch both arms and divide his weight equally between them. The effect of treatment increases if massage, heat, and pressure are combined with rotations and right-left twistings of the head and neck.

6. BL-38 (膏肓, *Kao-huang*)
Three sun on either side of the spinal column at points below the fourth thoracic vertebra.

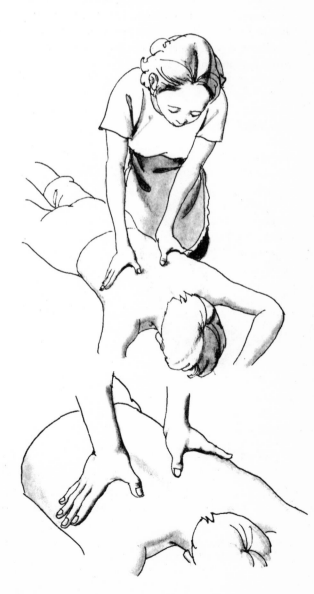

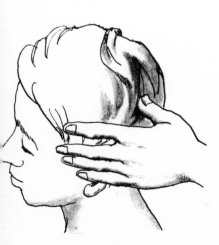

(6) Sore Throat

Some of the sicknesses affecting the throat are acute pharyngitis, laryngitis, throat cancer, diphtheria, tonsilitis, and swollen tonsils; the last is the most common. In light cases of swollen tonsils, the area on the inside of the throat in the vicinity of the tonsils becomes red, and swallowing is painful. In more serious cases, fever may develop; and, when matters grow still graver, pus may exude at the tonsils, and swallowing may become extremely difficult. Sometimes the muscle of deglutition may become paralyzed, making swallowing virtually impossible. These conditions may be accompanied by dryness in the throat, painful coughing, excessive phlegm, and discomfort in speech. In recent years, air pollution has caused many people to suffer from sore throat. In all of these cases, when the causes of the condition are physiological and pathological, consult a specialist.

But oriental therapy can be helpful in relieving soreness in the throat when the trouble arises from psychological causes. For instance, there are people who experience roughness and discomfort in the throat when they meet strangers because they have a fear of contact with people outside their ordinary circle of aquaintance. The major tsubo for treating such conditions are ST-9, ST-10, and ST-11 at the base of the throat and CV-22 (Fig. 20). CV-22 is easy to find: it is at the top of the sternum (at about the point where a man knots his necktie). Light digital pressure in the direction of the diaphragm applied to this tsubo arouses a sensation that can be felt from the throat to the lower jaw. Pressure on this tsubo is useful in relieving pain caused by swollen tonsils. In the past, acupuncture was used on CV-22 and on LI-4 (Fig. 21) for sore throat. A triangular-tipped needle was employed to produce hemorrhage. The treatment was highly effective.

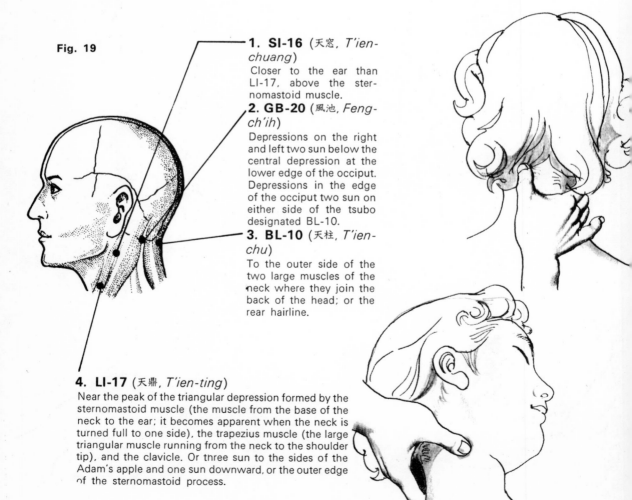

Fig. 19

1. SI-16 (天窓, *T'ien-chuang*)
Closer to the ear than LI-17, above the sternomastoid muscle.

2. GB-20 (風池, *Feng-ch'ih*)
Depressions on the right and left two sun below the central depression at the lower edge of the occiput. Depressions in the edge of the occiput two sun on either side of the tsubo designated BL-10.

3. BL-10 (天柱, *T'ien-chu*)
To the outer side of the two large muscles of the neck where they join the back of the head; or the rear hairline.

4. LI-17 (天鼎, *T'ien-ting*)
Near the peak of the triangular depression formed by the sternomastoid muscle (the muscle from the base of the neck to the ear; it becomes apparent when the neck is turned full to one side), the trapezius muscle (the large triangular muscle running from the neck to the shoulder tip), and the clavicle. Or three sun to the sides of the Adam's apple and one sun downward, or the outer edge of the sternomastoid process.

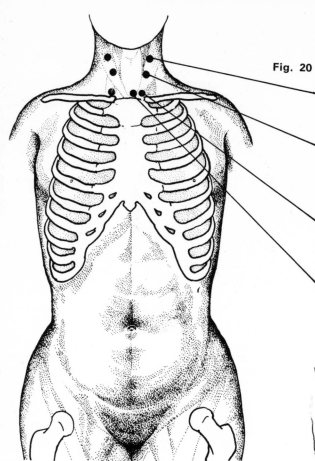

Fig. 20   *Sicknesses That Are Not Strictly Sicknesses* **73**

5. ST-9 (人迎, *Jen-ying*)
Points one sun and five bu on either side of the Adam's apple. The pulse is felt strongly in these places.

6. ST-10 (水突, *Shui-t'u*)
Points below and on the outer side of the Adam's apple on the front edge of the sternomastoid muscle. Directly below LI-17, on the top of the sterno-mastoid muscle.

7. ST-11 (気舎, *Ch'i-she*)
One sun and five bu on either side of the central point in the front of the neck. Inner tip of the clavicles and upper tip of the sternum.

8. CV-22 (天突, *T'ien-t'u*)
The depression immediately above the sternum or the depression above the midpoint between the clavicles.

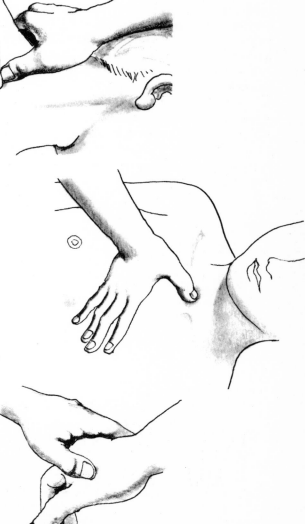

This is not, however, a practical domestic treatment. In its stead, use shiatsu pressure on CV-22 and LI-4 and combine this pressure with massage on SI-16, GB-20, BL-10, LI-17 (Fig. 19), ST-9, SI-10, and ST-11. Pressure on the throat must be light, for too much power can have adverse effects. Moxa combustion is effective in cases of this kind, though speedy results cannot be expected from it.

Fig. 21

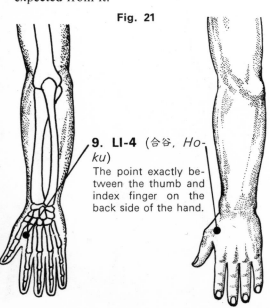

9. LI-4 (合谷, *Ho-ku*)
The point exactly between the thumb and index finger on the back side of the hand.

(7) Hot Flashes

Hot flashes to the neck and face are generally the result of psychological factors like having to appear before a large audience. They may, however, result from sudden transition from a very cold place to a warm one. The redness of the face that is experienced by people who have been exposed to the hot sun is usually confined to the skin alone and is the consequence of the expansion of the blood vessels. In addition, upsets in the autonomic nervous system can cause sudden flushing of the face and chilling of the feet, as can hyperactivity of the thyroid gland (Basedow's disease, in which greatly heightened metabolic activity keeps the body temperature high and the face flushed in a condition resembling the state the body is in shortly after a hot bath). Menopause in women sometimes causes chilling of the hands and feet and flushed face, accompanied by headaches, stiff shoulders, palpitations, dizziness, ringing in the ears, irritability, and other symptoms. Immediately before menstruation, women often experience flushing; and members of both sexes may be subject to this symptom in the early stages of such sicknesses as arteriosclerosis and high blood pressure. People suffering from rushes of blood to the face ought to avoid stress-causing situations and violent exercise. They must remain calm and quiet.

2. BL-10 (天柱, *T'ien-chu*)
To the outer side of the two large muscles of the neck where they join the back of the head.

Fig. 22

1. GV-20 (百会, *Pai-hui*)
At the point where a line directly upward from ear to ear crossing the top of the head and a line straight upward from the midpoint of the area between the shoulders to the top of the head intersect.

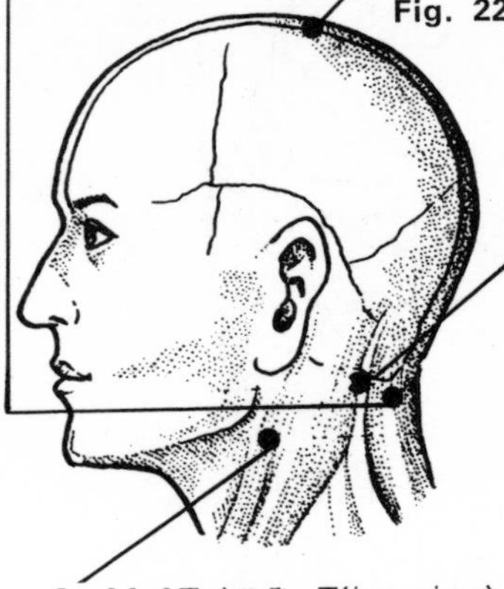

3. GB-20 (風池, *Feng-ch'ih*)
Depressions on the right and left two sun below the central depression at the lower edge of the occiput.

4. LI-17 (天鼎, *T'ien-ting*)
Near the peak of the triangular depression formed by the sternomastoid muscle (the muscle from the base of the neck to the ear; it becomes apparent when the neck is turned full to one side), the trapezius muscle (the large triangular muscle running from the neck to the shoulder tip), and the clavicle.

Massage or shiatsu therapy on the tsubo listed below will help avoid flushing and at the same time stabilize the blood pressure: first GV-20, BL-10, GB-20, and LI-17 (Fig. 22); then ST-11, CV-17, CV-12, CV-4, ST-27, CV-3 (Fig. 23) (apply only gentle pressure to the points from the side of the neck to throat, but apply ample pressure to the tsubo on the stomach).

Fig. 23

5. ST-11 (気舎, *Ch'i-she*)
Inner tips of the clavicles and upper tips of the sternum.
6. CV-17 (膻中, *Shang-chung*)
Middle of the front of the sternum at the midpoint between the nipples.

7. CV-12 (中脘, *Chung-wan*)
Four sun above the navel.
8. CV-4 (関元, *Kuan-yüan*)
Three sun below the navel.

9. ST-27 (大巨, *Ta-chü*)
Two sun below points two sun on either side of the navel.
10.   CV-3 (中極, *Chung-chi*)
Four sun below the navel.

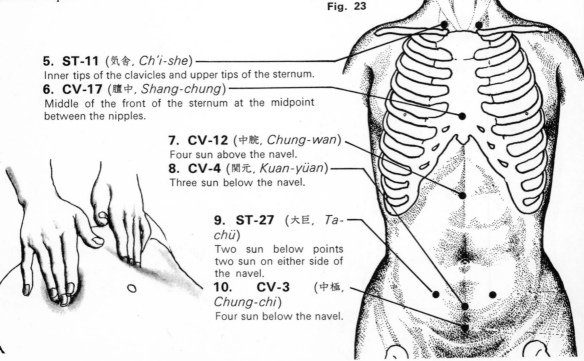

Fig. 24

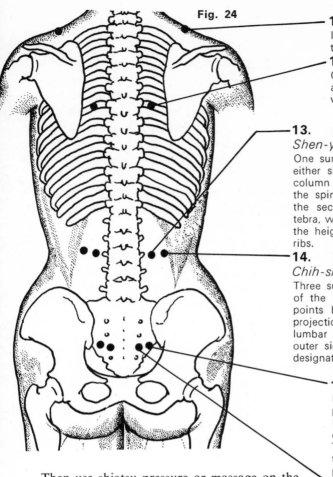

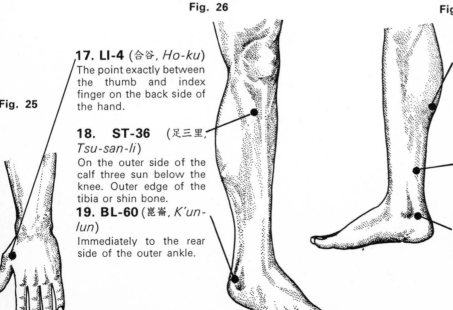

11. GB-21 (肩井, *Chien-ching*)
In the middle point between the base of the neck and the end of the shoulder.

12. BL-15 (心兪, *Hsin-yü*)
One sun and five bu on either side of the spinal column at points below the spinal projections of the fifth thoracic vertebra.

13. BL-23 (腎兪, *Shen-yü*)
One sun and five bu on either side of the spinal column at points below the spinal projections of the second lumbar vertebra, which is located at the height of the lowest ribs.

14. BL-47 (志室, *Chih-shih*)
Three sun on either side of the spinal column at points below the spinal projections of the second lumbar vertebra; on the outer sides of the tsubo designated BL-23.

15. BL-33 (中髎, *Chung-liao*)
Five sacral vertebrae are fused to form a rear wall for the pelvic cavity. The four tsubo BL-31, BL-32, BL-33, and BL-34 are located beside the openings on either side of the projections of the top four of these vertebrae. The pair of tsubo designated BL-31 is on the level of the topmost of the sacral vertebrae, and the others proceed downward in ascending numerical order.

16. BL-28 (膀胱兪, *P'ang-kuan-yü*)
One sun and five bu on either side of the projections of the second sacral vertebra.

Then use shiatsu pressure or massage on the following tsubo on the back: GB-21, BL-15, BL-23, BL-47, BL-33, and BL-28 (Fig. 24). Finally, treat these tsubo: LI-4 on the hands (Fig. 25), ST-36 and BL-60 on the feet, and KI-9, SP-6, and KI-3 (Figs. 26 and 27).

Fig. 25

Fig. 26

Fig. 27

17. LI-4 (合谷, *Ho-ku*)
The point exactly between the thumb and index finger on the back side of the hand.

18. ST-36 (足三里, *Tsu-san-li*)
On the outer side of the calf three sun below the knee. Outer edge of the tibia or shin bone.

19. BL-60 (崑崙, *K'un-lun*)
Immediately to the rear side of the outer ankle.

20. KI-9 (築賓, *Chu-pin*)
In the muscle that is the width of the index finger inward of the edge of the shin at a point five sun above the inner side of the ankle.

21. SP-6 (三陰交, *San-yin-chiao*)
Three sun upward on the side of the shin bone from the inner side of the ankle.

22. KI-3 (太谿, *T'ai-hsi*)
Rear part of the inside of the ankle.

(8) Motion Sickness

Some people who have suffered from motion sickness in the past find that the very recollection of the unpleasant experience acts as a suggestion causing recurrence of the distress whenever they ride in a vehicle. In other cases, motion sickness can be traced to upset stomach, lack of sleep, an empty stomach, or other purely physical causes. In general, motion stickness is related to the body's ability to sense equilibrium. This is governed by the semicircular ducts and the vestibule of the inner ear. These organs are related to both sight and smell. A deaf person never suffers from motion sickness.

Persons susceptible to this condition can prevent it by ensuring adequate sleep on the night before they must ride in a vehicle and by eating a suitable amount of easily digested food at least one hour before departure time. Such people should avoid clothes that bind at the neck and the waist. Parents of children who are likely to become motion sick should act as if nothing were wrong. If they fret, they will increase the danger of upsetting the child, who should ride in the part of the vehicle that shakes least and should be next to the window where he can be distracted by the scenery. Singing or doing amusing things to keep the child's mind occupied is an excellent preventative.

Should the person—adult or child—become motion sick, allow him to lie down in a comfortable position. Loosen his clothing. If he feels nauseous, he must be allowed to vomit. People prone to motion sickness should always prepare for the eventuality of an attack by carrying plastic bags or other suitable containers whenever they travel.

Since the most important cure is to develop a body that is no longer adversely affected by motion, about one week before a long trip—or regularly whenever free time is available—burn moxa on and massage the tsubo given below. You can expect effectiveness only if you persist in the treatment. Acupuncture is the most effective therapy, but you must apply to a specialist to have it done. These are the tsubo for treatment of motion sickness: GV-20 on the top of the head, BL-10 at the rear hairline, and GB-20 on either side of BL-10. Treatment on these tsubo calms the action of the heart. TH-17 below the earlobes and GB-11 immediately behind the ears are other tsubo used in treating this condition (Fig. 28).

Fig. 28

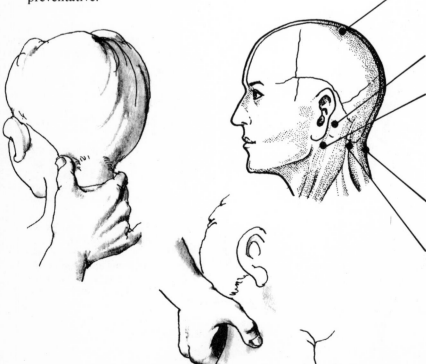

1. GV-20 (百会, *Pai-hui*)
At the point where a line directly upward from ear to ear crossing the top of the head and a line straight upward from the midpoint of the area between the shoulders to the top of the head intersect.

2. GB-11 (竅陰, *Ch'iao-yin*)
Point behind the ear directly opposite the ear hole.

3. TH-17 (翳風, *Yi-feng*)
In the depression between the lobe of the ear and the mastoid process.

4. BL-10 (天柱, *T'ien-chu*)
To the outer side of the two large muscles of the neck where they join the back of the head.

5. GB-20 (風池, *Feng-ch'ih*)
Depressions in the lower edge of the occiput two sun on either side of the tsubos designated BL-10.

In conjunction with therapy on these tsubo, treatment on BL-18 on the back (Fig. 29) and LV-14 on the abdomen (Fig. 30) helps prevent motion sickness. Once the person has become sick, it is too late for acupuncture or moxa combustion, but relief can be brought by pressing the tsubo on the stomach.

Fig. 29

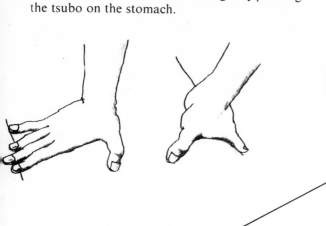

6. BL-18, (肝兪, *Kan-yü*)
One sun and five bu on either side of the spinal column at points below the spinal projections of the ninth thoracic vertebra.

Fig. 30

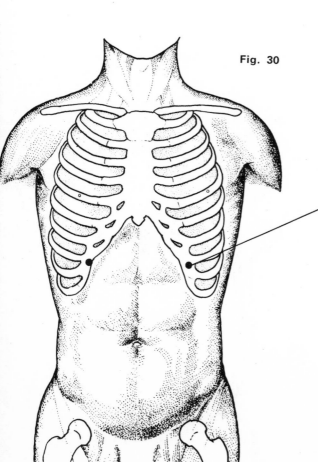

7. LV-14 (期門, *Ch'i-men*)
Extremities of the ninth ribs. Or a place located at the boundary between the rib and the abdomen directly below the nipple of the breast. The zone between the edge of the rib and the diaphragm.

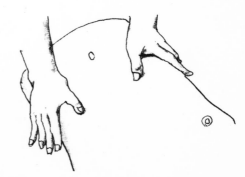

(9) Hangover

Young people can drink a little too much at night and wake in the morning with no ill effects. People who have already passed their mid-thirties, on the other hand, find that even a slight overindulgence leaves them with fierce hangovers, aching heads, nausea, and a general debility that makes work seem impossible. The symptoms gradually go away, and perhaps a day in bed is the best cure; but people who must work for a living cannot always afford such luxury. In these cases, simple massage and shiatsu performed before the person rises from bed can be effective in clearing up the head.

First apply firm, slow pressure with the thumbs to GV-20, GB-12, GB-20, and BL-10 (Fig. 31). Next, firmly grip the sternomastoid muscle with the thumb and four fingers and massage it in the direction shown by the arrows in the chart. This will relieve the flushed condition of the face.

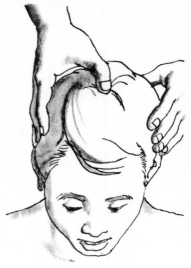

1. GV-20 (百会, *Pai-hui*)
At the point where a line directly upward from ear to ear crossing the top of the head and a line straight upward from the midpoint of the area between the shoulders to the top of the head intersect.

Fig. 31

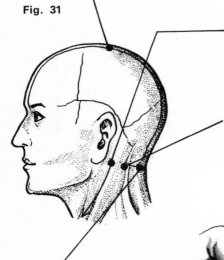

2. GB-12 (完骨, *Wan-ku*)
Depression in the back edge of the mastoid process behind the ear. In the depression that is located about the width of one finger above the mastoid process and about four bu from the hairline.

3. GB-20 (風池, *Feng-ch'ih*)
Depressions on the right and left two sun below the central depression at the lower edge of the occiput.

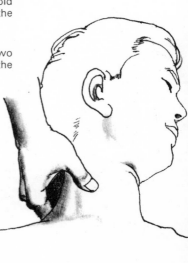

4. BL-10 (天柱, *T'ien-chu*)
To the outer side of the two large muscles of the neck where they join the back of the head; or the rear hairline.

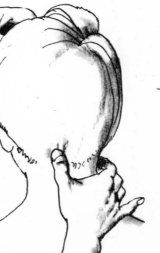

Then, folding a pillow and placing it under the patient's body, have him stretch his arms and legs out and arch his back. Using the four fingers, you must then press in a light, thrusting motion on CV-15, CV-14, CV-12, LV-14, and LV-13 (Fig. 32); work in the direction of the arrows. The person receiving the treatment must slowly open his mouth and relax his abdomen. Next, apply pressure to KI-16 and ST-25 (Fig. 32) for from five to six minutes. This will relieve the stiffness in the back and the sensation of nausea. The person suffering from the hangover will then feel surprisingly improved. He should stretch his entire body.

If the patient has felt very sick or extremely queasy, it is often a good idea to administer an emetic of baking soda and water or of salt water. If he suffers from severe headache, give him an ice pack. Once he feels better, he should further clear his head by drinking a cup of strong coffee or tea. The popular "hair of the dog"—that is, a small amount of alcohol taken as a curative—is in fact sometimes helpful. Finally, the patient should take a moderately warm bath. To prevent hangover, keep the feet cool while drinking.

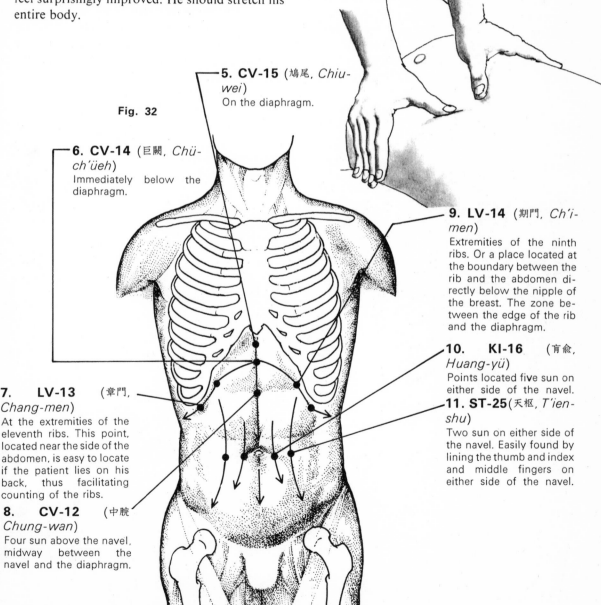

Fig. 32

5. CV-15 (鳩尾, *Chiu-wei*)
On the diaphragm.

6. CV-14 (巨闕, *Chü-ch'üeh*)
Immediately below the diaphragm.

9. LV-14 (期門, *Ch'i-men*)
Extremities of the ninth ribs. Or a place located at the boundary between the rib and the abdomen directly below the nipple of the breast. The zone between the edge of the rib and the diaphragm.

10.   KI-16 (肓俞, *Huang-yü*)
Points located five sun on either side of the navel.

11. ST-25 (天枢, *T'ien-shu*)
Two sun on either side of the navel. Easily found by lining the thumb and index and middle fingers on either side of the navel.

7.   LV-13 (章門, *Chang-men*)
At the extremities of the eleventh ribs. This point, located near the side of the abdomen, is easy to locate if the patient lies on his back, thus facilitating counting of the ribs.

8.   CV-12 (中脘, *Chung-wan*)
Four sun above the navel, midway between the navel and the diaphragm.

(10) Insomnia

The symptoms of this disorder are inability to fall asleep at night, shallow slumber, many dreams, early awakening, and so on. Most of the people who complain of insomnia are afflicted with psychological problems; but in some cases, disturbances of the autonomic nervous system, stomach upset, and other sicknesses can be the cause. In addition, itchiness of the skin, diarrhea, difficult breathing, stuffy nose, hunger, and pain make people easy victims of insomnia. Excess use of drugs and overconsumption of coffee can keep one awake.

The first thing to do is to discover why sleep is impossible and then to eliminate the cause. In the case of psychological factors, it is advisable to try to remove the troubling thing from the mind. Counting slowly—the old-fashioned counting sheep—often helps. It is important to avoid allowing the fear of insomnia to deprive you of sleep. Convince yourself that loss of one or even two nights of slumber will not kill you.

The members of the family can contribute to the creation of an environment in which the insomniac can sleep. If fever is the cause, the wife can prepare an ice pack. If the sufferer has a dry throat or a stuffy nose, adjustments in the temperature and humidity of the room ought to be made.

To treat the insomniac, first touch his back. You are likely to find a stiff area from the neck down the spine in the line of BL-10, BL-17, BL-18, and BL-23 (Fig. 33). Massage, shiatsu pressure, or moxa combustion on these tsubo can combat the stiffness. Combine slow shiatsu pressure with massage on these tsubo.

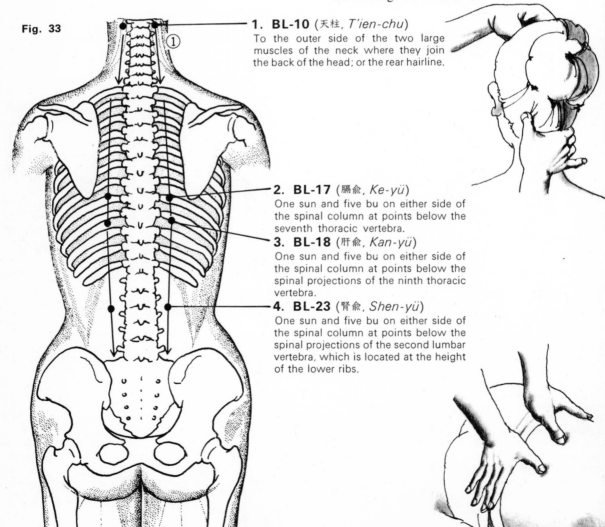

Fig. 33

1. BL-10 (天柱, *T'ien-chu*)
To the outer side of the two large muscles of the neck where they join the back of the head; or the rear hairline.

2. BL-17 (膈兪, *Ke-yü*)
One sun and five bu on either side of the spinal column at points below the seventh thoracic vertebra.

3. BL-18 (肝兪, *Kan-yü*)
One sun and five bu on either side of the spinal column at points below the spinal projections of the ninth thoracic vertebra.

4. BL-23 (腎兪, *Shen-yü*)
One sun and five bu on either side of the spinal column at points below the spinal projections of the second lumbar vertebra, which is located at the height of the lower ribs.

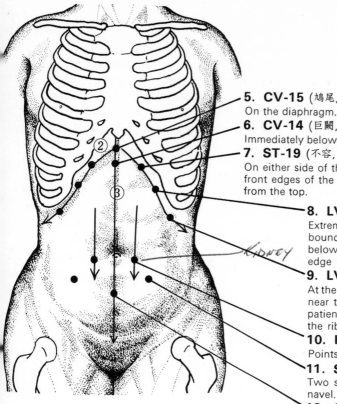

Fig. 34

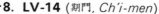

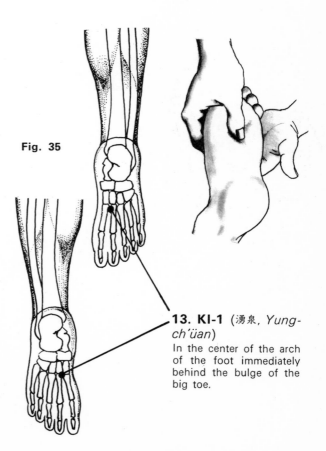

5. CV-15 (鳩尾, *Chiu-wei*)
On the diaphragm.
6. CV-14 (巨闕, *Chü-ch'üeh*)
Immediately below the diaphragm.
7. ST-19 (不容, *Pu-yung*)
On either side of the diaphragm at the front edges of the eighth ribs counted from the top.
8. LV-14 (期門, *Ch'i-men*)
Extremities of the ninth ribs. Or a place located at the boundary between the rib and the abdomen directly below the nipple of the breast. The zone between the edge of the rib and the diaphragm.
9. LV-13 (章門, *Chang-men*)
At the extremities of the eleventh ribs. This point, located near the side of the abdomen, is easy to locate if the patient lies on his back, thus facilitating counting of the ribs.
10. KI-16 (肓兪, *Huang-yü*)
Points located five sun on either side of the navel.
11. ST-27 (大巨, *Ta-chü*)
Two sun below points two sun on either side of the navel.
12. CV-4 (関元, *Kuan-yüan*)
Three sun below the navel, or midway between the navel and the pubis.

Next examine the front side of the body. There will probably be a zone where pressure creates sharp pain or causes the patient to cry out: CV-15, CV-14, ST-19, LV-14, LV-13, KI-16, ST-27, and CV-4 (Fig. 34). Treatment on these tsubo will gradually relieve pain and allow the patient to sleep.

Using the thumbs and the four fingers, massage lightly in the direction indicated by the arrows. Combine massage with adequate shiatsu pressure on the tsubo, or with moxa combustion.

When sluggishness of the feet and legs keeps you awake, first read the section on treating the feet and the hips. Then apply the method described there to relieve the weariness. A beer bottle rolled over the floor with the foot is effective. When the stiffness is removed from the tsubo KI-1 (Fig. 35), the patient will sleep well. Keeping the feet warm is important in preventing insomnia.

Fig. 35

13. KI-1 (湧泉, *Yung-ch'üan*)
In the center of the arch of the foot immediately behind the bulge of the big toe.

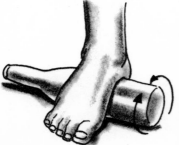

(11) Dizziness and Ringing in the Ears

Lack of sleep and protracted fatigue cause dizziness and metallic ringing in the ears when one rises suddenly to a standing position. The basic causes of the condition are various and include malfunctions in the ear, the cerebrum, and the cerebellum and resulting failure to maintain equilibrium. This can be traced to cerebral anemia, cephalemia, disturbances related to menopause, motion sickness, stomach or intestinal disorders, nervous ailments, and so on. In women in their forties and fifties, menopause is usually the cause; it produces a situation that sometimes becomes chronic. Knowledge of the simple massage and shiatsu therapies that can relieve this situation is extremely valuable. Since the treatments are simple, there is no excuse for being lax in performing them daily.

First using the palms of both hands, gently stroke the meridians and the tsubo listed below in the order given, then apply light shiatsu pressure three or four times to each tsubo in order. Use the fleshy balls of the index fingers and the thumbs. The tsubo and the meridians are as follows: meridian ① centering on GB-11, located behind the ear; meridian ② from the end of the eye, across the temple, and over the ear to TH-20; meridian ③ from the front hairline (GV-24) to GV-20 and GV-19 to BL-10; meridian ④ from BL-4 on the forehead to GB-20; meridian ⑤ from BL-10 to GB-20 to TH-17 (Figs. 36 and 37).

Fig. 36

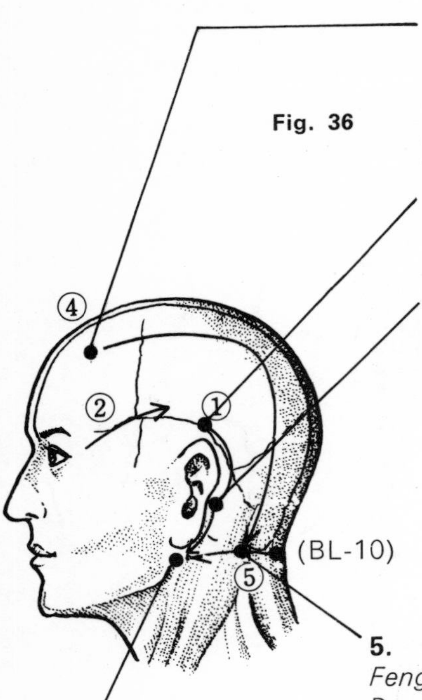

1. BL-4 (曲差, *Ch'ü-ch'a*)
Five bu above the hairline at points directly above the inner corners of the eyes.

2. TH-20 (角孫, *Chüe-hsun*)
Immediately above the ear.

3. GB-11 (竅陰, *Ch'iao-yin*)
Point behind the ear directly opposite the ear hole.

(BL-10)

4. TH-17 (翳風, *Yi-feng*)
In the depression between the lobe of the ear and the mastoid process. In the depression diagonally to the rear of the earlobe.

5. GB-20 (風池, *Feng-ch'ih*)
Depressions on the right and left two sun below the central depression at the lower edge of the occiput.

Fig. 37

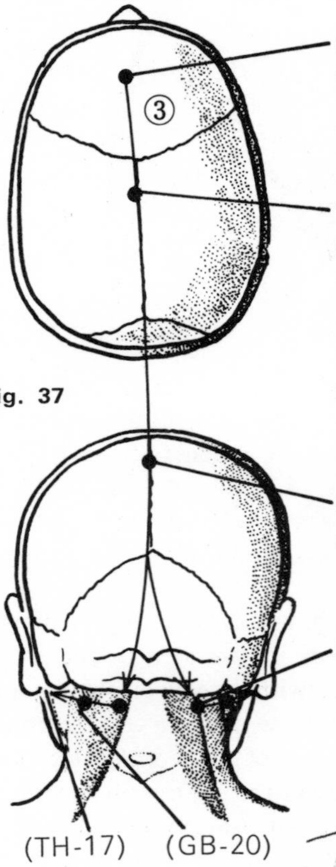

6. GV-24 (神庭 *Shen-t'ing*)
On a line passing through the center of the forehead five bu from the front hairline.

7. GV-20 (百会 *Pai-hui*)
At the point where a line directly upward from ear to ear crossing the top of the head and a line straight upward from the midpoint of the area between the shoulders to the top of the head intersect.

8. GV-19 (後頂 *Hou-ting*)
Behind and one suntive bu below the tsubo designated GV-20.

9. BL-10 (天柱 *Ti'en-chu*)
To the outer side of the two large muscles of the neck where they join the back of the head.

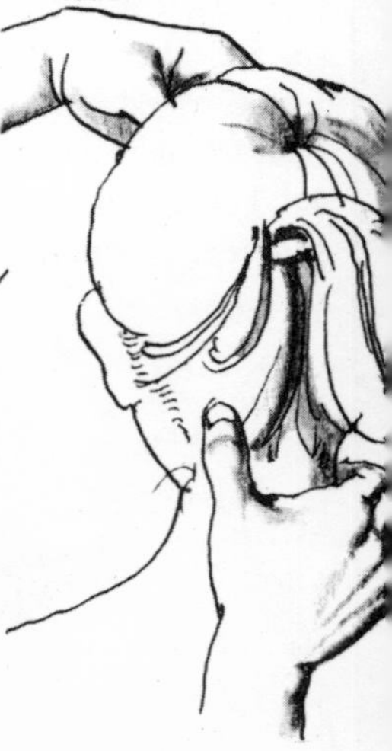

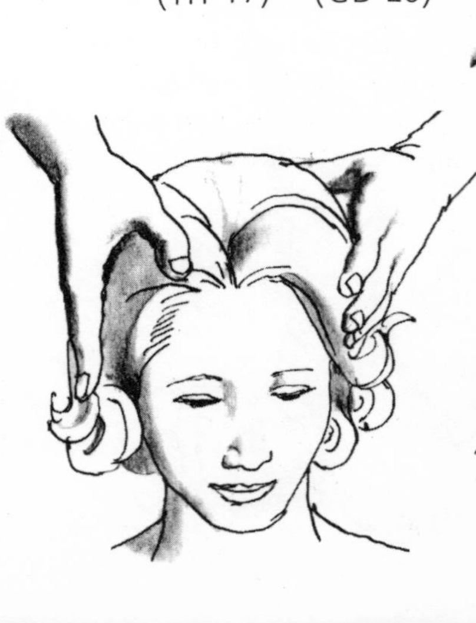

(TH-17) (GB-20)

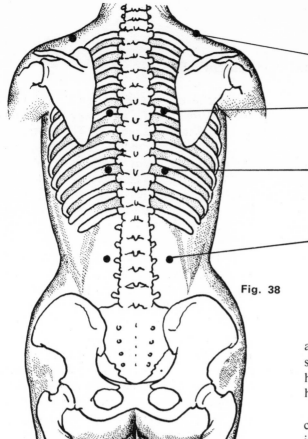

Fig. 38

10. GB-21 (肩井, *Chien-ching*)
In the point between the base of the neck and the end of the shoulder.

11. BL-15 (心兪, *Hsin-yü*)
One sun and five bu on either side of the spinal column at points below the spinal projections of the fifth thoracic vertebra.

12. BL-18 (肝兪, *Kan-yü*)
One sun and five bu on either side of the spinal column at points below the spinal projections of the ninth thoracic vertebra.

13. BL-23 (腎兪, *Shen-yü*)
One sun and five bu on either side of the spinal column at points below the spinal projections of the second lumbar vertebra, which is located at the height of the lowest ribs.

In Ménière's disease, paroxysms of dizziness and ringing in the ears occur at intervals of as short as thirty minutes and as long as four or five hours. Domestic treatment of the kind described here is powerless to cure this disease.

Although acupuncture and a weak electrical current prove especially effective in my laboratory in curing dizziness and ringing in the ears, these are not treatments for the home. Nevertheless, used regularly and carefully, massage and moxa combustion can ensure the changes in physical condition required to bring relief. Acupuncture is better in treating symptoms of the kind arising from anemia, high-blood pressure, sanguineous temperament, and nontypical conditions arising from neuroses and overwork. If there is the least suspicion of Ménières's disease, drug addiction, blockage of the blood in the brain, or brain tumor, the situation must be thoroughly discussed with a specialist before any home treatment is instituted.

Next apply shiatsu pressure to GB-21, BL-15, BL-18, and BL-23 (Fig. 38). Have the patient lie on his back so that you can apply shiatsu to GB-25, CV-12, KI-16 (Fig. 39), and KI-3 (Fig. 40). Finally massage BL-10 and GB-20 to the back of the neck.

Fig. 39

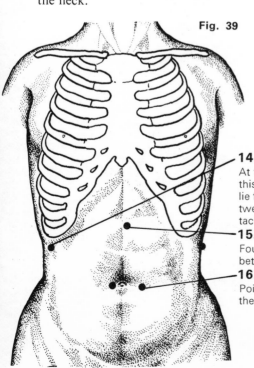

Fig. 40

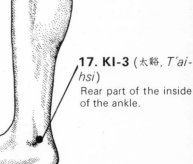

14. GB-25 (京門, *Ching-men*)
At the ends of the twelfth ribs. To find this have the patient kneel upright or lie facedown as you check his ribs. The twelfth ribs are short and are not attached at the small of the back.

15. CV-12 (中脘, *Chung-wan*)
Four sun above the navel; midway between the navel and the diaphragm.

16. KI-16 (肓兪, *Huang-yü*)
Points located five sun on either side of the navel.

17. KI-3 (太谿, *T'ai-hsi*)
Rear part of the inside of the ankle.

2. Illnesses of the Respiratory and Circulatory Systems

(1) High Blood Pressure

At first, it is difficult to diagnose high blood pressure by oneself. Usually, in the early stages, the person afflicted with this condition experiences headaches and dizziness upon arising in the morning. He may suffer from ringing in the ears, stiff shoulders, insomnia, palpitations, short breath, constipation, weariness, chills in the hands and feet, and so on. As the condition grows worse, hardening in the blood vessels in the vicinity of the heart and the brain begins. High blood pressure is declared when the blood pressure of a patient in a calm state is between a minimum of 90 and a maximum of 150. Other than heredity, the causes of the condition are difficult to pinpoint. It may be congenital, or it may be sporadic and caused by some disease. In addition to these causes, some young people of under thirty years of age and some women in menopause develop high blood pressure. But the overwhelming majority of cases is congenital and hereditary. The tendency to the condition is considered genetically dominant. If both parents have high blood pressure, roughly half of the offspring will be afflicted with it. If only one parent has the sickness, one-quarter of the offspring will have it as well.

The symptoms of congenital high blood pressure tend to manifest themselves most readily in people who suffer from frustrations, who become angry easily, who are irritable, and who are constantly in a state of psychological insecurity. Since business executives are its frequent victims, high blood pressure has come to be popularly known as the managerial complaint. It is likely to appear in people aged between forty and fifty, because this is the age bracket in which variations in blood pressure occur most commonly. Diet has an intimate connection with the manifestation of high blood pressure: too much salt or too much rice may contribute to its development.

Unfortunately, there is no single tsubo on the body where pressure can bring about sudden reductions in blood pressure. The treatment for this condition is gradually to relieve the symptoms that occur throughout the body as a result of it. To correct the headaches, stiff shoulders, and palpitations that invariably accompany high blood pressure, treat the following tsubo: GV-20, BL-10, ST-9, LI-17 (Fig. 1), GB-21, BL-15 (Fig. 2), LI-11, and LI-4 (Fig. 3).

If the patient suffers from insomnia, treat BL-17, and LV-14; if he tires easily, treat BL-23 and CV-4 (Figs. 4 and 5); if he has chills of the feet, treat GB-39 and SP-6 (Figs. 6 and 7).

Massage in the directions shown by the arrows along the meridians including the tsubo listed above. Moxa combustion (using finely cut moxa) three or four times on one place is effective. About one hundred taps with the right and one hundred taps with the left fist on KI-1 (Fig. 8) have an almost miraculously stimulating effect. Five minutes' application of an electric vibrator on KL-1 is effective.

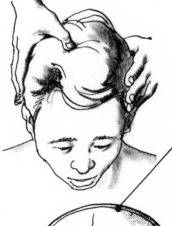

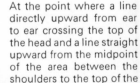

1. GV-20 (百会, *Pai-hui*)

At the point where a line directly upward from ear to ear crossing the top of the head and a line straight upward from the midpoint of the area between the shoulders to the top of the head intersect.

2. BL-10 (天柱, *T'ien-chu*)

To the outer side of the two large muscles of the neck where they join the back of the head.

3. ST-9 (人迎, *Jen-ying*)

Points one sun and five bu on either side of the Adams' apple. The pulse is felt strongly in these places.

4. LI-17 (天鼎, *T'ien-ting*)

Near the peak of the triangular depression formed by the sternomastoid muscle (the muscle from the base of the neck to the ear; it becomes apparent when the neck is turned full to one side), the trapezius muscle (the large triangular muscle running from the neck to the shoulder tip), and clavicle.

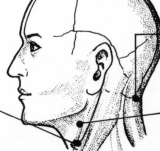

Fig. 1

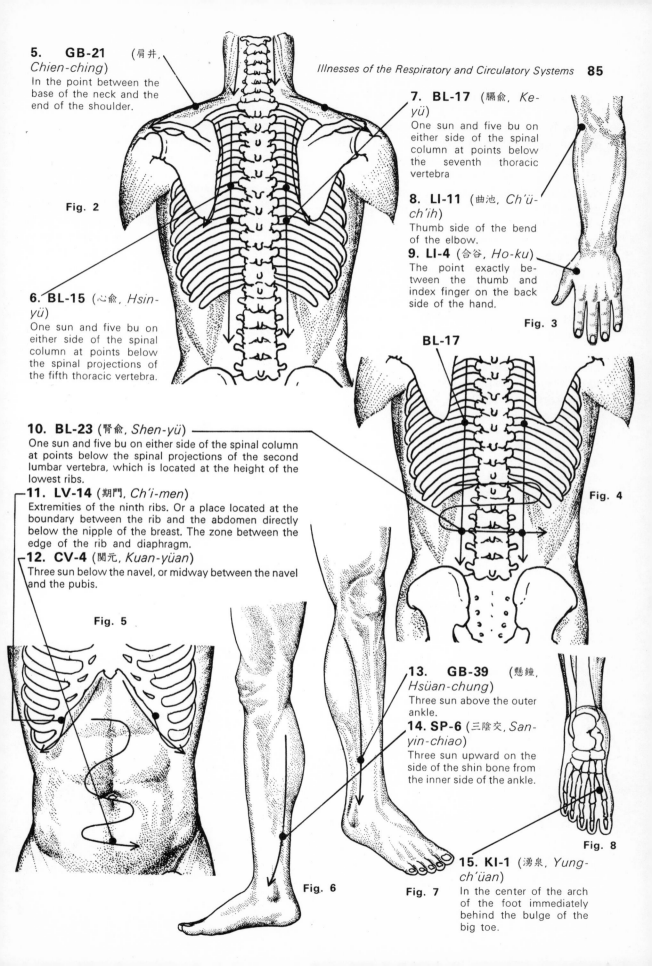

5. GB-21 (肩井, *Chien-ching*)
In the point between the base of the neck and the end of the shoulder.

Fig. 2

6. BL-15 (心兪, *Hsin-yü*)
One sun and five bu on either side of the spinal column at points below the spinal projections of the fifth thoracic vertebra.

7. BL-17 (膈兪, *Ke-yü*)
One sun and five bu on either side of the spinal column at points below the seventh thoracic vertebra

8. LI-11 (曲池, *Ch'ü-ch'ih*)
Thumb side of the bend of the elbow.

9. LI-4 (合谷, *Ho-ku*)
The point exactly between the thumb and index finger on the back side of the hand.

Fig. 3

BL-17

Fig. 4

10. BL-23 (腎兪, *Shen-yü*)
One sun and five bu on either side of the spinal column at points below the spinal projections of the second lumbar vertebra, which is located at the height of the lowest ribs.

11. LV-14 (期門, *Ch'i-men*)
Extremities of the ninth ribs. Or a place located at the boundary between the rib and the abdomen directly below the nipple of the breast. The zone between the edge of the rib and diaphragm.

12. CV-4 (関元, *Kuan-yüan*)
Three sun below the navel, or midway between the navel and the pubis.

Fig. 5

13. GB-39 (懸鐘, *Hsüan-chung*)
Three sun above the outer ankle.

14. SP-6 (三陰交, *San-yin-chiao*)
Three sun upward on the side of the shin bone from the inner side of the ankle.

Fig. 6

Fig. 7

Fig. 8

15. KI-1 (湧泉, *Yung-ch'üan*)
In the center of the arch of the foot immediately behind the bulge of the big toe.

(2) Low Blood Pressure

Generally speaking, a person's correct blood pressure should be the sum of his age plus ninety. Any blood pressure less than 100 can be considered abnormally low. The many causes of this condition can be divided into three large categories: symptomatic low blood pressure, orthostatic hypotensive low blood pressure, and congenital low blood pressure.

Symptomatic low blood pressure often occurs in patients who are undernourished; who suffer from cardiac conditions, cancer, or tuberculosis; or who have been forced to remain in bed for extended periods. Insufficiences in the hormones produced by the thyroid glands, the suprarenal glands, and the pituitary glands; hemorrhage; and shock can cause the condition. In all of these cases, the low blood pressure will be cured when the sickness causing it has been cured.

Orthostatic hypotensive low blood pressure is the name for a condition in which the blood pressure of the patient remains normal as long as he is in bed but drops suddenly when he gets up. This condition can be the cause of the dizziness and giddiness sometimes experienced by overly slender young women. Patients of high blood pressure and arteriosclerosis who take medication for their illnesses sometimes suffer from orthostatic hypotensive low blood pressure as an outcome.

The most common condition, however, is congenital low blood pressure, the cause of which is difficult to assign with any accuracy. The symptoms, which often manifest themselves in tall, slender people, resemble those of anemia: fatigue, sluggishness, lack of perseverence in work, headaches, dizziness, ringing in the ears, stiff shoulders, palpitations, shortness of breath, loss of appetite, heaviness in the stomach, constipation, chills of the hands and feet, menstrual irregularity, and so on. But, since the causes of anemia and those of low blood pressure are entirely different, it is best to consult a physician before attempting to diagnose a sickness of this kind.

People who suffer from congenital low blood pressure must eat plenty of easily digested proteins and fats. Oriental medical therapy concentrates on correcting abnormal symptoms in the body. To use it in cases of low blood pressure, use massage, shiatsu, or moxa combustion on and around the tsubo listed here: when the head aches, GV-20 and BL-10 (Fig. 9); for chills of the hands, HC-7, LU-9 (Fig. 10), LI-11, LI-5, and TH-4 (Fig. 11); for chills of the feet, SP-9, KI-3, and KI-6 (Fig. 12).

For dizziness, ringing in the ears, giddiness upon rising, weak stomach, and gastritis, consult the sections on those symptoms and apply moxa, massage, or shiatsu on the tsubo listed in Figs. 13 and 14.

In our clinic, we have achieved good effects by using ultrashort waves, supersonic waves, infrared lamps, and ultraviolet lamps on the tsubo listed above.

Fig. 9

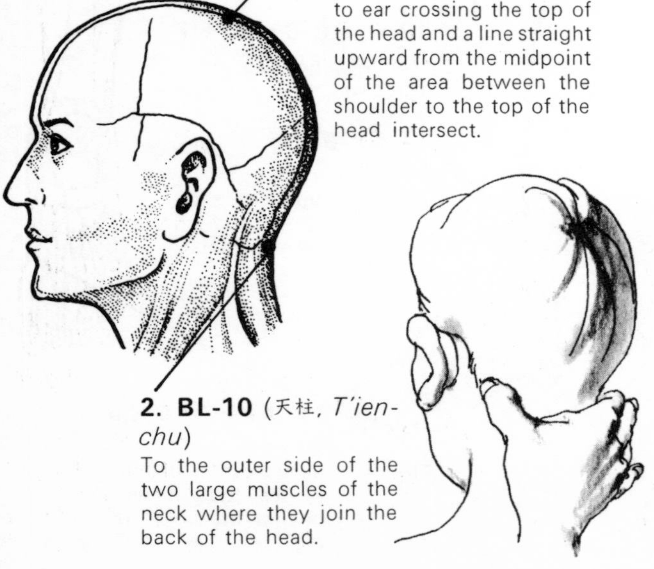

1. GV-20 (百会, *Pai-hui*)
At the point where a line directly upward from ear to ear crossing the top of the head and a line straight upward from the midpoint of the area between the shoulder to the top of the head intersect.

2. BL-10 (天柱, *T'ien-chu*)
To the outer side of the two large muscles of the neck where they join the back of the head.

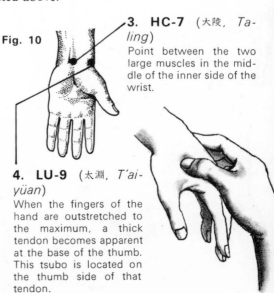

Fig. 10

3. HC-7 (大陵, *Ta-ling*)
Point between the two large muscles in the middle of the inner side of the wrist.

4. LU-9 (太淵, *T'ai-yüan*)
When the fingers of the hand are outstretched to the maximum, a thick tendon becomes apparent at the base of the thumb. This tsubo is located on the thumb side of that tendon.

5. LI-11 (曲池, *Ch'ü-ch'ih*)

Thumb side of the bend of the elbow.

6. LI-5 (陽谿, *Yang-hsi*)

Point between the two hard tendons on the back of the hand at the base of the thumb when the thumb is fully outstretched.

7. TH-4 (陽池, *Yang-ch'ih*)

When the palm is outstretched, on the back of the hand at the back of the wrist a hard, thick muscles becomes apparent. This tsubo is on the little-finger side of that muscle; that is, it is slightly to the little-finger side of the middle of the wrist.

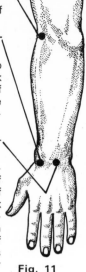

Fig. 11

Fig. 12

8. SP-9 (陰陵泉, *Yin-ling-ch'üan*)

Immediately below the large bone that protrudes just below the knee at the head of the shin.

9. KI-3 (太谿, *T'ai-hsi*)

Rear part of the inside of the ankle.

10. KI-6 (照海, *Chiao-hai*)

Depression immediately below the ankle.

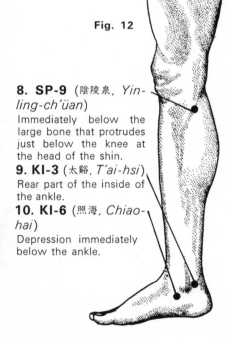

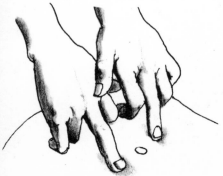

11. GB-21 (肩井, *Chien-ching*)

In the middle point between the base of the neck and the end of the shoulder.

Fig. 13

12. BL-38 (膏肓, *Kao-huang*)

Three sun on either side of the spinal column at points below the fourth thoracic vertebra.

13. BL-39 (神堂, *Shen-t'ang*)

Three sun on either side of the spinal column at points below the fifth thoracic vertebra. To the side of the tsubo designated BL-15, just inside the right and left shoulder blades.

14. BL-15 (心俞, *Hsin-yü*)

One sun and five bu on either side of the spinal column at points below the spinal projections of the fifth thoracic vertebra.

15. BL-23 (腎俞, *Shen-yü*)

One sun and five bu on either side of the spinal column at points below the spinal projections of the second lumbar vertebra, which is located at the height of the lowest ribs.

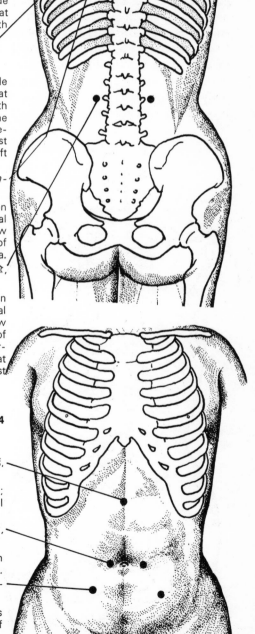

Fig. 14

16. CV-12 (中脘, *Chung-wan*)

Four sun above the navel; midway between the navel and the diaphragm.

17. KI-16 (肓俞, *Huang-yü*)

Points located five sun on either side of the navel.

18. ST-27 (大巨, *Ta-chü*)

Two sun below points two sun on either side of the navel.

(3) Heart Palpitations (Nervosum)

Many of the people who complain of this condition are nervous women aged from thirty to forty. Their symptoms are as follows: waking in the night with unexplainable palpitations of the heart that gradually produce a feeling of anxiety. This feeling in its turn prevents sleep; causes the pulse to race; and produces cardiac pain, chills, sweating, and shortness of breath. Palpitations may result both from conditions of the heart and from conditions unrelated to the heart. In the latter kind of case, sicknesses accompanied by high fevers and hypersecretion by the thyroid g lands (Basedow's disease) may be the causes. The hormone secreted by the thyroid glands governs the use of energy throughout the body. If this hormone is secreted in excessive amounts, the body uses too much energy, and the heart beat becomes too strong.

Sometimes anemia can cause palpitations. In cases of anemia, the oxygen in the blood is insufficient. This means that, even without using too much energy, the body makes extra demands on the amount of blood to compensate for the low oxygen content with the result that the person suffers from shortness of breath and palpitations.

Often the cause of palpitations cannot be traced to an organic heart condition, no matter how thoroughly specialists examine the body. The condition arises after extended periods of anger, anxiety, or irritability. And for this reason it is often described by the name *nervosum*, which means a kind of neurosis of the heart. In the past, tranquilizers, sleeping pills, and other medicines have been used to calm this condition; but the side effects by which such medicines are usually accompanied have gradually made it impossible to rely on them. In recent years, both acupuncture

Fig. 15

1. BL-14 (厥陰俞, *Chüeh-yin-yü*)
One sun and five bu on either side of the spinal column at points below the spinal projections of the fourth thoracic vertebra.

2. BL-15 (心俞, *Hsin-yü*)
One sun and five bu on either side of the spinal column at pints below the spinal projections of the fifth thoracic vertebra.

3. BL-39 (神堂, *Shen-t'ang*)
Three sun on either side of the spinal column at points below the fifth thoracic vertebra. To the side of the tsubo designated BL-15, just inside the right and left shoulder blades.

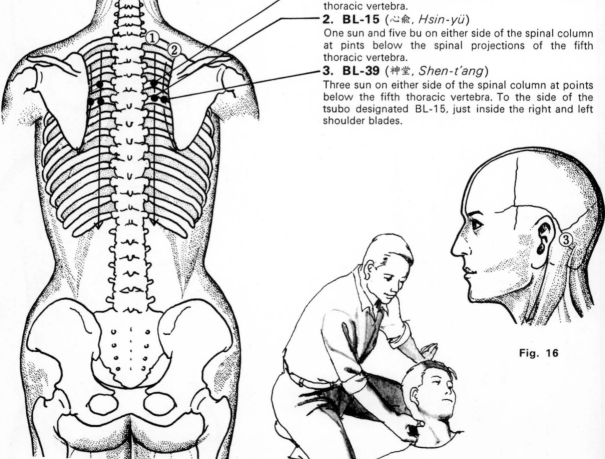

Fig. 16

and moxa combustion have been offering great hope of being therapeutic systems that calm the nerves and the heart while improving the general body condition. The most important tsubo in this treatment are BL-14, BL-15, CV-17, and CV-14 (Figs. 15 and 17). BL-39 (Fig. 15) is effective in calming palpitations. Thorough massage or shiatsu massage on the meridians shown in Figs. 15 through 19—meridians ① through ⑥—is effective.

is effective. Moxa combustion is good on these tsubo for chronic cases of heart palpitations; but for acute cases, massage on HC-4 and HT-7 (Fig. 18) is best.

This condition is difficult to cure entirely. Therapy requires the cooperation of the doctor and the home practitioner of oriental therapy. Since they are great enemies of the heart, such strong stimulants as coffee, liquor, and tobacco must be avoided.

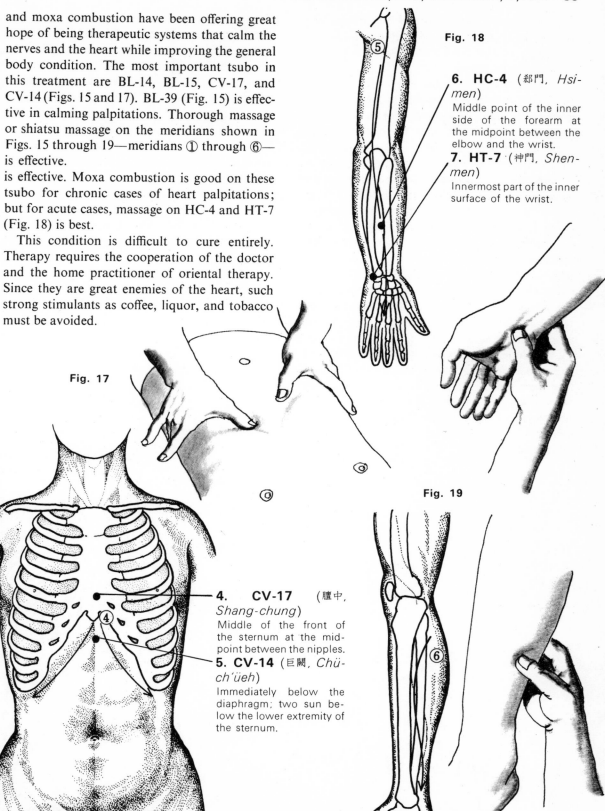

Fig. 18

6. HC-4 (郄門, *Hsi-men*)
Middle point of the inner side of the forearm at the midpoint between the elbow and the wrist.

7. HT-7 (神門, *Shen-men*)
Innermost part of the inner surface of the wrist.

Fig. 17

4. CV-17 (膻中, *Shang-chung*)
Middle of the front of the sternum at the mid-point between the nipples.

5. CV-14 (巨闕, *Chü-ch'üeh*)
Immediately below the diaphragm; two sun below the lower extremity of the sternum.

Fig. 19

(4)　Chronic Bronchitis (Coughing, Expectoration of Phlegm, and Difficulty in Breathing)

As soon as the chilly winds of fall begin to blow, some people resume the cough that they had forgotten in the heat of summer. For other people, coughing and phlegm that had presented no difficulty during the day become suddenly troublesome again in the cool of the evening.

Abnormalities in the respiratory tract are the cause of coughing, for which the following origins may be given. (1) Stimulus caused by breathing cold air, tobacco smoke, irritant gases, and so on. (2) Such obstructions as foreign matter—for instance, water—in the respiratory tract; in this instance, coughing is the body's way of trying to rid itself of the obstruction. (3) Abnormalities in the respiratory tract itself; these may take the form of soreness in the throat, swelling, fever, or secretions that the body is attempting to remove. Coughing may result from irritation of the throat cancer. (4) Accumulations of phlegm (the secretion of the mucous membrane of the respiratory tract) must be removed; coughing is the way this is achieved. (5) In the early stages of pleurisy, liquid exudations stimulate the pleura and cause coughing.

Diseases that cause fevers—colds, influenza, pleurisy, and pneumonia—can bring on coughing attacks. If the fever grows worse and the other symptoms do not abate, there is danger of whooping cough, asthma, heart sickness, pneumonia, or chronic bronchitis. In fact, coughs accompanied by phlegm are often a sign of chronic bronchitis. Malodorous phlegm resulting from the presence of pus organisms associated with chronic bronchitis are also associated with pneumonia, bronchial ecstasy, tuberculosis of the lungs, and influenza. People working in mines and in the woolens industry have come to consider chronic bronchitis an occupational disease. And, in recent years, environmental pollution has made it a common ailment among people living in industrial zones or along heavily trafficked highways. Heart sickness, kidney ailments, heavy drinking, and too much smoking can contribute to the appearance of this condition. If the sickness continues to grow worse, it

1. BL-13 (肺兪, *Fei-yü*)
One sun and five bu on either side of the spinal column at points below the spinal projections of the third thoracic vertebra.

Fig. 20

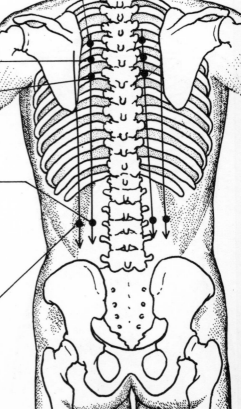

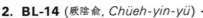
2. BL-14 (厥陰兪, *Chüeh-yin-yü*)
One sun and five bu on either side of the spinal column at points below the spinal projections of the fourth thoracic vertebra.
3. BL-15 (心兪, *Hsin-yü*)
One sun and five bu on either side of the spinal column at points below the spinal projections of the fifth thoracic vertebra.

4. BL-23 (腎兪, *Shen-yü*)
One sun and five bu on either side of the spinal column at points below the spinal projections of the second lumbar vertebra, which is located at the height of the lowest ribs.
5. BL-47 (志室, *Chih-shih*)
Three sun on either side of the spinal column at points below the spinal projections of the second lumbar vertebra; on the outer sides of the tsubo designated BL-23.

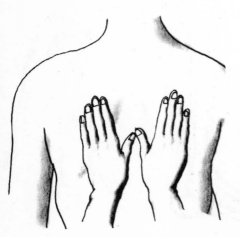

can involve danger of death; but massage, acupuncture, shiatsu, or moxa combustion can cure light cases.

In oriental medicine there is a special treatment for curing coughs and excess phlegm, conditions that tend to manifest themselves in people who are constitutionally weak. To check the condition, press BL-23 and BL-47 (Fig. 20) and KI-16 (Fig. 21). If there is stiffness at these tsubo or if pressing them causes pain, the person requires treatment, which must be applied to the following tsubo: BL-13, LU-1, LU-4, LU-6, and LU-9 to relieve coughing and excess phlegm; treatment on BL-14, BL-15, CV-17, and CV-14 removes pain and calms palpitations (Figs. 20 through 22). Massage with the thumbs on the meridians including these tsubo. (Massage must follow the direction indicated by the arrows in Figs. 20–23). At the same time, this treatment eliminates the slight stiffness that occurs in SP-9 and SP-6 (Fig. 23) in cases of this kind. Not all of these tsubo will manifest symptoms in all people. Check them, however; find the ones that are stiff; and treat accordingly. For chronic or stubborn cases, use moxa combustion.

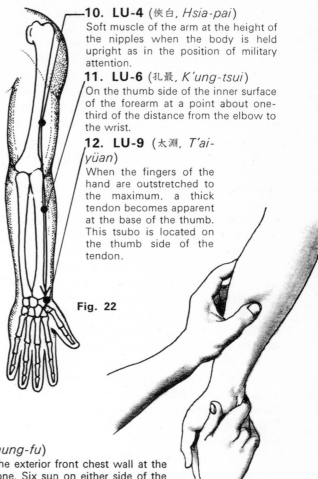

10. LU-4 (俠白, *Hsia-pai*)
Soft muscle of the arm at the height of the nipples when the body is held upright as in the position of military attention.

11. LU-6 (孔最, *K'ung-tsui*)
On the thumb side of the inner surface of the forearm at a point about one-third of the distance from the elbow to the wrist.

12. LU-9 (太淵, *T'ai-yüan*)
When the fingers of the hand are outstretched to the maximum, a thick tendon becomes apparent at the base of the thumb. This tsubo is located on the thumb side of the tendon.

Fig. 22

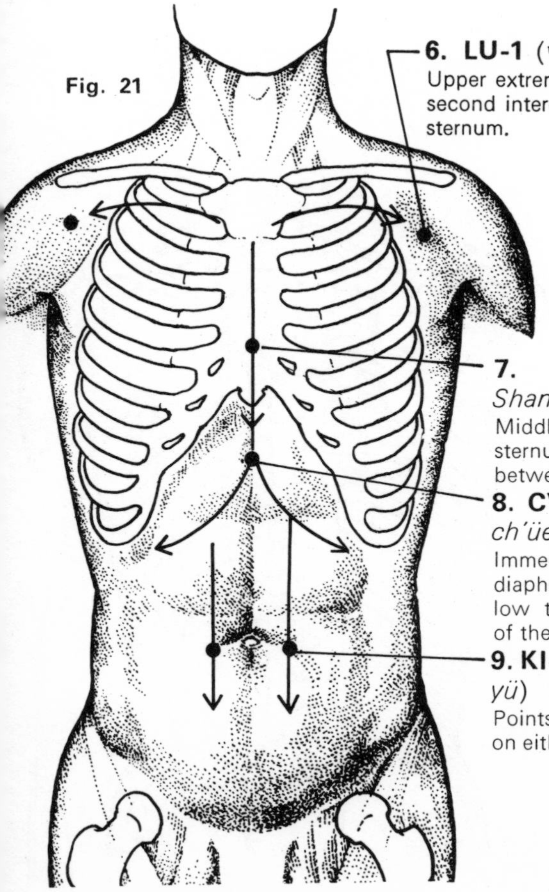

Fig. 21

6. LU-1 (中府, *Chung-fu*)
Upper extremity of the exterior front chest wall at the second intercostal zone. Six sun on either side of the sternum.

7. CV-17 (膻中, *Shang-chung*)
Middle of the front of the sternum at the midpoint between the nipples.

8. CV-14 (巨闕, *Chü-ch'üeh*)
Immediately below the diaphragm; two sun below the lower extremity of the sternum.

9. KI-16 (肓俞, *Huang-yü*)
Points located five bu on either side of the navel.

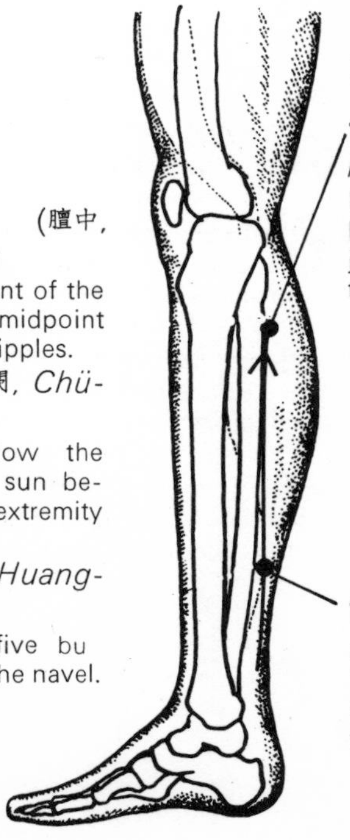

Fig. 23

13. SP-9 (陰陵泉, *Yin-ling-ch'üan*)
Immediately below the large bone that protrudes just below the knee at the head of the shin.

14. SP-6 (三陰交, *San-yin-chiao*)
Three sun upward on the side of the shin bone from the inner side of the ankle.

(5) Asthma (Infantile Asthma)

Only a person who suffers from asthma can know how distressing the disease is. Under ordinary conditions, the asthmatic patient is perfectly normal; but when an attack strikes, he coughs —a distinctive asthmatic cough—until he turns blue in the face and until his lips turn purple. Unable to lie down in comfort, he sits and waits for the attack to pass. This may require from as little as thirty minutes to as much as several hours—or even several days. People around the sufferer must suffer too since they are forced to watch, helpless to be of any assistance. When the coughing has ceased, the patient spits up thick, sticky phlegm.

About 30 percent of all sufferers and half of all male sufferers are under the age of ten. The cause of the attacks may be something in the air, or it may be an allergy to some kind of food or medicine. Pollen from plants, animal hair, bird feathers, or even flour can call down an asthmatic attack. The list of foods to which asthmatics are allergic is very long and includes such things as eggs, fish, shellfish, berries, spices, chocolate, spinach, bamboo shoots, yams, and buckwheat. Suppuration and tonsilitis are often to blame in the occurrence of asthma; but since there are people for whom some or all of these things are dangerous and others who are perfectly immune to everything on the list, it is clear that much mystery is still associated with this sickness.

During an attack—and even before it—pain will be felt when GV-14, BL-13, BL-15, (Fig. 24), CV-22, and LU-1 (Fig. 25) are pressed. These are the tsubo that have been long recognized as the locations where moxa combustion is effective in treating asthma. In addition however, hot water applications, and magnetic metal balls produce therapeutic effects when used on GB-21 (Fig. 24) and LU-4 and LU-6 (Fig. 26), if treatment is continued for about three weeks. Moxa should be applied from three to five times for each tsubo at each treatment session.

During an attack, leaving the patient in whatever position he is in, massage or apply shiatsu as shown by the arrows in Fig. 24; and his breathing will become easier. Then, using the thumbs of both hands, apply shiatsu massage to the meridians on the thick muscles running from the sides of the neck diagonally forward and downward (Fig. 27). Next make small circular motions on the flesh with the fingers.

Slowly massage in the directions of the arrows in Fig. 25. Gently rub the line running along the collarbone with the balls of the four fingers. Apply shiatsu pressure to LU-4 and LU-6. Hot hand baths for about ten minutes relieve blood congestion in the chest and make breathing more comfortable.

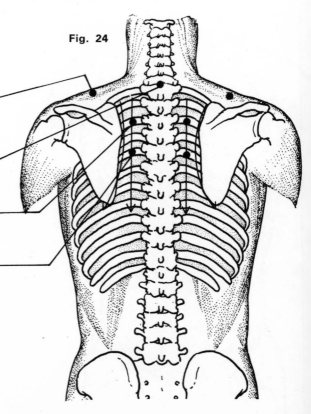

Fig. 24

1. GB-21 (肩井, *Chien-ching*)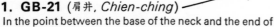
In the point between the base of the neck and the end of the shoulder.

2. GV-14 (大椎, *Ta-ch'ui*)
At the base of the neck in the back between the spinal projections of the seventh cervical and the first thoracic vertebra.

3. BL-13 (肺兪, *Fei-yü*)
One sun and five bu on either side of the spinal column at points below the spinal projections of the third thoracic vertebra.

4. BL-15 (心兪, *Hsin-yü*)
One sun and five bu on either side of the spinal column at points below the spinal projections of the fifth thoracic vertebra.

Fig. 25

5. CV-22 (天突, *T'ien-t'u*)
The depressions immediately above the sternum or the depression above the midpoint between the clavicles.

6. LU-1 (中府, *Chung-fu*)
Upper extremity of the exterior front chest wall at the second intercostal zone. Six sun on either side of the sternum.

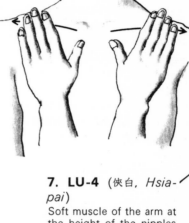

7. LU-4 (俠白, *Hsia-pai*)
Soft muscle of the arm at the height of the nipples when the body is held upright as in the position of military attention.

8. LU-6 (孔最, *K'ung-tsui*)
On the thumb side of the inner surface of the forearm at a point about one-third of the distance from the elbow to the wrist.

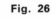

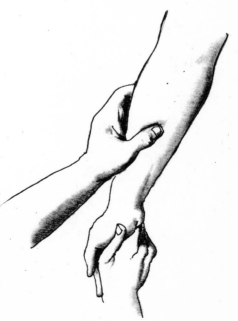

Fig. 26

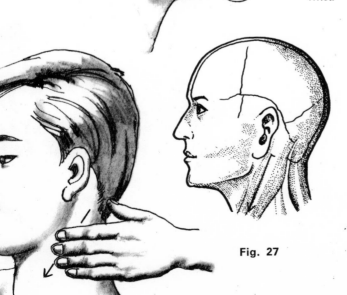

Fig. 27

(6) Colds

Probably everyone has had a cold at one time or another. Some people disparage the sickness as too trifling to require the attention of a physician; other people argue that the cold is the source of all illness. No matter which is the correct attitude, it is always better to cure a slight cold oneself. The usual cold is a minor respiratory condition frequently brought on by chills, cold air, or dampness. The nasal mucous membranes become inflamed and swollen. The nose may be runny, and the patient may sneeze frequently. When the condition grows worse, laryngitis may set in, the throat may become rough, and the patient may cough. Further aggravated, the cold may become bronchitis or pneumonia, both of which require the attention of a specialist. The treatment prescribed here is not intended for influenza or other bacteria-caused sicknesses.

According to oriental medical thought, colds are caused by evils that enter the body from the outside and that, in the early stage of the ailment, concentrate at the following tsubo: BL-12 (Fig. 29), GV-16, and GB-20 (Fig. 28). When a person thinks that he may have caught cold, he ought to have someone perform thorough shiatsu massage on GV-16 and GB-20. After massaging the occipital area, the masseur must apply shiatsu pressure to BL-13, LU-1 (Fig. 30), and LU-6 (Fig. 31). Special attention must be paid to LU-6 because it is very important in treating coughs.

If you are using moxa combustion, purchase medium moxa and apply it from three to five times to each tsubo daily. In conjunction with these therapeutic treatments, it is, of course, important to keep warm, eat nourishing food, rest, and get adequate sleep.

The symptoms of the cold are various and occur differently in different people. For instance 40 percent of all cold sufferers complain of coughs, 30 percent of sore throat and pain in the tonsils, 12 percent of sneezing and runny or stuffy nose, 10 percent of fever and chills, and 3 percent of headaches. Consequently, in treating colds, discover the symptoms and apply treatment to the appropriate tsubo. One must be cautious in making diagnoses, however, since sneezing, runny nose, and stuffy nose—major symptoms of the common cold—accompany such more serious illnesses as virus infections, asthma, and contagious sicknesses. If any of these seems to be possible, consult a physician before instituting home therapy.

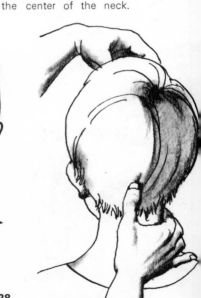

1. GV-16 (風府, *Feng-fu*)
One sun below the external occipital protuberance; about three bu below the depression in the center of the neck.

2. GB-20 (風池, *Feng-ch'ih*)
At the point where a line directly upward from ear to ear crossing the top of the head and a line straight upward from the midpoint of the area between the shoulders to the top of the head intersect.

Fig. 28

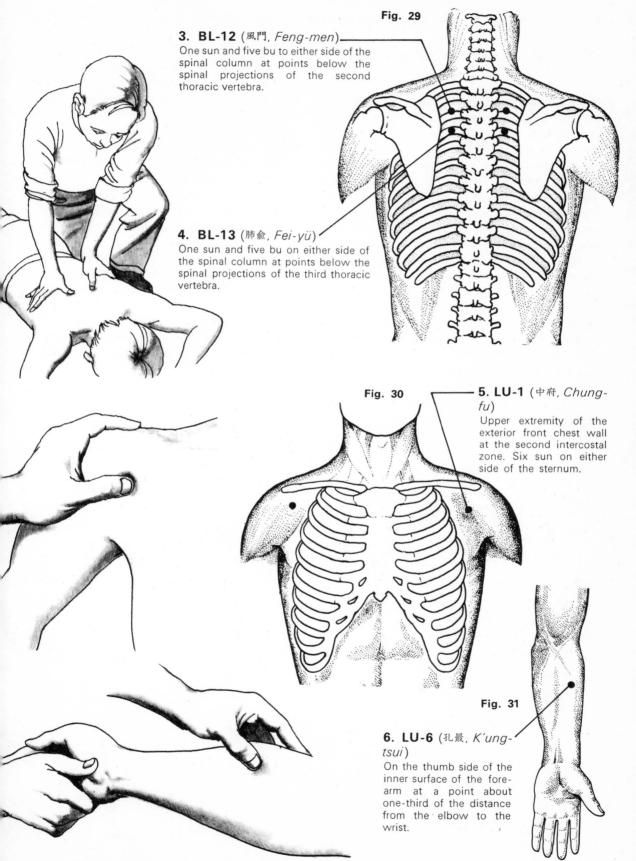

Fig. 29

3. BL-12 (風門, *Feng-men*)
One sun and five bu to either side of the spinal column at points below the spinal projections of the second thoracic vertebra.

4. BL-13 (肺俞, *Fei-yü*)
One sun and five bu on either side of the spinal column at points below the spinal projections of the third thoracic vertebra.

Fig. 30

5. LU-1 (中府, *Chung-fu*)
Upper extremity of the exterior front chest wall at the second intercostal zone. Six sun on either side of the sternum.

Fig. 31

6. LU-6 (孔最, *K'ung-tsui*)
On the thumb side of the inner surface of the forearm at a point about one-third of the distance from the elbow to the wrist.

3. Illnesses of the Alimentary System

(1) Weak Stomach (Heaviness on the Stomach or Heartburn)

Weak stomach and *heartburn* are words used to describe certain kinds of discomfort occurring after meals in some people; they are not, however, accurate names of sicknesses. Most often the conditions referred to in these ways are nervous stomach, gastroatonia, gastroptosis, and so on. Nervous stomach is not a congenital condition; it is usually caused by protracted stress in work or daily life. Almost all businessmen in their thirties or forties have experienced it. Gastroatonia and gastroptosis, on the other hand, are common in people who are thin and weak from birth; in other words, in atonic people. Sometimes, people who have been weakened by other illness or women who have been pregnant and have born children often suffer from gastroatonia, a slackness and lack of tone in the stomach muscles. Even a small amount of food fills the stomachs of people suffering from this condition; indeed, heavy meals cause them distress and heartburn.

Gastroptosis, also called fallen stomach, is an advanced state of gastroatonia. It causes pain in the stomach and an indescribable sensation of heaviness and oppression in the region from the diaphragm to the stomach. Gastroptosis is frequently accompanied by a fallen condition in the intestines and the kidneys.

Both gastroatonia and gastroptosis tend to be chronic and constitutional and to resist stomach medicines and pain killers. Oriental medical therapy is the best way to treat for them.

Have the patient lie on his back. Using both hands, held one on top of the other, gently rub the entire abdomen. Using both palms, rub meridian ① (Fig. 1) five or six times. Then rub meridian ② with the palms of both hands. Next have the patient lie on his stomach. With the thumbs of both hands, making small circular motions in the directions shown by the arrows (Fig. 2), massage and apply shiatsu massage to meridian ③.

Fig. 1

1. CV-14 (巨闕, *Chü-ch'üeh*)
Immediately below the diaphragm.
2. ST-19 (不容, *Pu-yung*)
On either side of the diaphragm at the edges of the eighth ribs counted from the top.
3. LV-14 (期門, *Ch'i-men*)
Extremities of the ninth ribs. Or a place located at the boundary between the rib and the abdomen directly below the nipple of the breast. The zone between the edge of the rib and the diaphragm.
4. LV-13 (章門, *Chang-men*)
At the extremities of the eleventh ribs. This point, located near the side of the abdomen, is easy to locate if the patient lies on his back, thus facilitating counting of the ribs.
5. CV-12 (中脘, *Chuang-wan*)
Four sun above the navel.
6. ST-25 (天枢, *T'ien-shu*)
Two sun on either side of the navel. Easily found by lining the thumb and index and middle fingers on either side of the navel.

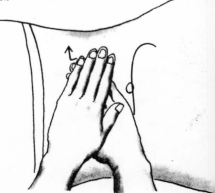

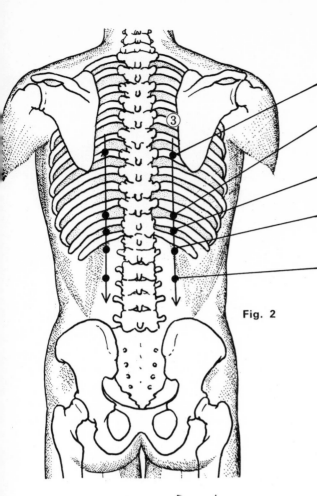

Fig. 2

7. BL-17 (膈俞, *Ke-yü*)
One sun and five bu on either side of the spinal column at points below the seventh thoracic vertebra.

8. BL-19 (胆俞, *Tan-yü*)
One sun and five bu on either side of the spinal column at points below the spinal projections of the tenth thoracic vertebra.

9. BL-20 (脾俞, *P'i-yü*)
One sun and five bu on either side of the spinal column at points below the eleventh thoracic vertebra.

10. BL-21 (胃俞, *Wei-yü*)
One sun and five bu on either side of the spinal column at points below the spinal projections of the twelfth thoracic vertebra.

11. BL-23 (腎俞, *Shen-yü*)
One sun and five bu on either side of the spinal column at points below the spinal projections of the second lumbar vertebra, which is located at the height of the lowest ribs.

When it is especially desirable to relieve symptoms of indigestion, apply gentle shiatsu to ST-34 and ST-36 (Fig. 3). If this fails to have the effect wanted, apply moxa to the tsubo mentioned above. Use medium moxa and apply it from three to five times to a tsubo daily for from three to five weeks. Acupuncture and other forms of moxa combustion too are effective in relieving heartburn and indigestion and in restoring the stomach to good functioning order. While employing these therapeutic systems, it is important to put the body in good general condition. Situps to strengthen the abdominal muscles should be done regularly. In cases of atonia, it is better to have the patient eat several light meals a day than to have him try to consume large amounts of food at the usual three meals. It is said that lying on one side after eating brings comfort to people in this condition. Have a specialist take X-ray photographs to ascertain the nature of the condition before beginning a course of home treatment.

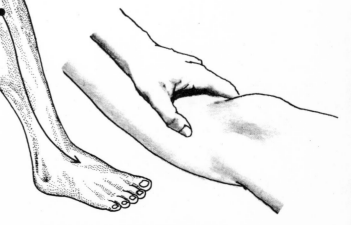

Fig. 3

12. ST-34 (梁丘, *Liang-chiu*)
Two sun above the upper edge of the kneecap. This can be easily located by fully extending the knee and finding the upper end of the groove formed on the outside of the kneecap. In other words, it is on the front of the thigh, two sun above the upper outer edge of the patella.

13. ST-36 (足三里, *Tsu-san-li*)
On the outer side of the calf three sun below the knee. Outer edge of the tibia or shin bone.

(2) Chronic Gastritis

Inflammation of the mucous membrane lining the stomach, or chronic gastritis, is a frequent cause of a condition in which one loses appetite, experiences constant oppressive feelings in the area between the stomach and diaphragm, belches acid liquid, has heartburn, and feels nauseous. In the past, when victims of this condition coughed up blood, they were immediately thought to have stomach ulcers. Today, however, it is known that chronic gastritis can be accompanied by considerable hemorrhage.

Although overindulgence and gluttony are causes of acute gastritis, the things that bring on chronic gastritis are not known for certain; and the condition is difficult to cure. Some people argue that too much alcohol and too much smoking cause chronic gastritis; and it is undeniably true that these things can be related to attacks of the sickness, though a definite causal relation has not yet been established. In many instances, acute gastritis degenerates into a chronic condition. When this happens, it is imperative to consult a physician who will use stomach cameras; X-ray photography; and examinations of stomach liquids, stool, and urine to make a diagnosis. In light cases, however, cures can be effected without this kind of treatment.

Practical experience has proved that moxa combustion on the six so-called stomach tsubo —BL-19, BL-20, and BL-21 (Fig. 4)—is effective in treating gastric conditions. Stiffness in these tsubo, located on large muscles on either side of the central spinal column and stiffness and hypersensitivity to pressure in CV-12 (Fig. 5) at the diaphragm are classic indications of chronic gastritis. To treat, using the palms or the thumbs, lightly massage meridian ① (Fig. 4) from BL-17 to BL-21. You may apply shiatsu massage to this zone. In performing shiatsu massage on the back, use the balls of the thumbs to knead and rub in small, circular motions.

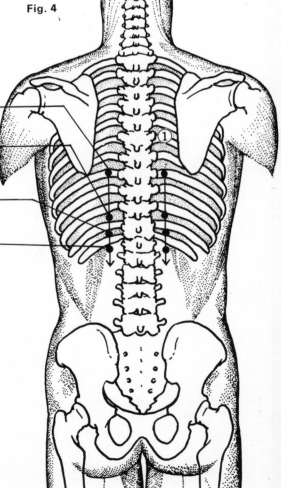

Fig. 4

1. BL-17 (膈俞, *Ke-yü*)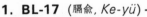
One sun and five bu on either side of the spinal column at points below the seventh thoracic vertebra.
2. BL-19 (胆俞, *Tan-yü*)
One sun and five bu on either side of the spinal column at points below the spinal projections of the tenth thoracic vertebra.
3. BL-20 (脾俞, *P'i-yü*)
One sun and five bu on either side of the spinal column at points below the eleventh thoracic vertebra.
4. BL-21 (胃俞, *Wei-yü*)
One sun and five bu on either side of the spinal column at points below the spinal projections of the twelfth thoracic vertebra.

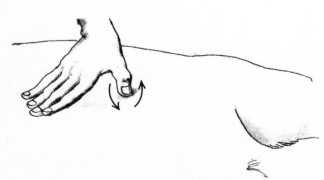

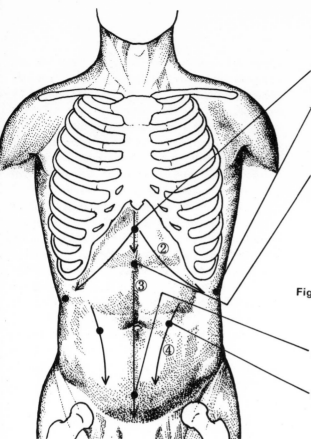

5. CV-14 (巨闕, *Chü-ch'üeh*)
Immediately below the diaphragm; two sun below the lower extremity of the sternum.

6. GB-25 (京門, *Ching-men*)
At the ends of the twelfth ribs. To find this have the patient kneel upright or lie facedown as you check his ribs. The twelfth ribs are short and are not attached at the small of the back.

7. CV-12 (中脘, *Chung-wan*)
Four sun above the navel; midway between the navel and the diaphragm.

Fig. 5

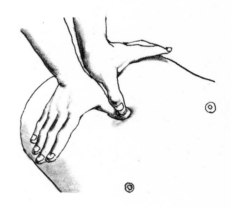

8. CV-2 (曲骨, *Ch'ü-ku*)
Directly below the navel and at the juncture of the pubis.

9. ST-25 (天枢, *T'ien-shu*)
Two sun on either side of the navel. Easily found by lining the thumb and index and middle fingers on either side of the navel.

The meridians for treatment on the front of the body are the following (Fig. 5): meridian ② from the diaphragm along the lines of the ribs to the sides (GB-25); meridian ③ from the diaphragm to the navel and from the navel to the lower abdomen (CV-2); and meridian ④, the lines passing through ST-25 on either side of the navel. Using the palms or the thumbs, massage these places in the order given and in the directions indicated by the arrows in the charts.

Moxa combustion—medium-grade moxa applied from three to five times on each tsubo—may be used on these places as well. In three weeks, the oppressive feeling in the stomach will have disappeared; and appetite will have greatly improved.

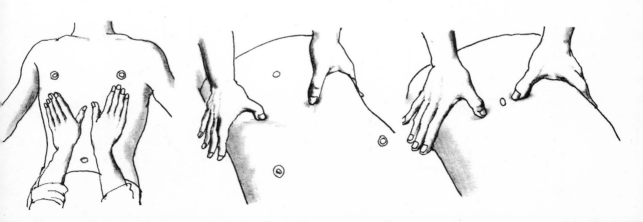

(3) Stomach Cramps

Today referred to as stomach neuralgia, spasmodic attacks of pain in the stomach may be mild; or they may be so sudden and shockingly painful that the patient faints. They may last from as little as two or three minutes to as long as two or three hours. The patient lies down with his back bent and his knees and thighs brought upward against his stomach. In addition to pain, he may experience chills, sweating fits, and attacks of nausea. He will, however, be perfectly normal once the cramps have stopped.

Cramps may be psychological; or they may be brought on by such things as consumption of spoiled or indigestible foods, gallstones, stomach or duodenal ulcers, disorders of the pyloris, brain or spinal conditions, or female troubles. People of weak nervous constitution are frequently the victims of these cramps. Merely seeing or hearing something disagreeable can bring on sudden attacks of nausea and spasmodic contractions of the stomach muscles caused by hyperactivity of the nerves in the stomach lining. Keeping a record of the duration of the cramp, its relation to the nearest mealtime, the kind of pain the patient experienced, and the nature of the material vomited can be of great help to the person attempting a diagnosis.

Specialist attention is required to treat the kinds of cramps that are caused by definite pathological conditions, though home tsubo therapy is helpful in treating those that are largely psychological in derivation. Acupuncture, moxa combustion, shiatsu massage, and ordinary massage are all effective, though the last two are the easiest to use in domestic emergencies.

First have the patient lie on his stomach. Using either the thumbs or the four fingers, perform shiatsu or ordinary massage on BL-17, BL-18. BL-19, and BL-20 (Fig. 6).

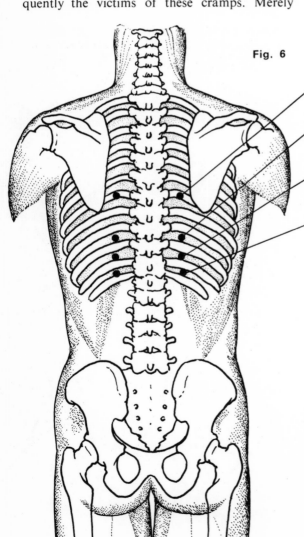

Fig. 6

1. BL-17 (膈俞, *Ke-yü*)
One sun and five bu on either side of the spinal column at points below the seventh thoracic vertebra.

2. BL-18 (肝俞, *Kan-yü*)
One sun and five bu on either side of the spinal column at points below the spinal projections of the ninth thoracic vertebra.

3. BL-19 (胆俞, *Tan-yü*)
One sun and five bu on either side of the spinal column at points below the spinal projections of the tenth thoracic vertebra.

4. BL-20 (脾俞, *P'i-yü*)
One sun and five bu on either side of the spinal column at points below the eleventh thoracic vertebra.

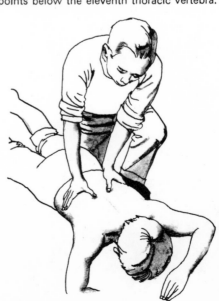

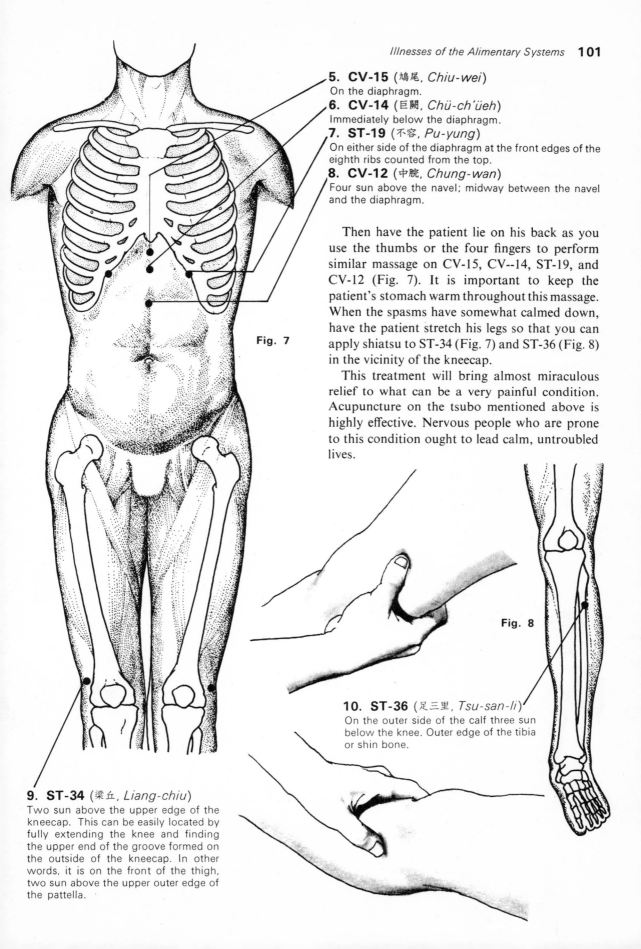

5. CV-15 (鳩尾, *Chiu-wei*)
On the diaphragm.

6. CV-14 (巨闕, *Chü-ch'üeh*)
Immediately below the diaphragm.

7. ST-19 (不容, *Pu-yung*)
On either side of the diaphragm at the front edges of the eighth ribs counted from the top.

8. CV-12 (中脘, *Chung-wan*)
Four sun above the navel; midway between the navel and the diaphragm.

Then have the patient lie on his back as you use the thumbs or the four fingers to perform similar massage on CV-15, CV-14, ST-19, and CV-12 (Fig. 7). It is important to keep the patient's stomach warm throughout this massage. When the spasms have somewhat calmed down, have the patient stretch his legs so that you can apply shiatsu to ST-34 (Fig. 7) and ST-36 (Fig. 8) in the vicinity of the kneecap.

This treatment will bring almost miraculous relief to what can be a very painful condition. Acupuncture on the tsubo mentioned above is highly effective. Nervous people who are prone to this condition ought to lead calm, untroubled lives.

Fig. 7

Fig. 8

10. ST-36 (足三里, *Tsu-san-li*)
On the outer side of the calf three sun below the knee. Outer edge of the tibia or shin bone.

9. ST-34 (梁丘, *Liang-chiu*)
Two sun above the upper edge of the kneecap. This can be easily located by fully extending the knee and finding the upper end of the groove formed on the outside of the kneecap. In other words, it is on the front of the thigh, two sun above the upper outer edge of the pattella.

(4) Chronic Diarrhea

Watery and frequent bowel movements are signs of diarrhea in adults. (It must be mentioned here that infants who are raised on mother's milk tend to have more liquid stools than children fed on artificial diets.) The signs of good health in human beings are pleasant eating, pleasant sleeping, and pleasant evacuation. Consequently, everyone should be aware of the times and ways in which they defecate (too often or not often enough) and of the nature of the fecal matter (too hard or too soft).

The causes of acute diarrhea are usually localized. They may include such things as food poisoning, overeating, or dysentery. But the causative factors of chronic diarrhea can range over a much wider field to include sicknesses of the stomach and intestines, disorders of the liver or kidneys, upsets in hormone secretions (Basedow's disease or Addison's disease), and other conditions. Advanced cancer in the organs of the digestive system can manifest itself in a diarrhetic condition.

But there are cases of diarrhea that cannot be described as sickness. Middle-aged men who drink alcohol every night sometimes suffer from diarrhea and become accustomed to one or two loose bowel movements a day. Some people of middle age or more suffer from diarrhea caused by a loss of stomach acidity.

All of these sicknesses must be given proper medical attention. The kind of diarrhea that responds to oriental tsubo therapy is that which is the result of psychological stress and irregular living habits. Even when the person suffering from this kind of condition consults a physician, he is generally told that there is nothing physical wrong with him. This kind of person is often thin and nervous. When he hears rumbling in his stomach, it may mean that the diarrhea is giving way to constipation. His condition cannot be cured with one or two hasty treatments. As a matter of fact, if he is frantically eager for a quick cure, he may find that his very frenzy only contributes to the aggravation of his state.

Begin treatment with thorough shiatsu massage on GV-14, BL-23, and BL-25 (Fig. 9). Next, have the patient turn over on his back to enable you to massage CV-12, and ST-25 (Fig. 10). After massaging LI-11, LI-10, and LI-1 (Fig. 11), move on the ST-34 (Fig. 10), then slightly farther downward to ST-36 (Fig. 12). Moxa combustion too is effective on these tsubo. Using commercially available, medium-grade moxa, burn it from five to seven times on each tsubo.

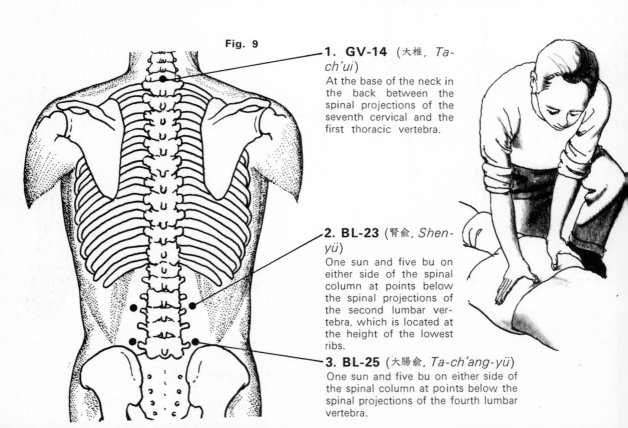

Fig. 9

1. GV-14 (大椎, Ta-ch'ui)
At the base of the neck in the back between the spinal projections of the seventh cervical and the first thoracic vertebra.

2. BL-23 (腎兪, Shen-yü)
One sun and five bu on either side of the spinal column at points below the spinal projections of the second lumbar vertebra, which is located at the height of the lowest ribs.

3. BL-25 (大腸兪, Ta-ch'ang-yü)
One sun and five bu on either side of the spinal column at points below the spinal projections of the fourth lumbar vertebra.

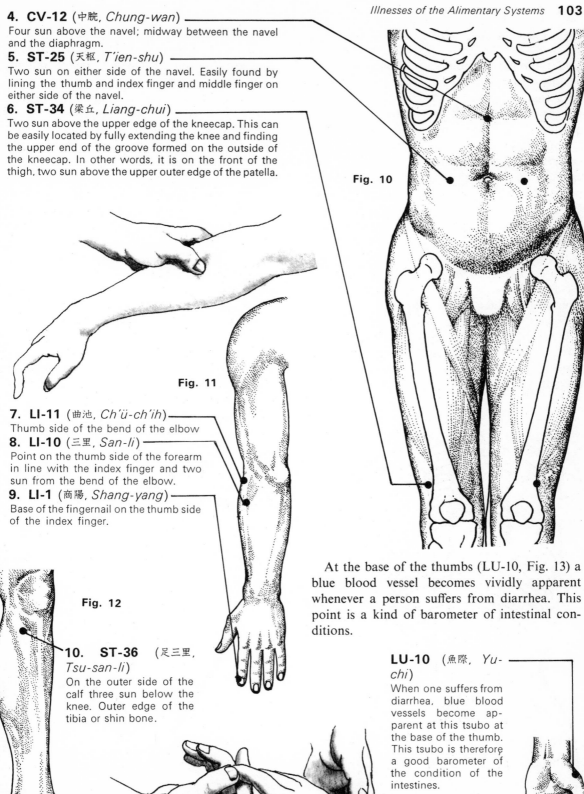

4. CV-12 (中脘, *Chung-wan*)
Four sun above the navel; midway between the navel and the diaphragm.

5. ST-25 (天枢, *T'ien-shu*)
Two sun on either side of the navel. Easily found by lining the thumb and index finger and middle finger on either side of the navel.

6. ST-34 (梁丘, *Liang-chui*)
Two sun above the upper edge of the kneecap. This can be easily located by fully extending the knee and finding the upper end of the groove formed on the outside of the kneecap. In other words, it is on the front of the thigh, two sun above the upper outer edge of the patella.

Fig. 10

Fig. 11

7. LI-11 (曲池, *Ch'ü-ch'ih*)
Thumb side of the bend of the elbow

8. LI-10 (三里, *San-li*)
Point on the thumb side of the forearm in line with the index finger and two sun from the bend of the elbow.

9. LI-1 (商陽, *Shang-yang*)
Base of the fingernail on the thumb side of the index finger.

Fig. 12

10. ST-36 (足三里, *Tsu-san-li*)
On the outer side of the calf three sun below the knee. Outer edge of the tibia or shin bone.

At the base of the thumbs (LU-10, Fig. 13) a blue blood vessel becomes vividly apparent whenever a person suffers from diarrhea. This point is a kind of barometer of intestinal conditions.

LU-10 (魚際, *Yu-chi*)
When one suffers from diarrhea, blue blood vessels become apparent at this tsubo at the base of the thumb. This tsubo is therefore a good barometer of the condition of the intestines.

Fig. 13

(5) Loss of Appetite

Under ordinary conditions, the appetite of a healthy person drops in the summer, when blood circulates in great abundance close to the surface of the body. In the autumn, when large quantities of blood once again nourish the internal organs to stimulate their activity—especially that of the stomach and intestines—the appetite usually picks up again. There are people, however, in whom this change in desire for food fails to occur. Such people remain tired and listless much of the time. One cause of this lack of appetite is a way of life in which the person remains indoors most of the time and does not exercise. Lack of movement dulls the actions of the stomach and intestines and causes poor blood circulation. These conditions in turn reduce appetite.

Overwork, lack of sleep, worry, and frustrations can produce tensions that reduce appetite. Most people, have no desire for food when they are worried, suffering, or in some kind of trouble.

Although this condition is psychological in nature, if it becomes pathological, it can make the person lose too much weight. Such conditions, often seen in young girls at the age of puberty, sometimes cause menstrual failure. Melancholia can produce stubborn loss of appetite.

Almost all sickness—stomach ailments, gastritis, stomach cancer, early acute hepatits, and so on—is accompanied by loss of appetite in combination with such other symptoms as nausea, pain, and jaundice. People suffering from fever and fever-associated illnesses rarely want food. The same is true of patients of kidney ailments, weak heart, tuberculosis of the lungs, constipation, alcoholism, parasites, anemia, morning sickness, and so on and of people who abuse medicines. As this impressive list suggests, loss of appetite must not be treated lightly since it can be related to serious conditions. When a person suffers from it, he ought to consult a specialist. After a thorough examination has shown that the loss of appetite is not the result of a serious disorder but arises from psychological causes, fatigue, or constipation, use the oriental tsubo therapy described below.

Fig. 14

1. BL-18 (肝兪, *Kan-yü*)
One sun and five bu on either side of the spinal column at points below the spinal projections of the ninth thoracic vertebra.

2. BL-20 (脾兪, *P'i-yü*)
One sun and five bu on either side of the spinal column at points below the eleventh thoracic vertebra.

3. BL-21 (胃兪, *Wei-yü*)
One sun and five bu on either side of the spinal column at points below the spinal projections of the twelfth thoracic vertebra.

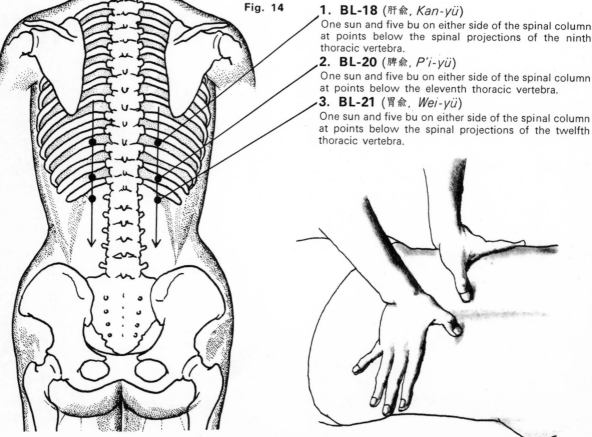

To calm the irritability that may be causing loss of appetite, to improve digestion and assimilation, and to rid the body of excess gas, perform shiatsu on the tsubo shown in Figs. 14 through 16. Then, using the four fingers, massage in the directions indicated by the arrows. It is essential that the shiatsu be performed gently and regularly. Great pressure must not be exerted. trolling energy in the stomach. BL-21 (Fig. 20), CV-14, ST-19, and CV-12 (Fig. 21) too are very important. Using either fine- or medium-grade moxa, apply it from three to five times once a day regularly. If this treatment is continued in moderation every day, the patient will come to await mealtime with eagerness. Meals must contain easily digested, highly nutritious foods. They must be attractive to the eye as well as to the palate.

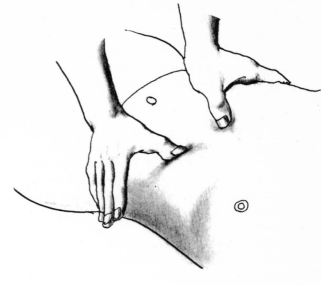

Fig. 15

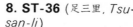

4. CV-12 (中脘, *Chung-wan*)
Four sun above the navel; midway between the navel and the diaphragm.

5. LV-14 (期門, *Ch'i-men*)
Extremities of the ninth ribs. Or a place located at the boundary between the rib and the abdomen directly below the nipple of the breast. The zone between the edge of the rib and the diaphragm.

6. KI-16 (肓兪, *Huang-yü*)
Points located five sun on either side of the navel.

7. ST-27 (大巨, *Ta-chü*)
Two sun below points two sun on either side of the navel.

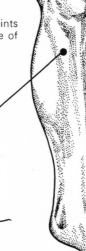

8. ST-36 (足三里, *Tsu-san-li*)
On the outer side of the calf three sun below the knee. Outer edge of the tibia or shin bone.

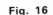

Fig. 16

(6) Nausea

The disagreeable sensation of nausea may be mild; or it may involve a severe, sudden contraction of the muscles of the throat, esophagus, stomach, duodenum, diaphragm, and intestinal walls. This contraction may threaten to empty the contents of the stomach through the mouth with violent force. The basic cause is a signal from the brain, which may arise as the outcome of any of a number of things. It may be caused by chemicals or poisons in the body, hypersensitivity in the brain, some nervous cause, too much tobacco or alcohol, or the stimulation brought on by such drugs as morphine. In addition, edocrinological upsets, diabetes, morning sickness, uremic poison, high brain pressure, cerebral hemorrhage, cerebral tumor, encephalitis, and meningitis can bring on nausea, as can worry, fear, shock, neurosis, and motion sickness. In addition, reflex causes, most common in such illness as stomach cancer, stomach ulcers, and gastritis, can produce nausea.

Early-morning nausea, at times when the stomach is empty, is usually the result of chronic gastritis or morning sickness. Nausea from one to four hours after a meal may be caused by stomach or duodenal cancer. Nausea during a period from thirteen and forty-eight hours after a meal suggests the possibility of stomach or duodenal ulcers. Chronic pancreatitis or nephritis too can produce a nauseous condition. Modern medicine explains the sensation of nausea as arising from a disorder in the vagus nerve, which runs from the head along the back and down the side of the neck to the front of the chest. Interestingly enough, from ancient times, oriental medicial theory has held that the tsubo SI-17 and ST-11 (Fig. 17), located on the thick muscle from the back of the neck to the front of the chest, are very important in treating nausea.

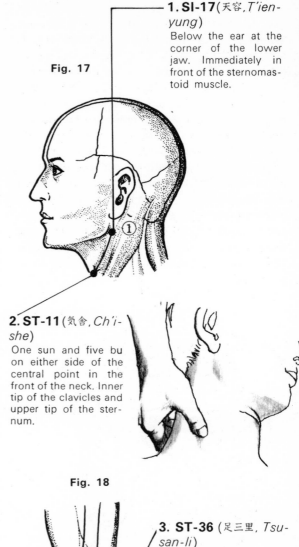

Fig. 17

1. SI-17(天容, *T'ien-yung*)
Below the ear at the corner of the lower jaw. Immediately in front of the sternomastoid muscle.

2. ST-11(気舎, *Ch'i-she*)
One sun and five bu on either side of the central point in the front of the neck. Inner tip of the clavicles and upper tip of the sternum.

Fig. 18

3. ST-36 (足三里, *Tsu-san-li*)
On the outer side of the calf three sun below the knee. Outer edge of the tibia or shin bone.

4. ST-45 (厲兌, *Li-tui*)
Side of the nail of the second toe.

Fig. 19

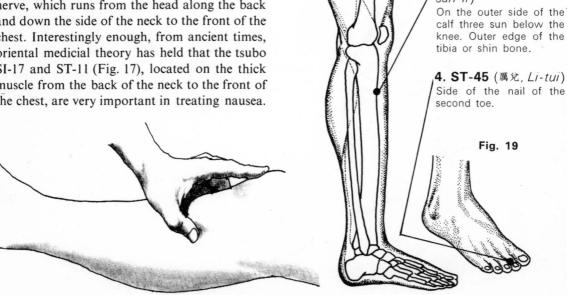

5. BL-21 (胃兪, *Wei-yü*) ─────
One sun and five bu on either side of
the spinal column at points below the
spinal projections of the twelfth thoracic
vertebra.

In addition, it is imperative to treat ST-36
and ST-45 (Figs. 18 and 19) on the meridian controlling energy in the stomach. BL-21 (Fig. 20),
CV-14, ST-19, and CV-12 (Fig. 21) too are very
important.

Although moxa combustion is the most effective treatment on these tsubo, when an attack
of nausea strikes, the necessary materials may
not be on hand. In such instances, massage the
tsubo as shown. Using the thumbs or the palms
of the hands, rub and stroke meridians ① through
④ in the directions shown by the arrows. Since
motion and cold are likely to aggravate the condition, the patient should be kept still and in a warm
place.

If the consumption of something that disagrees
with the body is the cause, it is best to allow the
patient to vomit. Patting on the back may
induce gagging; if this fails, the patient may put
his finger down his throat. If the condition is
accompanied by high fever or severe stomach
pains, a physician must be consulted.

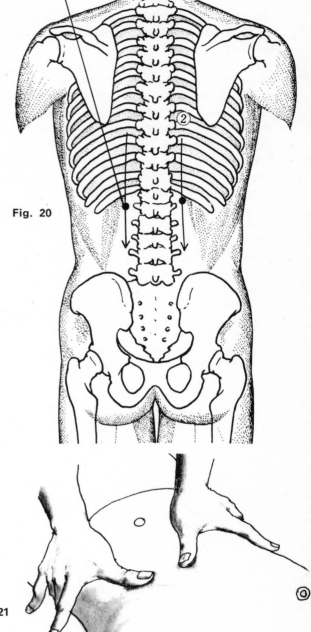

Fig. 20

Fig. 21

6. CV-14 (巨闕, *Chü-ch'üeh*)
Immediately below the diaphragm;
two sun below the lower extremity of
the sternum.

7. ST-19 (不容, *Pu-yung*)
On either side of the diaphragm at the
front edges of the eighth ribs counted
from the top.

8. CV-12 (中脘, *Chung-wan*)
Four sun above the navel; midway
between the navel and the diaphragm.

(7) Constipation

Since there are differences in the physical make-ups of all individuals, it is difficult to set a limit that unfailingly establishes the nature of the constipated condition. But, in general, it may be described as a feeling that bowel movements are incomplete and that fecal matter remains in the body even after evacuation. If this condition continues over a long time and there is no actual physical disorder in the system, it is called habitual constipation. It often manifests itself in young women, for whom it is a great distress. Not going to the toilet when the urge is felt, lack of roughage in the diet, insufficient liquids, lack of exercise, stomach and intestinal illnesses, obstructions in the sexual organs, pregnancy, physical constitution, and an irregular way of life can all be causes of this condition. Sometimes fecal matter reaches the rectum but, for some reason or another, cannot pass out of the body. This occurs in people who are physically weak, in people with weak anal sphincters, and in poorly nourished women who have recently born children. Psychological stress, too, can be a cause.

Habitual constipation may arise from sluggishness of the intestines or from hypertension of the intestines. It may also arise from a disorder in the autonomic nervous system. The former kind of constipation results in distention of the lower abdomen and no serious obstruction. In the case of the latter kind, the lower abdomen is distended; and there is a general feeling of heaviness and discomfort. Dull pain in the abdomen may result. The person will have no appetite, he will have an unpleasant taste in his mouth, he will lack sleep, and he will suffer from headaches and dizziness and may be very nervous. The fecal matter will be hard and dark in color. This condition could be serious and could require the attention of a specialist. But the constipation resulting from intestinal sluggishness responds to domestic treatment such as hot compresses, cold packs, massage, and shiatsu massage.

1. BL-20 (脾兪, *P'i-yü*)
One sun and five bu on either side of the spinal column at points below the eleventh thoracic vertebra.

Fig. 22

2. BL-22 (三焦兪, *San-chiao-yü*)
One sun and five bu on either side of the spinal column at points below the first lumbar vertebra.

3. BL-25 (大腸兪, *Ta-ch'ang-yü*)
One sun and five bu on either side of the spinal column at points below the spinal projections of the fourth lumbar vertebra.

4. BL-27 (小腸兪, *Hsiao-ch'ang-yü*)
The sacral vertebra are fused and formed into the rear wall of the pelvic cavity. These tsubo are located one sun and five bu on either side of the spinal column on either side of the first sacral vertebra.

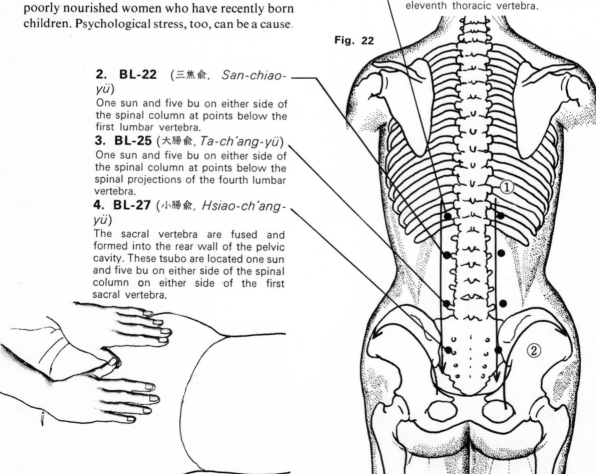

Fig. 23

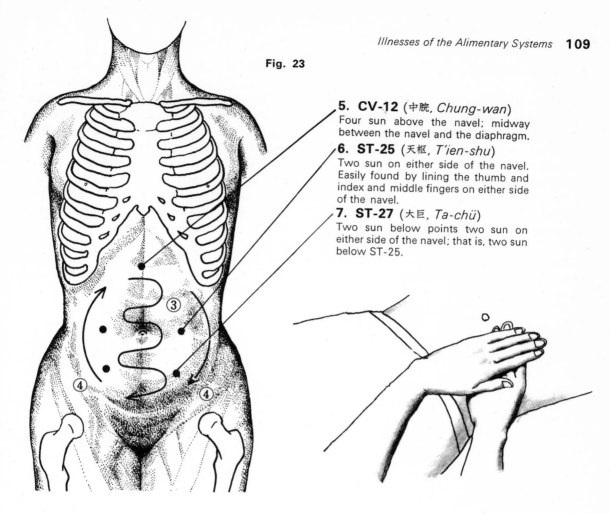

5. CV-12 (中脘, *Chung-wan*)
Four sun above the navel; midway between the navel and the diaphragm.
6. ST-25 (天枢, *T'ien-shu*)
Two sun on either side of the navel. Easily found by lining the thumb and index and middle fingers on either side of the navel.
7. ST-27 (大巨, *Ta-chü*)
Two sun below points two sun on either side of the navel; that is, two sun below ST-25.

To stimulate bowel movement, have the patient lie on his stomach as you massage meridians ① and ② (Fig. 22) in small, circular motions of the palms or the thumbs. Next, have the patient lie on his back. With the right hand on the left, make rowing motions as you massage meridian ③ and meridian ④ (Fig. 23). The patient must raise his knees and relax his abdominal muscles.

Moxa combustion too is effective treatment. To select the tsubo requiring therapy, press the ones shown in the figures and apply moxa to those that are stiff and to those that are sensitive to pressure. Pressure may be applied to these tsubo with the top of a beer bottle, preferably a bottle that is full. The patient must be treated in these ways daily. Moreover, he must lead a well ordered life and eat wholesome foods.

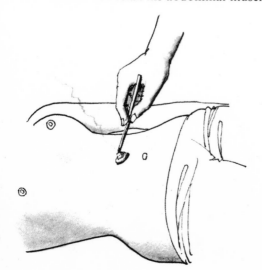

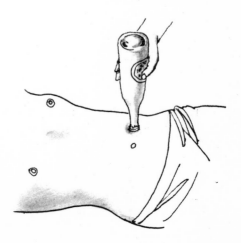

(8) Distended Stomach

A sense of strong tension in the lower abdomen and sharp pains in the sides of the stomach often accompany stomach disorders. When this condition afflicts women, they frequently have very cold feet that are virtually impossible to warm. To treat this condition, first apply warm compresses to meridians ① and ② from BL-15 to BL-25 (Fig. 24). Next have the patient lie on his stomach, leaving the hot compress in place. Then place another hot compress on the back and, lightly, in the direction of the arrows, massage meridians ① and ②. With the thumbs, perform shiatsu massage on BL-15, BL-19, BL-20, BL-21, and BL-25. Be especially careful in massaging BL-25, which, in this instance, is the most important in the group. It would be very good to use moxa or acupuncture on this tsubo.

Having the patient lie on his back again, with one hand on the other, use the balls of the fingers to massage meridian ③ (Fig. 25) in large, circular motions. Then, in the line of the small intestine, massage meridian ④, which centers on CV-12 and CV-4. Massage the area of the large intestine in the same way. This is meridian ⑤, which centers on CV-14 and LV-14. In this case CV-4 is the most important tsubo; it would be a good idea to use moxa combustion and acupuncture on it. Apply medium-grade moxa to it from five to seven times. In cases of severe chilling of the feet, massage ST-36 (Fig. 26), SP-6, KI-3, and SP-5 (Fig. 27). Wrap the feet entirely in warm compresses.

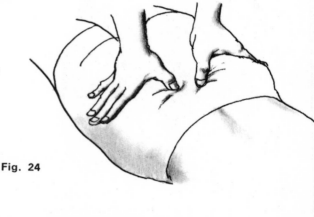

Fig. 24

1. BL-15 (心兪, *Hsin-yü*)
One sun and five bu on either side of the spinal column at points below the spinal projections of the fifth thoracic vertebra.

2. BL-19 (胆兪, *Tan-yü*)
One sun and five bu on either side of the spinal column at points below the spinal projections of the tenth thoracic vertebra.

3. BL-20 (脾兪, *P'i-yü*)
One sun and five bu on either side of the spinal column at points below the eleventh thoracic vertebra.

4. BL-21 (胃兪, *Wei-yü*)
One sun and five bu on either side of the spinal column at points below the spinal projections of the twelfth thoracic vertebra.

5. BL-25 (大腸兪, *Ta-ch'ang-yü*)
One sun and five bu on either side of the spinal column at points below the spinal projections of the fourth lumbar vertebra.

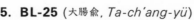

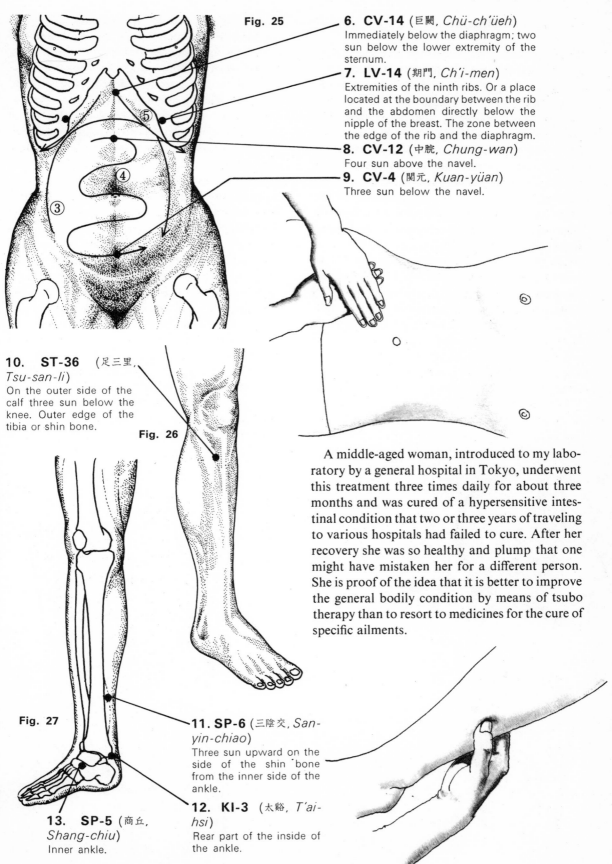

Fig. 25

6. CV-14 (巨闕, *Chü-ch'üeh*)
Immediately below the diaphragm; two sun below the lower extremity of the sternum.

7. LV-14 (期門, *Ch'i-men*)
Extremities of the ninth ribs. Or a place located at the boundary between the rib and the abdomen directly below the nipple of the breast. The zone between the edge of the rib and the diaphragm.

8. CV-12 (中脘, *Chung-wan*)
Four sun above the navel.

9. CV-4 (関元, *Kuan-yüan*)
Three sun below the navel.

10. ST-36 (足三里, *Tsu-san-li*)
On the outer side of the calf three sun below the knee. Outer edge of the tibia or shin bone.

Fig. 26

A middle-aged woman, introduced to my laboratory by a general hospital in Tokyo, underwent this treatment three times daily for about three months and was cured of a hypersensitive intestinal condition that two or three years of traveling to various hospitals had failed to cure. After her recovery she was so healthy and plump that one might have mistaken her for a different person. She is proof of the idea that it is better to improve the general bodily condition by means of tsubo therapy than to resort to medicines for the cure of specific ailments.

Fig. 27

11. SP-6 (三陰交, *San-yin-chiao*)
Three sun upward on the side of the shin bone from the inner side of the ankle.

12. KI-3 (太谿, *T'ai-hsi*)
Rear part of the inside of the ankle.

13. SP-5 (商丘, *Shang-chiu*)
Inner ankle.

(9) Liver Ailments

Since the liver acts as a purifier and remover of harmful substances from the body, it often comes into contact with poisons. Furthermore, it encounters the bacteria of the small intestine by way of the bile ducts; and sometimes such bacteria invade the liver and cause a condition known as hepatitis, which is a liver inflammation. In most cases, this condition develops in one of two ways. It may cause acute and sudden destruction of liver tissue (acute yellow atrophy of the liver). Or it may become a chronic condition slowly producing atrophy or hardening (cirrhosis) of the liver.

There are no definite symptoms that may be said to characterize the early stages of liver ailments. The patient merely loses appetite, suffers from abundant intestinal gas, and feels generally sluggish and rundown. Although, in some cases, the sickness is cured naturally before the patient is aware of being ill, recently it has been shown that such possible symptoms of liver illness as constant weariness can, if allowed to go unattended, develop into serious conditions. If the liver, which is a central organ in metabolism, is heavily invaded, weariness increases; and the nutritional values of the foods consumed are largely lost. At first, the patient may suffer from jaundice. He will certainly lose appetite and feel tired most of the time. As the illness progresses, he will suffer fits of rage and loss of consciousness and will be unable to sleep. Finally, his arms and legs will tremble; and he will fall into a coma.

Although many causes have been advanced for liver sickness, no definite causative factor has ever been pinned down. Some of the things that are said to produce the condition are food poisoning, malnutrition, infection, contact with parasite carriers, obstruction in the circulatory system, and so on. Although excess consumption of alcohol is sometimes given as a cause, it seems more likely that poor nourishment accompanying bad living habits associated with too much drinking is the basic cause in many instances.

It is difficult to cure liver sickness with tsubo therapy, but the oriental systems may be employed to bring relief from the symptoms. In addition to applying oriental therapy, it is essential to seek the advice of a specialist.

To bring relief from the symptoms of liver sickness, first apply shiatsu pressure to BL-10 (Fig. 28). Then have the patient lie on his stomach as you apply shiatsu massage to BL-18, GV-8, and BL-23 (Fig. 29). Next have the patient lie

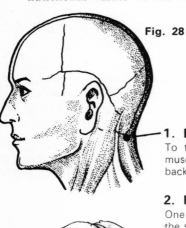

Fig. 28

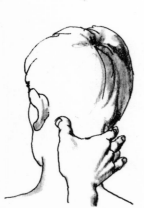

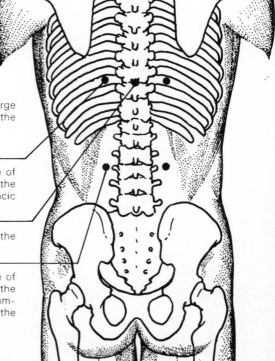

Fig. 29

1. BL-10 (天柱, *T'ien-chu*)
To the outer side of the two large muscles of the neck where they join the back of the head.

2. BL-18 (肝兪, *Kan-yü*)
One sun and five bu on either side of the spinal column at points below the spinal projections of the ninth thoracic vertebra.

3. GV-8 (筋縮, *Chin-so*)
Below the spinal projections of the ninth thoracic vertebra.

4. BL-23 (腎兪, *Shen-yü*)
One sun and five bu on either side of the spinal column at points below the spinal projections of the second lumbar vertebra, which is located at the height of the lowest ribs.

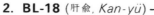

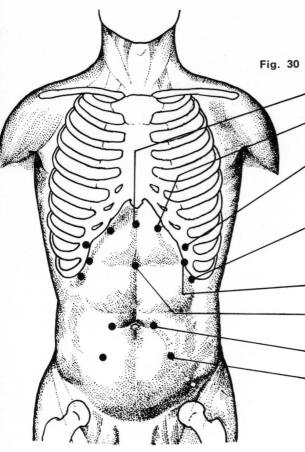

Fig. 30

5. CV-14 (巨闕, *Chü-ch'üeh*)
Two sun below the lower extremity of the sternum.
6. ST-19 (不容, *Pu-yung*)
On either side of the diaphragm at the front edges of the eighth ribs counted from the top.
7. LV-14 (期門, *Ch'i-men*)
Extremities of the eleventh ribs. Or a place located at the boundary between the rib and the abdomen directly below the nipple of the breast. The zone between the edge of the rib and the diaphragm.
8. LV-13 (章門, *Chang-men*)
At the extremities of the eleventh ribs. This point, located near the side of the abdomen, is easy to find if the patient lies on his back, thus facilitating counting of the ribs.
9. GB-24 (日月, *Jin-yueh*)
Immediately below the lower edge of the ninth rib.
10. CV-12 (中脘, *Chung-wan*)
Four sun above the navel; midway between the navel and the diaphragm.
11. KI-16 (肓兪, *Huang-yü*)
Points located five sun on either side of the navel.
12. ST-27 (大巨, *Ta-chü*)
Two sun below points two sun on either side of the navel.

on his back so that you can treat the tsubo on the abdominal region. Using both thumbs, thoroughly massage, in the shiatsu fashion, the following tsubo: ST-19, CV-14, LV-14, LV-13, GB-24, CV-12, KI-16, and ST-27 (Fig. 30). This treatment should be combined with therapy on LI-11 and LI-4 (Fig. 31) on the hands and ST-36 and LV-3 (Fig. 32) and LV-8 (Fig. 33) on the feet.

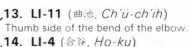

Fig. 31

13. LI-11 (曲池, *Ch'ü-ch'ih*)
Thumb side of the bend of the elbow.
14. LI-4 (合谷, *Ho-ku*)
The point exactly between the thumb and index finger on the back of the hand.

Fig. 32

15. ST-36 (足三里, *Tsu-san-li*)
On the outer side of the calf three sun below the knee. Outer edge of the tibia or shin bone.
16. LV-3 (太衝, *T'ai-ch'ung*)
Two sun upward on the instep from the crotch between the first and second toes.

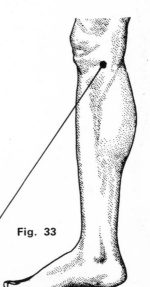

17. LV-8 (曲泉, *Ch'ü-ch'üan*)
In the depression on the innerside of the knee joint. The extremity of the groove formed when the knee is bent.

Fig. 33

(10) Indigestion

The human body ingests food through the mouth. The food then passes through the esophagus; to the stomach; then to the small and large intestines; and finally, as waste, to the rectum, from which it is removed from the body through the anus. Along the alimentary canal, as this tract is called, various juices are secreted to bring about the digestion and assimilation of nutrients. All of the parts of the alimentary canal are important, but the most important are the stomach, intestines, and liver. Because it comes into direct contact with the exterior world at both ends, the alimentary canal is more susceptible to damage from outside than any of the other bodily organs. For this reason, upsets in it are very common.

The most significant of such upsets are those in the stomach and intestines. These are followed in importance by liver complaints. Many different kinds of sicknesses, some of which are quite serious, afflict the digestive organs. Loss of appetite and diarrhea, both the result of upsets in the stomach or intestines, are complaints that one hears frequently. Indeed, almost everyone has upsets in the intestines have adverse effects on the operations of the stomach.

Digestion is the result of both physical and chemical actions. In the first place, the peristaltic, segmental, and pendulum motions of the stomach and intestines act on foods to break them down. In the second place such juices as those secreted by the stomach, intestines, and pancreas act chemically on foods to put them into forms in which the body can assimilate them. Reactions to emotional stress or pathological change in the stomach and intestines affect the autonomic nerves controlling the digestive tract and cause indigestion, which is represented by such symptoms as loss of appetite, loss of weight, constipation, heartburn, and so on. When this kind of condition is accompanied by severe side effects, sudden and violent diarrhea, or organic change, as is often the case, a physician must be consulted at once.

Tsubo therapy is effective in treating the kind of indigestion that has psychological or emotional causes. Furthermore, it can be helpful in dealing with children who demonstrate the unnatural phenomenon of eating adequately without gaining weight. The cause of this condition is failure of the digestive tract to make use of and to assimilate the foods the body takes in. Such a disorder is of great concern in growing children. To treat them, first determine whether the cause of the condition is an organic illness. If there is no organic disturbance requiring the attention of a physician, apply oriental tsubo therapy. A word of caution is needed however, for, although tsubo treatment can help regulate the functioning of the liver, stomach, and intestines, to bring about a complete cure, the patient must get adequate exercise and must eat regularly and wisely.

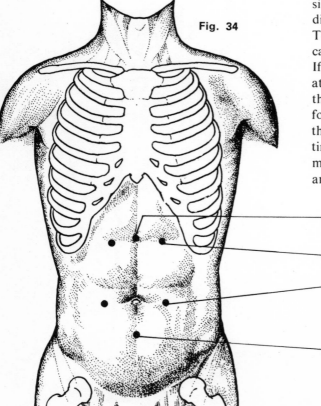

Fig. 34

1. CV-12 (中脘, *Chung-wan*)
Four sun above the navel; midway between the navel and the diaphragm.

2. ST-21 (梁門, *Liang-men*)
Two sun on either side of CV-12.

3. ST-25 (天枢, *T'ien-shu*)
Two sun on either side of the navel. Easily found by lining the thumb and index and middle fingers on either side of the navel.

4. CV-4 (関元, *Kuan-yüan*)
Three sun below the navel.

First, have the patient lie on his back as you suffered from this kind of distress at one time or another. But, in many instances, upsets of the stomach and intestines occur when there is nothing physically the matter with these organs. Since their operations are very delicate, even changes in the environment, emotional distress, or other kinds of sickness or unpleasantness can affect the functioning of the stomach and intestines. Because of the intimate relation between the two, when the stomach is in poor condition, the intestines usually fail to function properly. Similarly,

massage CV-12, ST-21, ST-25, and CV-4 (Fig. 34). The massage must be synchronized with the patient's breathing: when he exhales, you apply pressure. Then have the patient lie on his stomach so that you may massage GV-12, BL-18, BL-19, and BL-20 (Fig. 35). Once again, synchronize massage with the patient's breathing. Finally, massage LI-11 and LI-7 (Fig. 36), which are related to the functioning of the intestines, and ST-36 (Fig. 37), which is related to the functioning of the stomach.

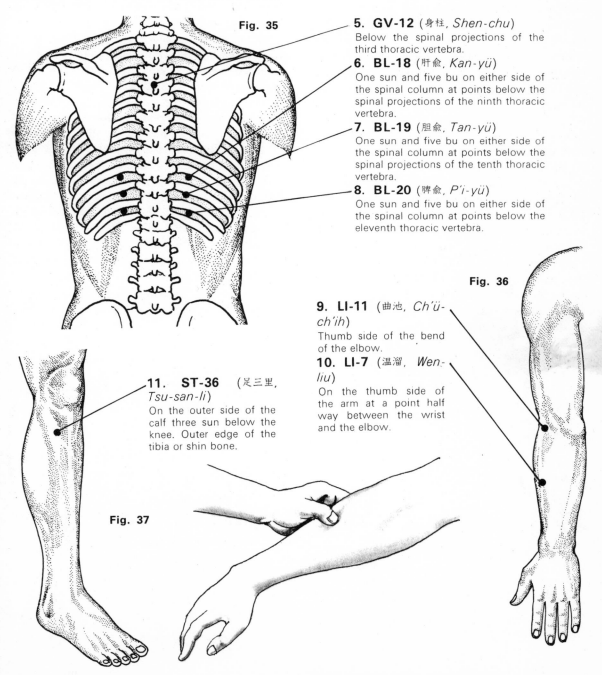

Fig. 35

5. GV-12 (身柱, *Shen-chu*)
Below the spinal projections of the third thoracic vertebra.

6. BL-18 (肝兪, *Kan-yü*)
One sun and five bu on either side of the spinal column at points below the spinal projections of the ninth thoracic vertebra.

7. BL-19 (胆兪, *Tan-yü*)
One sun and five bu on either side of the spinal column at points below the spinal projections of the tenth thoracic vertebra.

8. BL-20 (脾兪, *P'i-yü*)
One sun and five bu on either side of the spinal column at points below the eleventh thoracic vertebra.

Fig. 36

9. LI-11 (曲池, *Ch'ü-ch'ih*)
Thumb side of the bend of the elbow.

10. LI-7 (温溜, *Wen-liu*)
On the thumb side of the arm at a point half way between the wrist and the elbow.

11. ST-36 (足三里, *Tsu-san-li*)
On the outer side of the calf three sun below the knee. Outer edge of the tibia or shin bone.

Fig. 37

Sicknesses of the Metabolic System

(1) Diabetes

The classical symptoms of diabetes are weariness, dryness in the mouth, and loss of weight in spite of adequate food consumption. Anyone who experiences these conditions ought to call on the services of a specialist who will conduct a thorough, painstaking physical examination. Some of the other symptoms of diabetes, which need not necessarily all occur in any given case, are the following: increased urination, blurred vision, skin sicknesses, numbness in the hands and feet, loss of sexual urge in males, and menstrual irregularities in females. Diabetes is sometimes considered the basis of many other diseases since, unless treated and cured quickly, it can so weaken the body that susceptibility to arteriosclerosis, hemorrhage in the eyes, cataracts, cardiac infarction, kidney diseases, neuralgia, bacterial infection, skin diseases, pneumonia, and tuberculosis of the lungs greatly increases.

A certain amount of sugar in the blood stream provides the energy needed for the functioning of the muscles and internal organs. Should the amount of sugar in the blood exceed the needed amount, a condition called glykohemia arises. Sugar is then found in the urine. This is the definitive characteristic of diabetes. Insulin, a hormone produced by the pancreas, is essential to the use in the body of sugar and other nutrients. In diabetics, a lack of this hormone makes it impossible for the body to use all of the sugar in the bloodstream. The condition may be hereditary; or it may be caused by excess eating, insufficient exercise, or stress. In middle-aged people who lead irregular lives with too many parties and too much alcohol, the condition is not uncommon. To cure the sickness, the supply of insulin in the body must be reinforced. This is, of course, impossible to do with oriental therapy alone, but massage and shiatsu on the tsubo can relieve the discomfort caused by the symptoms of diabetes.

Massage and shiatsu on BL-20 (Fig. 1) can remove the dryness in the mouth and the tendency to loss of weight because this tsubo is related to the pancreas, the insufficient activity of which is the cause of the symptoms. To stimulate digestion and absorption in the stomach and intestines, massage and apply shiatsu pressure to BL-21. Sometimes headaches and forgetfulness accompany diabetes. In such cases, use massage and shiatsu on BL-10 and GB-20 (Fig. 2). To relieve sluggishness in the hands and feet, treat the following tsubo: ST-36 and GB-34 (Fig. 4); and SP-9 and SP-6 (Fig. 5); LI-11 (Fig. 6). Massage these tsubo in the directions shown by the arrows. In cases of constipation, massage ST-25 and ST-27 (Fig. 3).

Fig. 1

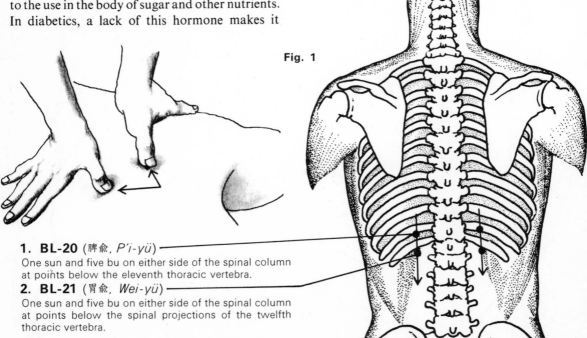

1. BL-20 (脾兪, *P'i-yü*)
One sun and five bu on either side of the spinal column at points below the eleventh thoracic vertebra.
2. BL-21 (胃兪, *Wei-yü*)
One sun and five bu on either side of the spinal column at points below the spinal projections of the twelfth thoracic vertebra.

Fig. 2

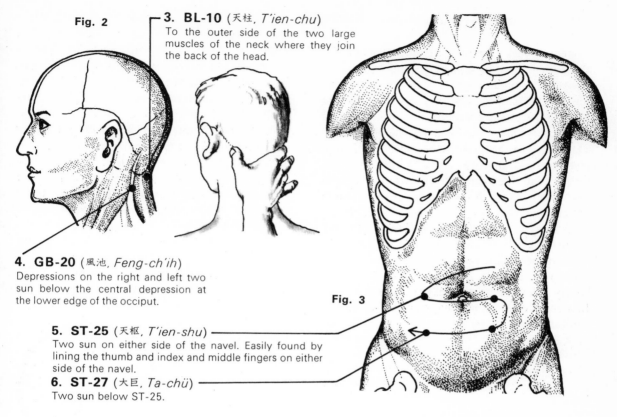

3. BL-10 (天柱, *T'ien-chu*)
To the outer side of the two large muscles of the neck where they join the back of the head.

Fig. 3

4. GB-20 (風池, *Feng-ch'ih*)
Depressions on the right and left two *sun* below the central depression at the lower edge of the occiput.

5. ST-25 (天枢, *T'ien-shu*)
Two *sun* on either side of the navel. Easily found by lining the thumb and index and middle fingers on either side of the navel.

6. ST-27 (大巨, *Ta-chü*)
Two *sun* below ST-25.

In all instances, massage must be performed in the directions of the arrows and must be centered on these tsubo. Shiatsu, moxa combustion, and application of magnetic steel balls too are effective on these tsubo.

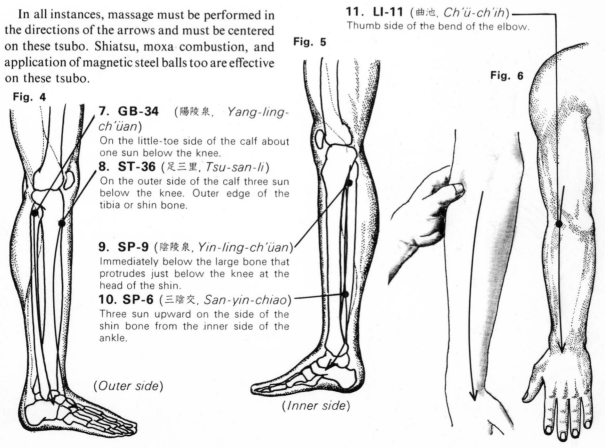

11. LI-11 (曲池, *Ch'ü-ch'ih*)
Thumb side of the bend of the elbow.

Fig. 5

Fig. 6

Fig. 4

7. GB-34 (陽陵泉, *Yang-ling-ch'üan*)
On the little-toe side of the calf about one *sun* below the knee.

8. ST-36 (足三里, *Tsu-san-li*)
On the outer side of the calf three *sun* below the knee. Outer edge of the tibia or shin bone.

9. SP-9 (陰陵泉, *Yin-ling-ch'üan*)
Immediately below the large bone that protrudes just below the knee at the head of the shin.

10. SP-6 (三陰交, *San-yin-chiao*)
Three *sun* upward on the side of the shin bone from the inner side of the ankle.

(Outer side)

(Inner side)

(2) Chronic Thyropathy

The commonest thyroid disease is goiter, of which the patient may be completely unaware unless the swelling of the thyroid gland, which causes the condition, becomes very great. Since the early stages of the condition cannot be detected visibly, it is imperative to have someone perform a tactile test on the throat in the area of the thyroid gland to try to detect swelling. A swelling in the throat that does not move when the patient swallows is likely to result from swollen lymph vessels. Swollen thyroid glands move during swallowing. Sometimes goiter may be chronic; in such cases, the entire thyroid gland swells without serious alteration of its general outline. The swelling, may, however, be localized and knotty. Chronic goiter may be the result of Basedow's disease, or it may be a chronic inflammation. Acute knotty goiter may be cancerous.

These symptoms must be diagnosed and treated by a specialist; but, once the condition has been stabilized, a design for wholesome living becomes imperative. In this connection, tsubo therapy can be of great significance.

People afflicted with Basedow's disease are listless and slightly feverish. Their pulse is fast, their hearts palpitate, they cannot sleep, and they lose weight. These symptoms result from hyperactivity of the thyroid. Underactivity of the thyroid brings about excess gain of weight, which is not fat, but an accumulation of water. In this situation, the patient's memory is likely to fail.

According to oriental medical thought, the heart, liver, and kidneys control the flow of energy throughout the body. This consideration is important in selecting tsubo for treatment since the aim is to improve energy circulation and thus to increase the patient's powers of resistance.

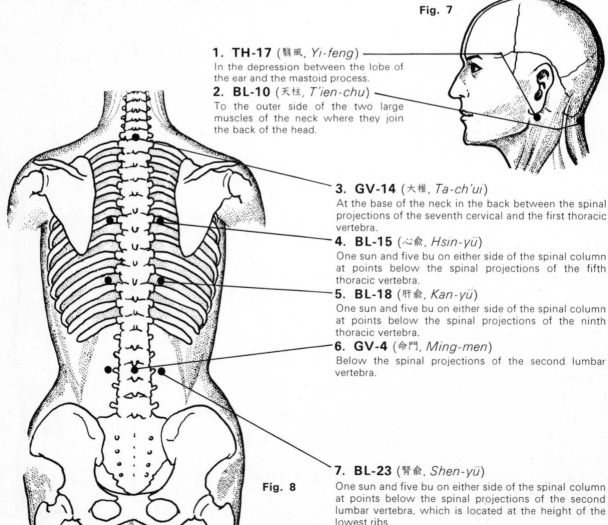

Fig. 7

1. TH-17 (翳風, *Yi-feng*)
In the depression between the lobe of the ear and the mastoid process.
2. BL-10 (天柱, *T'ien-chu*)
To the outer side of the two large muscles of the neck where they join the back of the head.

3. GV-14 (大椎, *Ta-ch'ui*)
At the base of the neck in the back between the spinal projections of the seventh cervical and the first thoracic vertebra.
4. BL-15 (心兪, *Hsin-yü*)
One sun and five bu on either side of the spinal column at points below the spinal projections of the fifth thoracic vertebra.
5. BL-18 (肝兪, *Kan-yü*)
One sun and five bu on either side of the spinal column at points below the spinal projections of the ninth thoracic vertebra.
6. GV-4 (命門, *Ming-men*)
Below the spinal projections of the second lumbar vertebra.

Fig. 8

7. BL-23 (腎兪, *Shen-yü*)
One sun and five bu on either side of the spinal column at points below the spinal projections of the second lumbar vertebra, which is located at the height of the lowest ribs.

First have the patient lie on his stomach so that you may apply gentle, slow shiatsu therapy to TH-17, BL-10 (Fig. 7), GV-14, BL-15, BL-18, GV-4, BL-23 (Fig. 8). Next have the patient lie on his back as you treat ST-9 (Fig. 9), ST-36 (Fig. 10), LI-11, and LI-4 (Fig. 11). Because the aim of this tsubo therapy is to improve the total body functions, it must be performed regularly every day. Treatment on CV-22, ST-11, CV-17, CV-14, CV-12, KI-16, and CV-4 (Fig. 9) is useful in these cases.

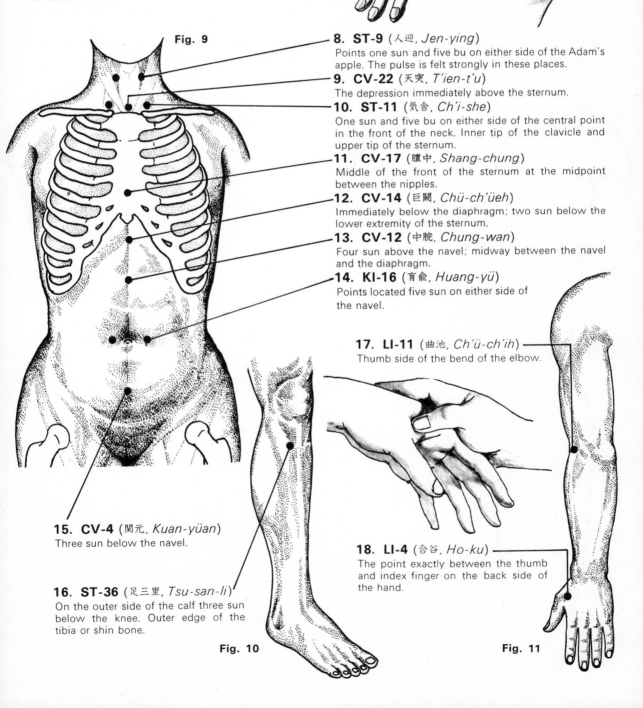

Fig. 9

8. ST-9 (人迎, *Jen-ying*)
Points one sun and five bu on either side of the Adam's apple. The pulse is felt strongly in these places.

9. CV-22 (天突, *T'ien-t'u*)
The depression immediately above the sternum.

10. ST-11 (気舎, *Ch'i-she*)
One sun and five bu on either side of the central point in the front of the neck. Inner tip of the clavicle and upper tip of the sternum.

11. CV-17 (膻中, *Shang-chung*)
Middle of the front of the sternum at the midpoint between the nipples.

12. CV-14 (巨闕, *Chü-ch'üeh*)
Immediately below the diaphragm; two sun below the lower extremity of the sternum.

13. CV-12 (中脘, *Chung-wan*)
Four sun above the navel; midway between the navel and the diaphragm.

14. KI-16 (肓俞, *Huang-yü*)
Points located five sun on either side of the navel.

17. LI-11 (曲池, *Ch'ü-ch'ih*)
Thumb side of the bend of the elbow.

15. CV-4 (関元, *Kuan-yüan*)
Three sun below the navel.

16. ST-36 (足三里, *Tsu-san-li*)
On the outer side of the calf three sun below the knee. Outer edge of the tibia or shin bone.

18. LI-4 (合谷, *Ho-ku*)
The point exactly between the thumb and index finger on the back side of the hand.

Fig. 10

Fig. 11

(3) Beriberi

Constant weariness and lack of will to work or do anything is a frequently heard complaint. There can be many organic and pathological reasons for this condition; one of them is beriberi.

Beriberi arises as a result of a deficiency of vitamin B_1 and thiamin in the diet. It is characterized by disorders in the nervous system and the blood vessels and by swelling. The sickness is found most often in temperate and tropical Asian zones where rice is a staple food. It has largely been eliminated from Japan, though it is encountered sometimes in large cities. Strong people between the ages of fifteen and thirty-five are susceptible to attacks of beriberi, which strikes most often in the summertime. In the early stages, the patient experiences numbness and perhaps paralysis of the sensory nerves in the back of the feet, the fingers, and the navel zone. His legs may become weak and may tire easily. In addition, he may suffer from palpitations, shortness of breath, lack of appetite, constipation, and swellings. To relieve fatigue and weariness, massage or use shiatsu pressure on ST-36 (Fig. 17), SP-8 (Fig. 18), and BL-23 (Fig. 14). For improved general physical condition, massage as shown in Figs. 12 through 18.

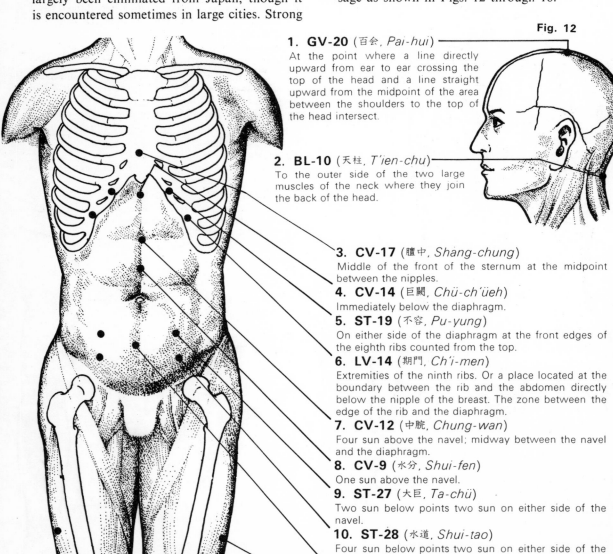

Fig. 12

1. GV-20 (百会, *Pai-hui*)
At the point where a line directly upward from ear to ear crossing the top of the head and a line straight upward from the midpoint of the area between the shoulders to the top of the head intersect.

2. BL-10 (天柱, *T'ien-chu*)
To the outer side of the two large muscles of the neck where they join the back of the head.

3. CV-17 (膻中, *Shang-chung*)
Middle of the front of the sternum at the midpoint between the nipples.

4. CV-14 (巨闕, *Chü-ch'üeh*)
Immediately below the diaphragm.

5. ST-19 (不容, *Pu-yung*)
On either side of the diaphragm at the front edges of the eighth ribs counted from the top.

6. LV-14 (期門, *Ch'i-men*)
Extremities of the ninth ribs. Or a place located at the boundary between the rib and the abdomen directly below the nipple of the breast. The zone between the edge of the rib and the diaphragm.

7. CV-12 (中脘, *Chung-wan*)
Four sun above the navel; midway between the navel and the diaphragm.

8. CV-9 (水分, *Shui-fen*)
One sun above the navel.

9. ST-27 (大巨, *Ta-chü*)
Two sun below points two sun on either side of the navel.

10. ST-28 (水道, *Shui-tao*)
Four sun below points two sun on either side of the navel.

11. CV-4 (関元, *Kuan-yüan*)
Three sun below the navel.

12. GB-31 (風市, *Feng-shih*)
Seven sun above the knees on the outsides of the thighs, at a point where there are two muscles.

Fig. 13

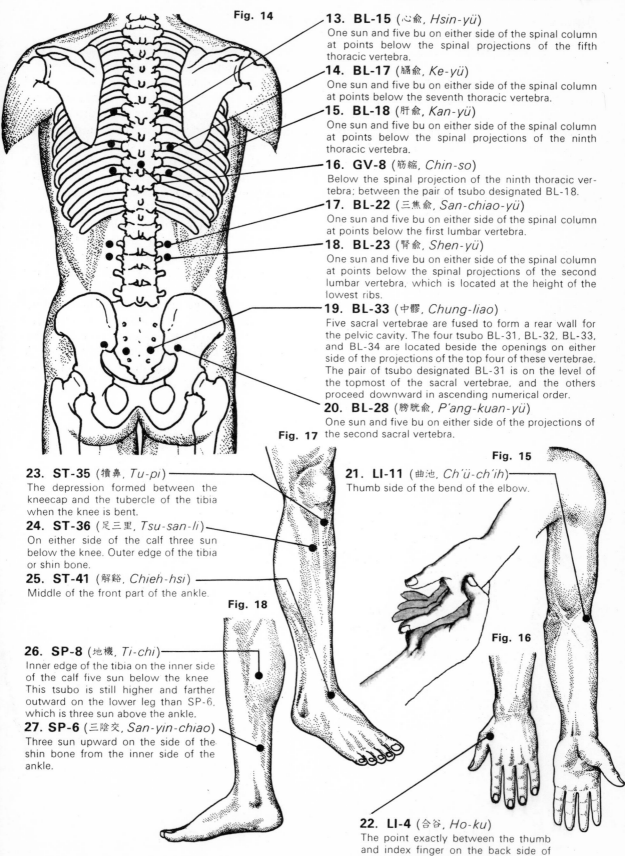

Fig. 14

13. BL-15 (心兪, *Hsin-yü*)
One sun and five bu on either side of the spinal column at points below the spinal projections of the fifth thoracic vertebra.

14. BL-17 (膈兪, *Ke-yü*)
One sun and five bu on either side of the spinal column at points below the seventh thoracic vertebra.

15. BL-18 (肝兪, *Kan-yü*)
One sun and five bu on either side of the spinal column at points below the spinal projections of the ninth thoracic vertebra.

16. GV-8 (筋縮, *Chin-so*)
Below the spinal projection of the ninth thoracic vertebra; between the pair of tsubo designated BL-18.

17. BL-22 (三焦兪, *San-chiao-yü*)
One sun and five bu on either side of the spinal column at points below the first lumbar vertebra.

18. BL-23 (腎兪, *Shen-yü*)
One sun and five bu on either side of the spinal column at points below the spinal projections of the second lumbar vertebra, which is located at the height of the lowest ribs.

19. BL-33 (中髎, *Chung-liao*)
Five sacral vertebrae are fused to form a rear wall for the pelvic cavity. The four tsubo BL-31, BL-32, BL-33, and BL-34 are located beside the openings on either side of the projections of the top four of these vertebrae. The pair of tsubo designated BL-31 is on the level of the topmost of the sacral vertebrae, and the others proceed downward in ascending numerical order.

20. BL-28 (膀胱兪, *P'ang-kuan-yü*)
One sun and five bu on either side of the projections of the second sacral vertebra.

Fig. 17

23. ST-35 (犢鼻, *Tu-pi*)
The depression formed between the kneecap and the tubercle of the tibia when the knee is bent.

24. ST-36 (足三里, *Tsu-san-li*)
On either side of the calf three sun below the knee. Outer edge of the tibia or shin bone.

25. ST-41 (解谿, *Chieh-hsi*)
Middle of the front part of the ankle.

Fig. 18

26. SP-8 (地機, *Ti-chi*)
Inner edge of the tibia on the inner side of the calf five sun below the knee. This tsubo is still higher and farther outward on the lower leg than SP-6, which is three sun above the ankle.

27. SP-6 (三陰交, *San-yin-chiao*)
Three sun upward on the side of the shin bone from the inner side of the ankle.

21. LI-11 (曲池, *Ch'ü-ch'ih*)
Thumb side of the bend of the elbow.

Fig. 15

Fig. 16

22. LI-4 (合谷, *Ho-ku*)
The point exactly between the thumb and index finger on the back side of the hand.

Illnesses of the Brain and Nervous System

(1) Neuralgia in the Arms

The nerves of the arms arise from between the fifth cervical and the first lumbar vertebrae and pass under the armpits to the arms, forearms, and hands. Three nerves branch from the forearm to travel to the fingers: the radial nerve leading to the thumb, the median nerve leading to the middle fingers, and the ulnar nerve leading to the little finger. Usually, the sharp, violent pains sometimes felt along these nerves have no pathological origins. The things that bring them on are cold, moisture, sudden chilling, overwork, and constipation. Middle-aged and old people experience this condition together with arteriosclerosis. In women, it occurs during pregnancy or at the conclusion of the menstrual period. Nervous people, hysterical people, and girls at the age of puberty are susceptible to it. This complaint usually affects either the right or the left arm, but not both at once. The condition causing pain and weakness in both arms at the same time is rheumatism or a high form of cervical neuralgia. Muscular inflammation, food poisoning, gout, and diabetes can produce symptoms much like those of neuralgia of the arms, except that the condition will be accompanied by fever and flushing. When these symptoms manifest themselves or whenever there is indication of a serious illness, consult a specialist immediately. Depending on the nerve affected, neuralgia of the arms is called radial, median, or ulnar. To treat, using the thumbs to make small circular motions, massage from the arm to the base of the arm along the nerve in pain. The case is radial neuralgia when the pain moves along the line from the cervical vertebra and the base of the neck, to the armpit, the arm, the forearm, and then to the thumb. It is median neuralgia if the pain runs along the same path and then from the forearm moves to the middle of the palm of the hand. If, at the forearm, the pain moves to the little finger, it is ulnar neuralgia.

Fig. 1

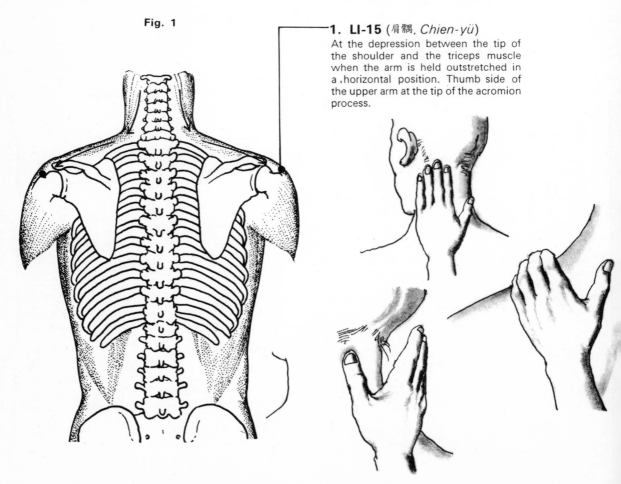

1. LI-15 (肩髃, *Chien-yü*)
At the depression between the tip of the shoulder and the triceps muscle when the arm is held outstretched in a ‚horizontal position. Thumb side of the upper arm at the tip of the acromion process.

In slight cases, heat treatment is sufficient to relieve pain. Wrapping the neck in a thick towel soaked in hot water and the arm in another thick towel, treat with a hair dryer. If you press along the nerve of the patient and find points that are hypersensitive to pressure, you will have located the tsubo that must be treated with massage or shiatsu to relieve the symptoms: LI-15 (Fig. 1), LI-14, LI-11, LI-10, LI-4 (Fig. 2), LU-4, HT-3, LU-5, HC-4, HT-7, HC-7, LU-9 (Fig. 3). Massage or shiatsu on these points increases the effectiveness of the heat treatment. Acupuncture too is excellent therapy on these tsubo, but a specialist's assistance is needed to apply it.

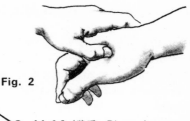

Fig. 2

2. LI-14 (臂臑, *Pi-nao*)
About seven sun above LI-11 on the thumb side of the upper arm; at the place in the upper arm where the triceps muscle gradually narrows to a tendon.

3. LI-11 (曲池, *Ch'ü-ch'ih*)
Thumb side of the bend of the elbow.

4. LI-10 (三里, *San-li*)
Point on the thumb side of the forearm in line with the index finger and two sun from the bend of the elbow.

5. LI-4 (合谷, *Ho-ku*)
The point exactly between the thumb and index finger on the back side of the hand.

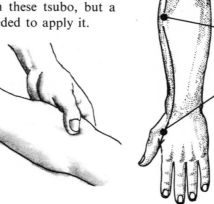

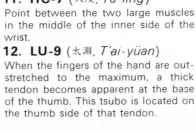

Fig. 3

6. LU-4 (俠白, *Hsia-pai*)
Soft muscle of the arm at the height of the nipples when the body is held upright as in the position of military attention.

7. HT-3 (少海, *Shiao-hai*)
Innermost point on the little-finger side of the large bone of the elbow joint.

8. LU-5 (尺沢, *Chi-tse*)
The hard tendon that is apparent in the inner side of the elbow when the wrist is bent, or the place at which pulse can be seen in the inner depression of the elbow joint.

9. HC-4 (郤門, *Hsi-men*)
Middle point of the inner side of the forearm at the midpoint between the elbow and the wrist.

10. HT-7 (神門, *Shen-men*)
Innermost part of the inner surface of the wrist.

11. HC-7 (大陵, *Ta-ling*)
Point between the two large muscles in the middle of the inner side of the wrist.

12. LU-9 (太淵, *T'ai-yüan*)
When the fingers of the hand are outstretched to the maximum, a thick tendon becomes apparent at the base of the thumb. This tsubo is located on the thumb side of that tendon.

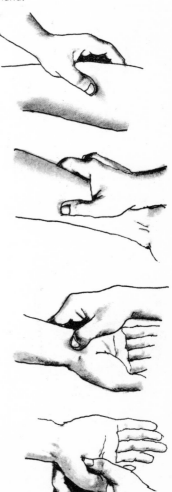

(2) Trigeminal Neuralgia

The trigeminal—three from the same origin—nerves are on the sides of the face. Each of them is triple-branched: one branch of each runs to the forehead, one from the cheek to the upper jaw, and one to the lower jaw. In middle-aged people of both sexes and in women pain occurs in these nerves that may, if violent, affect the eyes, the cheeks, the upper jaw, the back of the head, and the shoulders. In slight cases, there is pain for a few seconds in the face. The pain may, however, last for minutes or even hours. In severe cases, even the patient who remains perfectly still feels burning, cutting pains throughout the face, head, and shoulders. He is unable to speak, eat, or sleep. As the illness progresses, both the hypersensitive nerves and the body become exhausted.

Although other conditions—colds, influenza, sore eyes, earaches, nasal disturbances, food poisoning, diabetes, and syphilis—can cause trigeminal neuralgia, in most cases the causes are unknown. Consequently, modern medicine has no proved cure for it; and the person suffering an attack may become neurotic because of the insecurity of an apparently incurable condition. Since, in addition to physical causes, psychological factors seem to play an important part in these attacks, people susceptible to them should lead calm daily lives.

If the attack is severe, call on the services of a trained acupuncture specialist. If it is slight, however, relief from pain can be had from massage and shiatsu therapy. The branches of the trigeminal nerves are clearly shown in Figs. 4 through 7. Massage and shiatsu should be performed in the vicinity of the tsubo on these

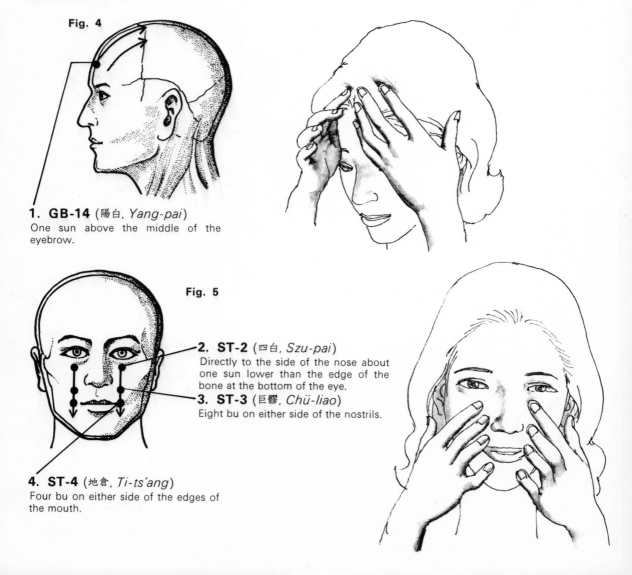

Fig. 4

1. GB-14 (陽白, *Yang-pai*)
One sun above the middle of the eyebrow.

Fig. 5

2. ST-2 (四白, *Szu-pai*)
Directly to the side of the nose about one sun lower than the edge of the bone at the bottom of the eye.

3. ST-3 (巨髎, *Chü-liao*)
Eight bu on either side of the nostrils.

4. ST-4 (地倉, *Ti-ts'ang*)
Four bu on either side of the edges of the mouth.

nerve branches. First, using the balls of the thumbs or of the index fingers, lightly massage GB-14 (Fig. 4) above the eyes in the direction of the arrows. The nerves branch below the eyes. Following the arrows, apply shiatsu massage, laying special emphasis on the tsubo in Figs. 5 and 6. Massage from TH-17 to LI-17 (Fig. 7) on the lower jaw.

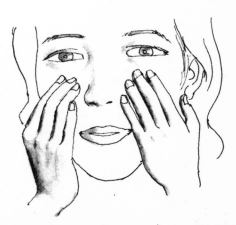

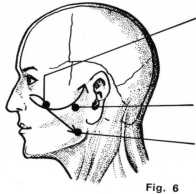

5. ST-7 (下関, *Hsia-kuan*)
The depression in front of the part of the lower jaw that passes in front of the ear hole. Lower edge of the zygomatic arch. Depression under the cheek bone (zygomatic arch) opposite the nostrils.

6. SI-18 (顴髎, *Ch'üan-liao*)
The cheek projections immediately below the outer ends of the eyes.

7. ST-6 (頬車, *Chia-ch'e*)
Depression fromed between the corner of the lower jaw and the earlobe when the mouth is open wide.

Fig. 6

Fig. 7

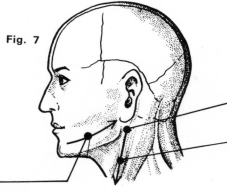

8. TH-17 (翳風, *Yi-feng*)
In the depression between the lobe of the ear and the mastoid process.

9. LI-17 (天鼎, *T'ien-ting*)
Three sun to the sides of the Adam's apple and one sun downward, or to the outer edge of the sternomastoid muscle.

10. ST-5 (大迎, *Ta-ying*)
Depression in the lower jaw one sun and three bu from its corner.

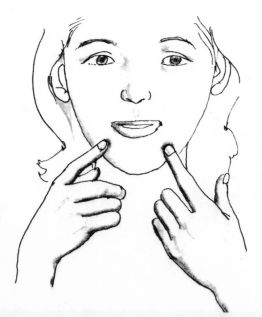

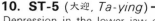

Finally rub the entire face lightly with the palms of the hands. Heat treatments with hot packs or hair dryer are effective in these cases.

(3) Facial Cramps

Two systems of nerves control the movements of the facial muscles and the sensations of pain, heat, and cold in the face. These are the trigeminal nerves and the facial nerves. In the preceding section, I discussed the symptoms of trigeminal neuralgia. When the facial nerves are affected, the entire face becomes paralyzed, and cramps cause the skin to twitch. But because, unlike the skin of the rest of the human body, that of the face is united with the musculature, hypersensitivity in the facial nerves causes cramping in the skin and the muscles simultaneously. Sometimes these cramps take the form of twitching around the eyes or the mouth. This is especially the case with irritable and emotionally unsettled people. When such a condition arises, it is the result of hyperfunctioning of the facial nerves and consequent loss of control of the muscles around the eyes and mouth.

To bring relief from this condition, apply shiatsu massage to TH-17 (Fig. 8). Have the patient gently close his eyes as you press on this point with the thumbs and the index fingers. Then use shiatsu massage on TH-23 and GB-1 (Fig. 9); BL-2 and BL-1 (Fig. 10). For cramps and twitching around the mouth, apply shiatsu massage to TH-17, ST-2, ST-4, and CV-24 (Fig. 12). To bring relief from twitching and cramps in the cheeks, apply shiatsu to SI-18 (Fig. 11). In addition to shiatsu, hot compresses, moxa with garlic or ginger root, and mild moxa combustion bring relief from facial cramps.

Fig. 8

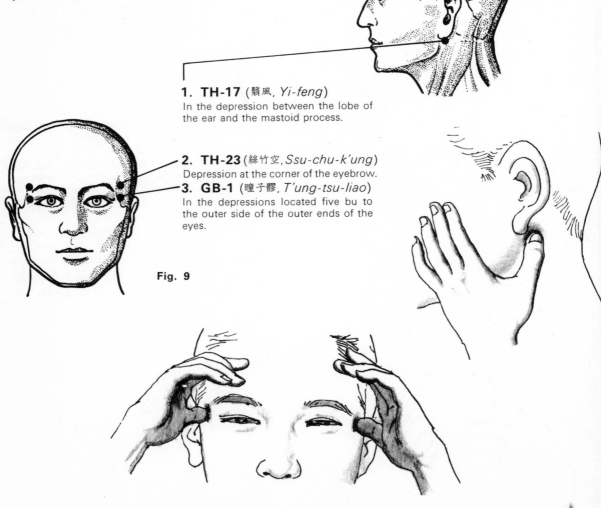

1. TH-17 (翳風, *Yi-feng*)
In the depression between the lobe of the ear and the mastoid process.

2. TH-23 (絲竹空, *Ssu-chu-k'ung*)
Depression at the corner of the eyebrow.
3. GB-1 (瞳子髎, *T'ung-tsu-liao*)
In the depressions located five bu to the outer side of the outer ends of the eyes.

Fig. 9

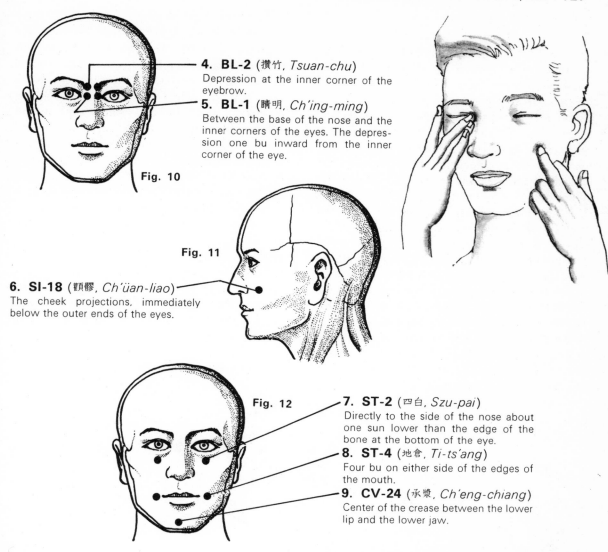

4. BL-2 (攢竹, *Tsuan-chu*)

Depression at the inner corner of the eyebrow.

5. BL-1 (睛明, *Ch'ing-ming*)

Between the base of the nose and the inner corners of the eyes. The depression one bu inward from the inner corner of the eye.

Fig. 10

Fig. 11

6. SI-18 (顴髎, *Ch'üan-liao*)

The cheek projections, immediately below the outer ends of the eyes.

Fig. 12

7. ST-2 (四白, *Szu-pai*)

Directly to the side of the nose about one sun lower than the edge of the bone at the bottom of the eye.

8. ST-4 (地倉, *Ti-ts'ang*)

Four bu on either side of the edges of the mouth.

9. CV-24 (承漿, *Ch'eng-chiang*)

Center of the crease between the lower lip and the lower jaw.

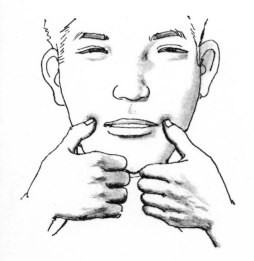

In the majority of cases, neuralgia of the trigeminal nerves, reflex reactions to disturbances in the reproductive organs, nervous tension, and emotional conditions cause facial cramps and spasms. When the condition is a reflex of another sickness, it is wise to combine treatment for both at the same time. Spasms in the muscles around the eyes (*orbicularis oculi*) can be of two kinds: a rigid condition occurring when the eyes are closed, and a spasm that makes the eyes wink. The latter kind can become habitual.

(4) Facial Paralysis

In the hot summertime, remaining too long in front of an electric fan can paralyze the muscles of the face, making it impossible to smile, frown, or give facial expression to any emotion. In very severe cases, the eyes remain open and staring, and the mouth is so slack and uncontrollable that eating is impossible. Naturally, for the sake of appearances, anyone afflicted with this condition wants to rectify it immediately. When both sides of the face are rigidly paralyzed, however, brain sickness may be the cause. In such instances, the care of a specialist must be sought at once. Many causes can be given for facial paralysis, but the passing kind that affects only one side of the face is most responsive to tsubo therapy. Cases that are the results of syphilis, meningitis, cerebral hemorrhage, and other serious illness require the treatment of a specialist. Since facial paralysis can make it difficult or impossible to close the eyes, it can be the indirect cause of conjunctivitis or corneitis. Should this danger exist, the eyes must be carefully washed.

In cases of mild facial paralysis, first apply a hot towel to the face. Then, using the thumbs and the four fingers, massage the meridians shown in Figs. 13, 14, and 15, in the directions of the arrows. When the massage has been performed, the patient should stand in front of a mirror and practice as many exaggerated facial expressions as he can think of to limber the facial muscles. If this treatment is carried out regularly daily in the morning and the evening, a moderate case of facial paralysis can be cured in three weeks.

In some cases, in combination with the tsubo already mentioned, it is necessary to treat CV-12, CV-4, BL-22, and BL-23 (Figs. 16 and 17). A patient who came to my laboratory after suffering for about six months from facial paralysis brought on by an all-night session of mahjong was cured in three weeks by means of the treatment outlined above. The most important thing is to persevere in the massage and the practice of exaggerated facial expressions. Successful treatment cannot be expected in a day.

Fig. 13

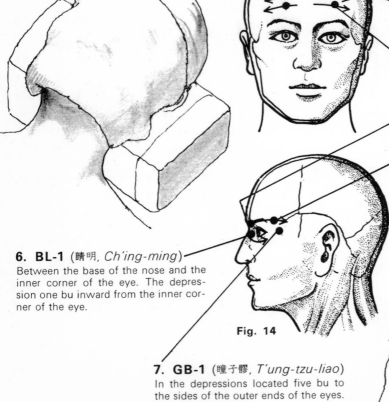

Fig. 14

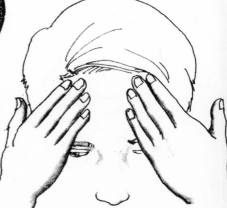

1. GV-24 (神庭, *Shen-t'ing*)
On a line passing through the center of the forehead five bu from the front hairline.

2. ST-8 (頭維, *T'ou-wei*)
Four sun and five bu on either side of a point five bu directly above the hairline in the center of the forehead.

3. GB-14 (陽白, *Yang-pai*)
One sun above the middle of the eyebrow.

4. BL-2 (攢竹, *Tsuan-chu*)
Depression at the inner corner of the eyebrow.

5. TH-23 (絲竹空, *Ssu-chu-k'ung*)
Depression at the outer tip of the eyebrow.

6. BL-1 (睛明, *Ch'ing-ming*)
Between the base of the nose and the inner corner of the eye. The depression one bu inward from the inner corner of the eye.

7. GB-1 (瞳子髎, *T'ung-tzu-liao*)
In the depressions located five bu to the sides of the outer ends of the eyes.

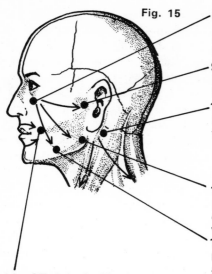

Fig. 15

8. ST-2 (四白, *Szu-pai*)
Directly to the side of the nose about one sun lower than the edge of the bone at the bottom of the eye.
9. SI-19 (聴宮, *T'ing-kung*)
Immediately below the soft projection in front of the ear.
10. TH-17 (翳風, *Yi--feng*)
In the depression between the lobe of the ear and the mastoid process.

11. ST-6 (頬車, *Chia-ch'e*)
Depression formed between the corner of the lower jaw and the earlobe when the mouth is open wide.
12. ST-5 (大迎, *Ta-ying*)
Depression in the lower jaw one sun and three bu from its corner.

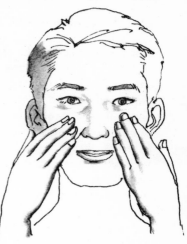

13. ST-4 (地倉, *Ti-ts'ang*)
Four bu on either side of the edges of the mouth.

Fig. 16

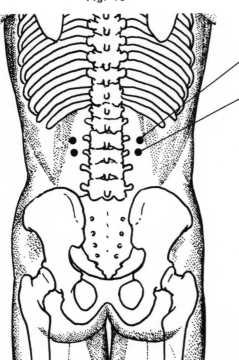

14. BL-22 (三焦兪, *San-chiao-yü*)
One sun and five bu on either side of the spinal column at points below the spinal projections of the third lumbar vertebra.
15. BL-23 (腎兪, *Shen-yü*)
One sun and five bu on either side of the spinal column at points below the spinal projections of the second lumbar vertebra, which is located at the height of the lowest ribs.

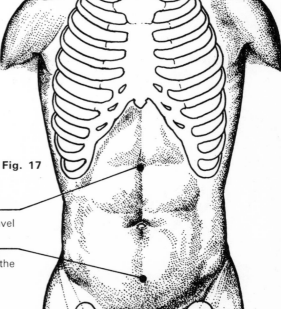

Fig. 17

16. CV-12 (中脘, *Chung-wan*)
Four sun above the navel; midway between the navel and the diaphragm.
17. CV-4 (関元, *Kuan-yüan*)
Three sun below the navel, or midway between the navel and the pubis.

(5) Occipital Neuralgia

Pains in the back of the head (occipital region), stiffness in the back of the neck and the shoulders, pain in the face, and hypersensitivity to touch in the vicinity of the hairline can be the result of faults in the circulatory system. If blood is overabundant in the head, the condition is called hyperemic headache; if blood is insufficient, it is known as anemic headache. In very slight cases, such moderate motion as twisting the neck to the right and left and bending the head forward and backward relieves the pain. Many people are willing to suffer slight pain in preference to calling on a physician. Such people will find massage on the meridians shown in the charts a highly convenient and effective kind of treatment.

First, using the palms of the hands, massage the meridians from GV-20 to GV-16 and BL-10 (Fig. 18). Next, thorough massage from BL-7 to GB-20 then from GB-4 to GB-12 (Fig. 19) is necessary. Then thoroughly massage the area behind the ears in the vicinity of GB-12. In all of this massage, the motions must be slow and of the kneading variety. Apply thorough shiatsu massage to GV-20, BL-10, GB-20, and GB-12. A kneading massage is needed to help relieve the pain at the hairline.

Should the condition become chronic, I recommend moxa combustion on the tsubo listed above. Part the hair carefully, massage the tsubo, and make an ink mark to indicate the location for moxa combustion to help you remember it for the next application. Apply moxa combustion to GV-20, GB-4, and GV-16 and to the tsubo listed above for reference. The treatment must be continued regularly and faithfully for at least three weeks if cure is to be expected. Since stiff shoulders often accompany this condition, refer to p. 152 for the treatment for that ailment.

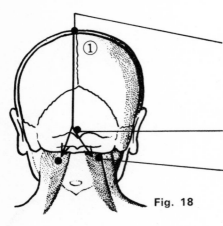

Fig. 18

1. GV-20 (百会, *Pai-hui*)
At the point where a line directly upward from ear to ear crossing the top of the head and a line straight upward from the midpoint of the area between the shoulders to the top of the head intersect.

2. GV-16 (風府, *Feng-fu*)
One sun below the external occipital protuberance.

3. BL-10 (天柱, *T'ien-chu*)
To the outer side of the two large muscles of the neck where they join the back of the head.

4. BL-7 (通天, *T'ung-t'ien*)
One sun and five bu from the very top of the head.

5. GB-20 (風池, *Feng-ch'ih*)
Depression in the lower edge of the occiput two sun on either side of BL-10.

6. GB-4 (頷厭, *Han-yen*)
Points located behind the hairline on either side of the forehead.

Fig. 19

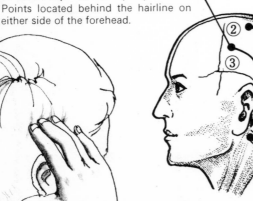

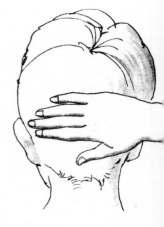

7. GB-12 (完骨, *Wan-ku*)
Depression in the back edge of the mastoid process behind the ear. In the depression that is located about the width of one finger above the mastoid process and about four bu from the hairline.

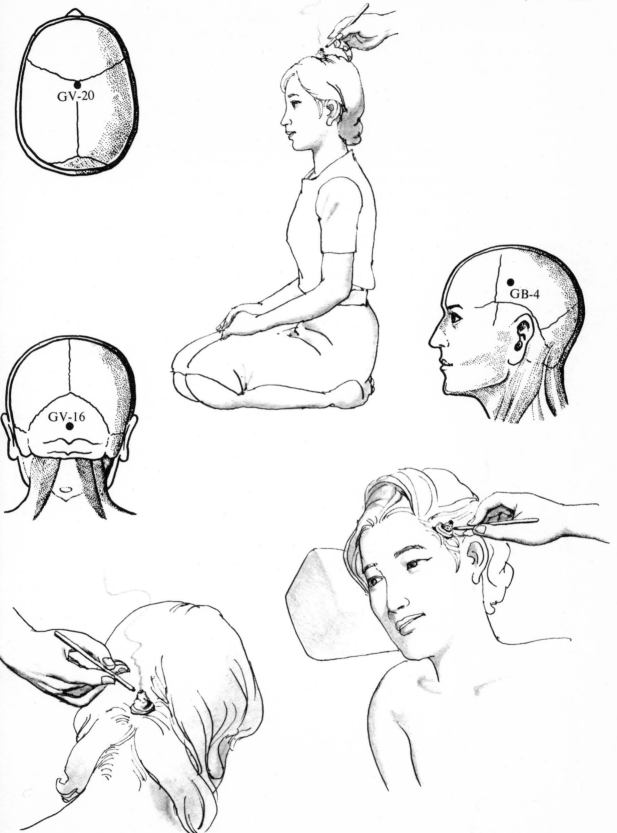

GV-20

GV-16

GB-4

(6) Epilepsy

Long regarded as a disease either divine or demonic in origin, epilepsy can now be treated with considerable hope of complete success. It nonetheless remains a serious illness. The symptoms are of two kinds: spasms and personality alterations apart from the spasms. When an attack of epilepsy strikes, the victim loses consciousness and collapses. For the first few moments, his body will be utterly rigid. Then his arms and legs will begin to tremble and to undergo periodic cramps and spasms. In the last few minutes of the attack, he will snore and appear to be asleep. It requires more than ten minutes for the patient to regain complete consciousness. Sometimes the attack is sudden and without unwarning. At other times, the patient may experience flashes in front of his eyes and numbness in the arms and legs; in other words, there are instances in which the epilepsy patient is aware that he is about to experience an attack.

There are two kinds of epilepsy: the true and the symptomatic. True epilepsy is the result of causes related to the brain but not fully understood. Symptomatic epilepsy, on the other hand, is caused by some other disease attacking the body at the same time. The only thing that is known for certain about true epilepsy is its hereditary nature.

Epilepsy attacking infants shortly after birth is usually caused by natal damage. This damage may result in cerebral paralysis, encephalitis, or meningitis. Epilepsy attacking children in their teens is usually true epilepsy. When the condition attacks people in their thirties or older people, it may be caused by faulty circulation in the brain or by cerebral tumor.

Tsubo therapy can be used to reduce the frequency and shorten the duration of attacks of true epilepsy. The major tsubo in treating epilepsy arue the ones used in curing headaches: GV-21, GV-20, GV-19 (Fig. 20), BL-10, and GB-20 (Fig. 21). To calm spasms in the arms and legs, treat BL-63 (Fig. 23), BL-13, BL-15, BL-22, and BL-23 (Fig. 25). To relieve the chilling that accompanies epileptic attacks, treat LI-11 (Fig. 24), ST-36, and SP-6 (Fig. 22). The most effective treatment on those tsubo is moxa combustion. Using medium-grade moxa, persist regularly in treatment. Hot compresses on the tsubo on the back, hips, and legs will relieve chills. Constipation can be an indirect cause of epileptic attacks. Prevent this condition from developing by massaging CV-12 and ST-27 (Fig. 26) regularly.

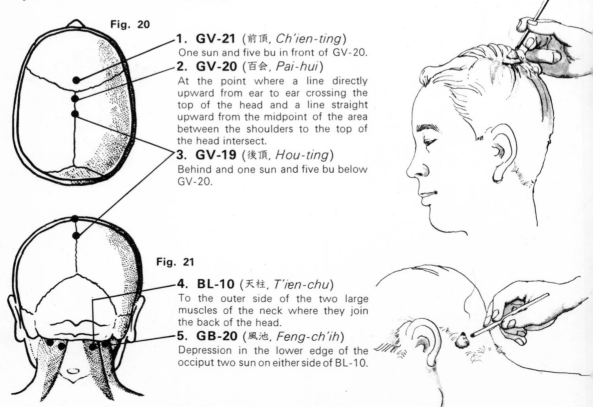

Fig. 20

1. GV-21 (前頂, *Ch'ien-ting*)
One sun and five bu in front of GV-20.
2. GV-20 (百会, *Pai-hui*)
At the point where a line directly upward from ear to ear crossing the top of the head and a line straight upward from the midpoint of the area between the shoulders to the top of the head intersect.
3. GV-19 (後頂, *Hou-ting*)
Behind and one sun and five bu below GV-20.

Fig. 21

4. BL-10 (天柱, *T'ien-chu*)
To the outer side of the two large muscles of the neck where they join the back of the head.
5. GB-20 (風池, *Feng-ch'ih*)
Depression in the lower edge of the occiput two sun on either side of BL-10.

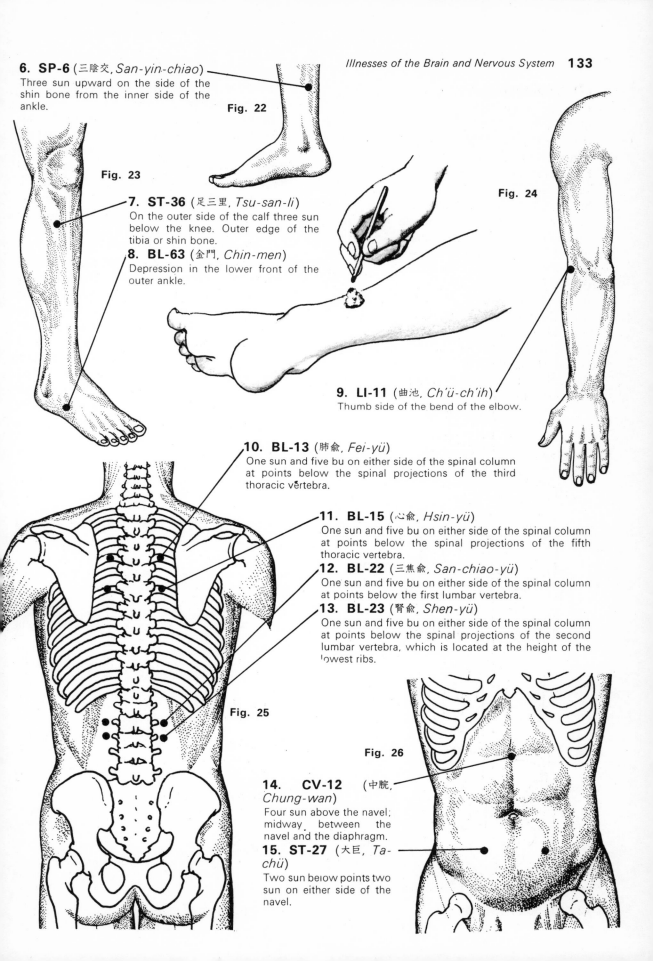

6. SP-6 (三陰交, *San-yin-chiao*)
Three sun upward on the side of the shin bone from the inner side of the ankle.

Fig. 22

Fig. 23

Fig. 24

7. ST-36 (足三里, *Tsu-san-li*)
On the outer side of the calf three sun below the knee. Outer edge of the tibia or shin bone.

8. BL-63 (金門, *Chin-men*)
Depression in the lower front of the outer ankle.

9. LI-11 (曲池, *Ch'ü-ch'ih*)
Thumb side of the bend of the elbow.

10. BL-13 (肺兪, *Fei-yü*)
One sun and five bu on either side of the spinal column at points below the spinal projections of the third thoracic vertebra.

11. BL-15 (心兪, *Hsin-yü*)
One sun and five bu on either side of the spinal column at points below the spinal projections of the fifth thoracic vertebra.

12. BL-22 (三焦兪, *San-chiao-yü*)
One sun and five bu on either side of the spinal column at points below the first lumbar vertebra.

13. BL-23 (腎兪, *Shen-yü*)
One sun and five bu on either side of the spinal column at points below the spinal projections of the second lumbar vertebra, which is located at the height of the lowest ribs.

Fig. 25

Fig. 26

14. CV-12 (中脘, *Chung-wan*)
Four sun above the navel; midway between the navel and the diaphragm.

15. ST-27 (大巨, *Ta-chü*)
Two sun below points two sun on either side of the navel.

(7) Semiparalysis

Paralysis of half of the body results from apoplexy, which may be caused by cerebral hemorrhage or by cerebral infarction. Cerebral hemorrhage occurs frequently in people with high blood pressure. In time of sudden excitement or sudden cold, blood rushes to the brain; but the blood vessels of such people have hardened and become too slender to withstand the onrush. Consequently, they burst, causing hemorrhage into the brain. When a clot or some foreign matter clogs the blood vessels in the brain and thus impairs the functioning of the brain cells, the condition is called either cerebral infarction or cerebral thrombosis. The former condition is commoner in old people, and the latter in young people. In both cases, an obstruction in the blood vessels blocks the flow of blood and nutrients to the brain tissues, which then become sluggish and gradually soften.

Cerebral hemorrhage strikes suddenly and paralyzes one side of the body. Victims find that they cannot speak clearly, that they have headaches, that they feel nauseous, and that they slowly lose consciousness or sink into a coma. When consciousness returns, one half of the body is likely to be completely paralyzed. Cerebral thrombosis often strikes at night when the person is in bed. Paralysis or numbness in half of the body and lack of clarity in speech occur. Sometimes the patient cannot speak at all.

Should someone in your family suffer cerebral hemorrhage, have the patient lie still without moving his head. Immediately have a doctor come or have the patient transported to a hospital in an ambulance. When he becomes conscious again, the patient must undergo a specialist's course of rehabilitation therapy, which will include training in moving the limbs, walking, crawling, turning over in bed, and other motions. Although curing paralysis is

Fig. 27

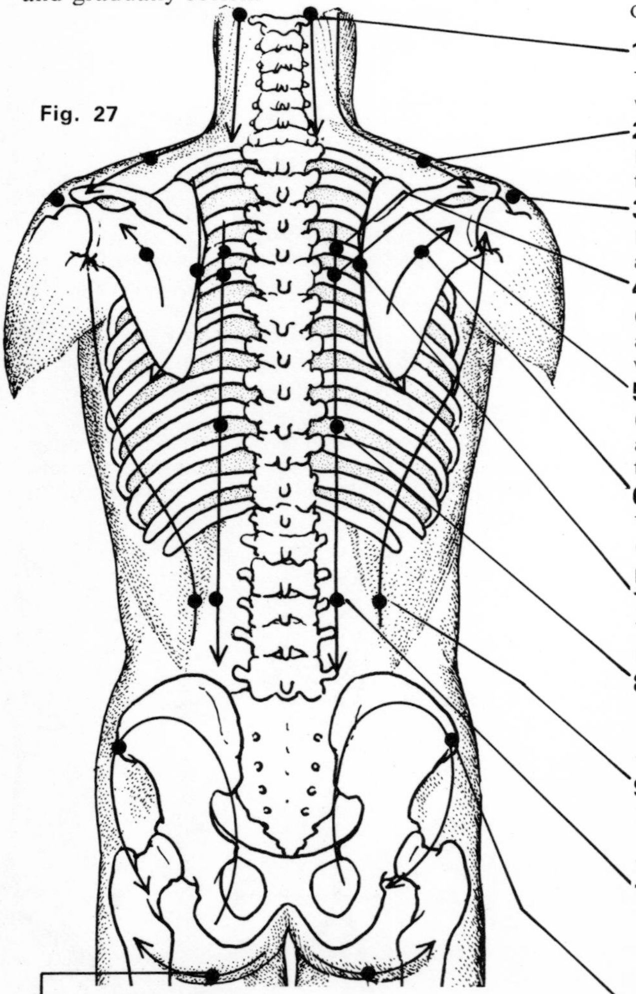

1. BL-10 (天柱, *T'ien-chu*)
To the outer side of the two large muscles of the neck where they join the back of the head.

2. GB-21 (肩井, *Chien-ching*)
In the middle point between the base of the neck and the end of the shoulder.

3. TH-14 (肩髎, *Chien-liao*)
Depression at the under edge of the external tip of the acromion process.

4. BL-13 (肺兪, *Fei-yü*)
One sun and five bu on either side of the spinal column at points below the spinal projections of the third thoracic vertebra.

5. BL-14 (厥陰兪, *Chüeh-yin-yü*)
One sun and five bu on either side of the spinal column at points below the spinal projections of the fourth thoracic vertebra.

6. SI-11 (天宗, *T'ien-tsung*)
The depression in the middle of the shoulder blade. One sun and five bu below the center of the scapular process.

7. BL-38 (膏肓, *Kao-huang*)
Three sun on either side of the spinal column at points below the fourth thoracic vertebra.

8. BL-18 (肝兪, *Kan-yü*)
One sun and five bu on either side of the spinal column at points below the spinal projections of the ninth thoracic vertebra.

9. BL-47 (志室, *Chih-shih*)
Three sun on either side of the spinal column at points below the spinal projections of the second lumbar vertebra.

10. BL-23 (腎兪, *Shen-yü*)
One sun and five bu on either side of the spinal column at points below the spinal projections of the second lumbar vertebra, which is located at the height of the lowest ribs.

12. BL-50 (承扶, *Ch'eng-fu*)
In the centers of the grooves that form below the buttocks when the body is in the military attention position.

11. GB-29 (居髎, *Chü-liao*)
Eight sun and three bu below the extremities of the eleventh ribs.

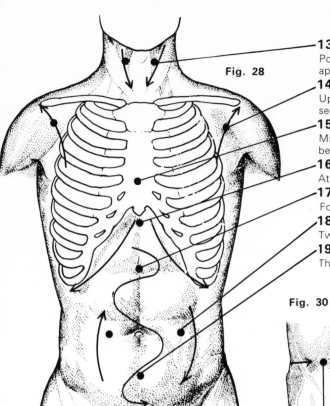

Fig. 28

13. ST-9 (人迎, *Jen-ying*)
Points one sun and five bu on either side of the Adam's apple.

14. LI-1 (中府, *Chung-fu*)
Upper extremity of the exterior front chest wall at the second intercostal zone.

15. CV-17 (膻中, *Shang-chung*)
Middle of the front of the sternum at the midpoint between the nipples.

16. CV-15 (鳩尾, *Chiu-wei*)
At the diaphragm.

17. CV-14 (中脘, *Chung-kuan*)
Four sun above the navel.

18. ST-25 (天枢, *T'ien-shu*)
Two sun on either side of the navel.

19. CV-4 (関元, *Kuan-yüan*)
Three sun below the navel.

Fig. 29

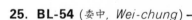

Fig. 30

21. TH-10 (天井, *T'ien-ching*)
On the back of the upper arm on the ulna about one sun from the elbow.

22. TH-4 (陽池, *Yang-ch'ih*)
When the palm is outstretched, on the back of the hand at the back of the wrist a hard, thick muscles becomes apparent. This tsubo is on the little-finger side of that muscle; that is, it is slightly to the little-finger side of the middle of the wrist.

23. LU-5 (尺沢, *Chi-tse*)
The hard tendon that is apparent in the inner side of the elbow when the wrist is bent, or the place at which pulse can be seen in the inner depression of the elbow joint.

24. HC-7 (大陵, *Ta-ling*)
Point between the two large muscles in the middle of the inner side of the wrist.

Fig. 31

beyond the limits of tsubo therapy, such treatment can relieve some of the unpleasant symptoms that arise in consequence of inability to move the limbs. In addition, in light cases of paralysis, tsubo therapy can be helpful in effecting a cure. Since neck movement is of the greatest importance, first massage the areas of the tsubo on the head and shoulders. Prolonged lying in one position reduces the circulation of blood to the muscles of the back. Those muscles therefore weaken. To prevent this, massage the meridians shown in Fig. 27. When the paralytic patient suffers from constipation, massage the meridians on the stomach (Fig. 28). Should the patient have pain in his sound arm or leg, massage the areas around the tsubo in Figs. 29 to 33. Move the paralyzed limbs often to prevent their stiffening.

25. BL-54 (委中, *Wei-chung*)
In the center of the groove formed behind the knee.

26. KI-3 (太谿, *T'ai-hsi*)
Rear part of the inside of the ankle.

27. BL-60 (崑崙, *k'un-lun*)
Immediately to the rear side of the outer ankle.

28. SP-9 (陰陵泉, *Yin-ling-ch'üan*)
Immediately below the large bone that protrudes just below the knee at the head of the shin.

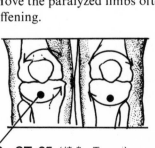

20. ST-35 (犢鼻, *Tu-pi*)
The depression formed between the kneecap and the tubercle of the tibia when the knee is bent.

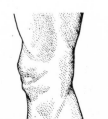

Figl 32

29. ST-36 (足三里, *Tsu-san-li*)
On the outer side of the calf three sun below the knee. Outer edge of the tibia or shin bone.

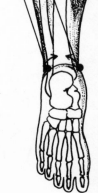

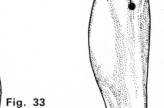

Fig. 33

(8) Irritability

The stress of modern living causes irritability and frustrations that mar the harmony of everyday living. In the brain of the human being are a new cortex and an old cortex that regulate emotions and actions. The new cortex governs reason, and the old cortex such animal instincts as the desire for food. Control of the old cortex by the new one sometimes gives rise to frustrations and irritability.

The oriental therapy for this kind of condition does not—surprisingly perhaps to the Western mind—involve treatment of the tsubo on the head. This is because, according to Eastern medical thought, the Zo and Fu organs, and not the brain, control the emotions. To treat irritability, massage the following tsubo: BL-13, BL-15, BL-18, BL-20, and BL-23 (Fig. 34), which are points for treating the Zo organs. At the same time, treat BL-37, BL-39, BL-44, and BL-47. The massage must be performed with the palms of the hands in the direction of the arrows in the chart. The pressure exerted by the hands must remain steady throughout the massage.

Other tsubo on which treatment calms irritability are these: LU-1, CV-17, CV-14, LV-14, GB-25, KI-16 (Fig. 37), GV-20 (Fig. 35), GB-21 (Fig. 36), ST-36. SP-6, and KI-3 (Fig. 38). From ancient times, KI-3 and ST-36 have been considered especially important in this connection. When massage on the back has been completed, have the patient lie face-up to allow you to massage his abdomen and legs. In addition to this kind of treatment, half closing the eyes and making a deliberate attempt to be calm is helpful in moments of emotional upset.

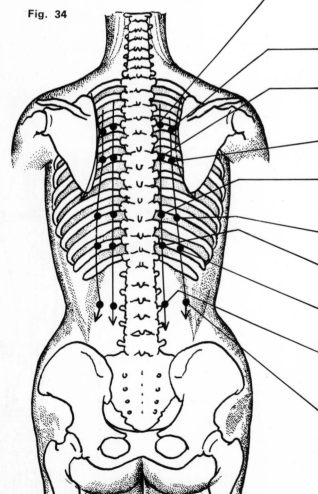

Fig. 34

1. BL-13 (肺俞, *Fei-yü*)
One sun and five bu on either side of the spinal column at points below the spinal projections of the third thoracic vertebra.

2. BL-37 (魄戸, *P'o-hu*)
On the right and left, three sun below the third thoracic vertebra.

3. BL-15 (心俞, *Hsin-yü*)
One sun and five bu on either side of the spinal column at points below the spinal projections of the fifth thoracic vertebra.

4. BL-39 (神堂, *Shen-t'ang*)
Three sun on either side of the spinal column at points below the fifth thoracic vertebra. To the side of BL-15.

5. BL-18 (肝俞, *Kan-yü*)
One sun and five bu on either side of the spinal column at points below the spinal projections of the ninth thoracic vertebra.

6. BL-42 (魂門, *Hun-men*)
Three sun on either side of the spinal column at points below the ninth thoracic vertebra; to the sides of BL-18.

7. BL-20 (脾俞, *P'i-yü*)
One sun and five bu on either side of the spinal column at points below the eleventh thoracic vertebra.

8. BL-44 (意舎, *Yi-she*)
Three sun on either side of the spinal column at points below the eleventh thoracic vertebra.

9. BL-23 (腎俞, *Shen-yü*)
One sun and five bu on either side of the spinal column at points below the spinal projections of the second lumbar vertebra, which is located at the height of the lowest ribs.

10. BL-47 (志室, *Chih-shih*)
Three sun on either side of the spinal column at points below the spinal projections of the second lumbar vertebra; on the outer side of the tsubo designated BL-23.

11. GV-20 (百会, *Pai-hui*)
At the point where a line directly upward from ear to ear crossing the top of the head and a line straight upward from the midpoint of the area between the shoulders to the top of the head intersect.

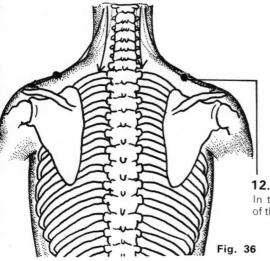

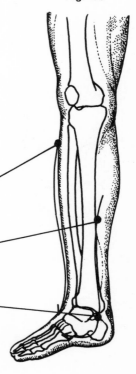

Fig. 35

12. GB-21 (肩井, *Chien-ching*)
In the middle point between the base of the neck and the end of the shoulder.

Fig. 36

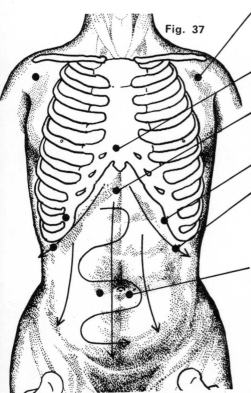

Fig. 37

13. LU-1 (中府, *Chung-fu*)
Upper extremity of the exterior front chest wall at the second intercostal zone. Six sun on either side of the sternum.

14. CV-17 (壇中, *Shang-chung*)
Middle of the front of the sternum at the midpoint between the nipples.

15. CV-14 (巨闕, *Chü-ch'üeh*)
Immediately below the diaphragm; two sun below the lower extremity of the sternum.

16. LV-14 (期門, *Ch'i-men*)
Extremities of the ninth ribs.

17. GB-25 (京門, *Ching-men*)
At the ends of the twelfth ribs. To find this, have the patient kneel upright or lie facedown as you check his ribs. The twelfth ribs are short and are not attached at the small of the back.

18. KI-16 (肓俞, *Huang-yü*)
Points located five sun on either side of the navel.

19. ST-36 (足三里, *Tsu-san-li*)
On the outer side of the calf three sun below the knee. Outer edge of the tibia or shin bone.

20. SP-6 (三陰交, *San-yin-chiao*)
Three sun upward on the side of the shin bone from the inner side of the ankle.

21. KI-3 (太谿, *T'ai-hsi*)
Rear part of the inside of the ankle.

Fig. 38

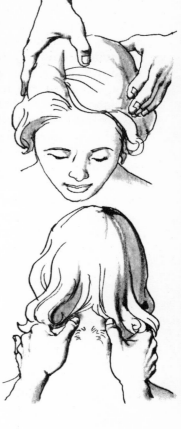

(9) Obsessive Fears

Excessive fear of other people is an obsessive neurosis related to what Sigmund Freud called metastatic neurosis and what Pierre Janet called neurasthenia. A person suffering from this condition is obsessed with actions and attitudes that he knows are without basis or that are meaningless but that he cannot prevent himself from performing or entertaining. Accompanying the obsession there is usually a fear. For instance, a person may be obsessed with the danger of knives and the possibility that, if he has one in his hands, he may harm someone. This obsession generates in him a terror of knives. Some of the kinds of symptoms of this condition include the following: obsessive ideas, obsessive acts, obses-

sive fears, fears of dirtiness, fears of being left alone, fears of open spaces, fears of sharp-pointed objects, erythrophobia, and fear of other people. The acts—repeated washing of the hands, for instance—that obsessed people perform are symbolic in nature and relieve the tensions caused by the obsession. In terms of physical and mental symptoms, obsessions often cause damage to the autonomic nervous system, palpitations, shortness of breath, chilling in the arms and legs, difficulty in sleeping muscular tensions, and so on. To relieve these symptoms, a planned way of wholesome living is necessary. In addition, massage or moxa combustion on the following tsubo is effective: BL-15, BL-23, (Fig. 40), CV-17, CV-12, and CV-4 (Fig. 4). Shiatsu massage on the tsubo shown in Figs. 39 to 43 is of great benefit.

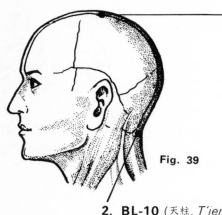

Fig. 39

1. GV-20 (百会, *Pai-hui*)
At the point where a line directly upward from ear to ear crossing the top of the head and a line straight upward from the midpoint of the area between the shoulders to the top of the head intersect.

2. BL-10 (天柱, *T'ien-chu*)
On the outer side of the two large muscles of the neck where they join the back of the head.

Fig. 40

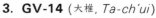
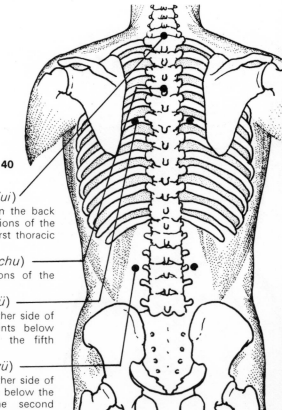

3. GV-14 (大椎, *Ta-ch'ui*)
At the base of the neck in the back between the spinal projections of the seventh cervical and the first thoracic vertebra.

4. GV-12 (身柱, *Shen-chu*)
Below the spinal projections of the third thoracic vertebra.

5. BL-15 (心兪, *Hsin-yü*)
One sun and five bu on either side of the spinal column at points below the spinal projections of the fifth thoracic vertebra.

6. BL-23 (腎兪, *Shen-yü*)
One sun and five bu on either side of the spinal column at points below the spinal projections of the second lumbar vertebra, which is located at the height of the lowest ribs.

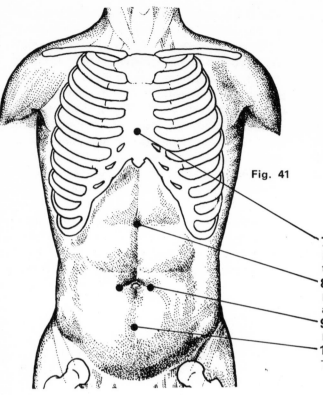

Fig. 41

7. CV-17 (膻中, *Shang-chung*)
Middle of the front of the sternum at the midpont between the nipples.

8. CV-12 (中脘, *Chung-wan*)
Four sun above the navel; midway between the navel and the diaphragm.

9. KI-16 (肓兪, *Huang-yü*)
Points located five sun on either side of the navel.

10. CV-4 (関元, *Kuan-yüan*)
Three sun below the navel.

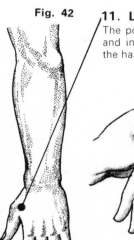

Fig. 42

11. LI-4 (合谷, *Ho-ku*)
The point exactly between the thumb and index finger on the back side of the hand.

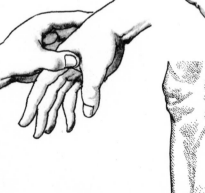

Fig. 43

12. KI-9 (築賓, *Chu-pin*)
In the muscle that is the width of the index finger inward of the edge of the shin at a point five sun above the inner side of the ankle.

13. SP-6 (三陰交, *San-yin-chiao*)
Three sun upward on the side of the shin bone from the inner side of the ankle.

14. KI-3 (太谿, *T'ai-hsi*)
Rear part of the inside of the ankle.

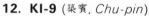

(10) Stammering

Of the various speech impediments—some physical, some psychological, and some results of no more than regional speech habits—stammering brings the victi the greatest mental suffering and embarrassment. It is estimated that, in Japan, about one percent of all children stammer and that the number of males so afflicted is greater than the number of females. Although the causes of the condition are by no means clearly understood, they seem to include mental elements, skills, and hereditary factors. It is deeply significant that stammering usually first arises before the age of three or, at the latest, before the age of eight; these are times when social influences and relations assume major importance.

Stammering results from spasms in the organs of enunciation. According to the generally accepted modern interpretation, social and environmental conditions and the child's ability to adapt to them cause what might be called mal-circuiting in the paths of transmission of information along the central nervous system. This mal-circuiting is manifest in the form of stammering. Hypertension in the organs of enunciation brings about stammering and, at the same time, causes tenseness in the muscles of the limbs and face. The question is what brings about the hypertension.

In many aspects of life, hypertension—tension beyond what is required for ordinary activities—can become an obstruction. For instance, many people find themselves virtually paralyzed when called upon to perform in public some act that

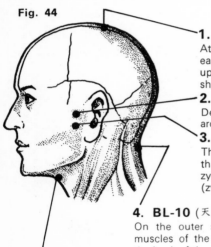

Fig. 44

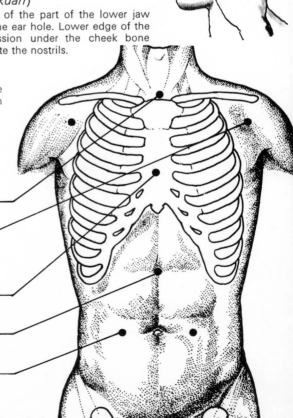

1. GV-20 (百会, *Pai-hui*)
At the point where a line directly upward from ear to ear crossing the top of the head and a line straight upward from the midpoint of the area between the shoulders to the top of the head intersect.

2. GB-3 (客主人, *K'e-chu-jen*)
Depression slightly above the middle of the zygomatic arch.

3. ST-7 (下関, *Hsia-kuan*)
The depression in front of the part of the lower jaw that passes in front of the ear hole. Lower edge of the zygomatic arch. Depression under the cheek bone (zygomatic arch) opposite the nostrils.

4. BL-10 (天柱, *T'ien-chu*)
On the outer side of the two large muscles of the neck where they join the back of the head.

5. CV-23 (廉泉, *Lien-ch'üan*)
Front upper part of the neck in the crease on the side of the Adam's apple.

6. CV-22 (天突, *T'ien-t'u*)
The depression immediately above the sternum or the depression above the midpoint between the clavicles.

7. LU-1 (中府, *Chung-fu*)
Upper extremity of the exterior front chest wall at the second intercostal zone. Six sun on either side of the sternum.

8. CV-17 (膻中, *Shang-chung*)
Middle of the front of the sternum at the midpoint between the nipples.

9. CV-12 (中脘, *Chung-wan*)
Four sun above the navel; midway between the navel and the diaphragm.

10. ST-25 (天枢, *T'ien-shu*)
Two sun on either side of the navel. Easily found by lining the thumb and index and middle fingers on either side of the navel.

Fig. 45

11. BL-13 (肺俞, *Fei-yü*)
One sun and five bu on either side of the spinal column at points below the spinal projections of the third thoracic vertebra.

12. BL-20 (脾俞, *P'i-yü*)
One sun and five bu on either side of the spinal column at points below the eleventh thoracic vertebra.

13. BL-23 (腎俞, *Shen-yü*)
One sun and five bu on either side of the spinal column at points below the spinal projections of the second lumbar vertebra, which is located at the height of the lowest ribs.

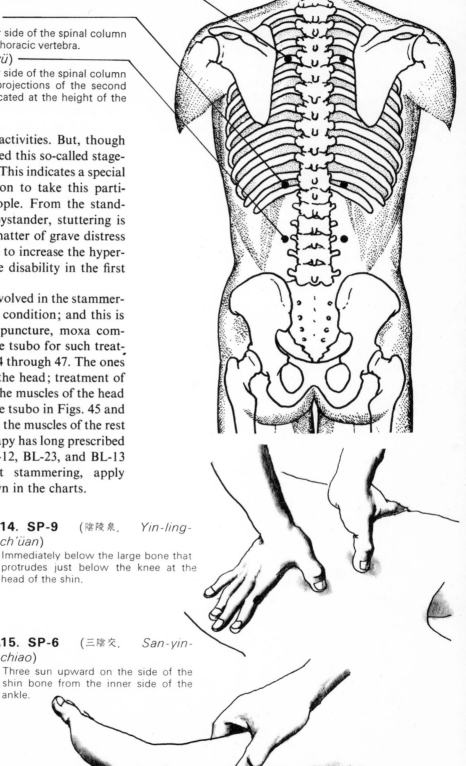

Fig. 46

is part of their everyday activities. But, though most of us have experienced this so-called stage-fright, few of us stammer. This indicates a special factor causing hypertension to take this particular form in certain people. From the standpoint of the unafflicted bystander, stuttering is unimportant; but it is a matter of grave distress for the sufferer and serves to increase the hypertension that brings on the disability in the first place.

Relaxing the muscles involved in the stammering is the way to cure the condition; and this is entirely feasible with acupuncture, moxa combustion, and massage. The tsubo for such treatment are shown in Figs. 44 through 47. The ones in Fig. 44 are located on the head; treatment of them is designed to relax the muscles of the head and face. Treatment on the tsubo in Figs. 45 and 46 relieves hypertension in the muscles of the rest of the body. Oriental therapy has long prescribed moxa combustion on CV-12, BL-23, and BL-13 for relaxation. To treat stammering, apply therapy to the tsubo shown in the charts.

14. SP-9 (陰陵泉, *Yin-ling-ch'üan*)
Immediately below the large bone that protrudes just below the knee at the head of the shin.

Fig. 47

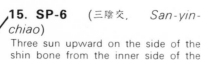

15. SP-6 (三陰交, *San-yin-chiao*)
Three sun upward on the side of the shin bone from the inner side of the ankle.

Sicknesses of the Muscles and Joints

(1) Rheumatism

Some of the complaints often voiced of aches in the joints are the outcome of overwork or unusual exercise. When the person complaining feels pain upon arising in the morning, on the other hand, he is probably suffering from rheumatism. Aching of the joints in the morning and swelling of the middle knuckles of the middle fingers are characteristics of this illness. The earliest symptoms are weakness, loss of weight, weariness, and anemia. As the condition progresses, the small joints of the fingers become sore; then the pain and stiffness move to the larger joints of the feet, legs, hands, and arms. In some instances, the pain reaches the joints of the neck. Chilling, fever, and sudden swelling or pain in the joints accompany the condition in some cases. As the condition becomes chronic, the joints refuse to function and develop the knots that are characteristic of rheumatism. Affected joints are covered with skin that is unnaturally smooth and glossy.

Viruses and still more complicated microscopic organisms are among the things suggested as causes of rheumatism, as are allergies; but the true cause remains uncertain. Wind, cold, moisture, and bad weather aggravate the condition or make one more susceptible to attacks of it. Women twenty years of age or older are the most frequent rheumatic victims. In fact, female patients of rheumatism are three times more numerous than male patients. Symptoms of rheumatism in children deserve the closest attention and the greatest caution as they often result from rheumatic fever, which is brought on by hemolytic streptococci. This disease causes inflammation of the heart.

Though the causes of rheumatism are uncertain, oriental tsubo therapy can bring relief from the pain it inflicts, because this kind of treatment improves the circulation of blood throughout the body. First, massage the tsubo in the vicinity of the joints that are most painful: LU-5, HC-3 HT-7, HC-7, LU-9, (Fig. 1), TH-10, LI-11 LI-5, and TH-4 (Fig. 2). To treat pain in the ankles, massage SP-5, KI-3 (Fig. 3), ST-41, and BL-60 (Fig. 4). In addition, massage around the aching joint. It is important to continue the massage daily. Hot compresses and paraffin baths provide benefit against rheumatism. Moxa combustion too is effective, but one must avoid strong shiatsu massage.

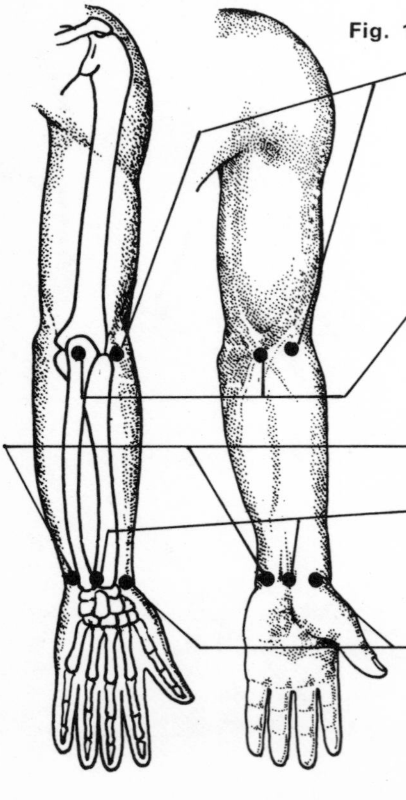

Fig. 1

1. LU-5 (尺沢, *Chi-tse*)
The hard tendon that is apparent in the inner side of the elbow when the wrist is bent.

2. HC-3 (曲沢, *Ch'ü-tse*)
Little-finger side of the hard tendon that becomes apparent at the middle of the elbow when the elbow is bent.

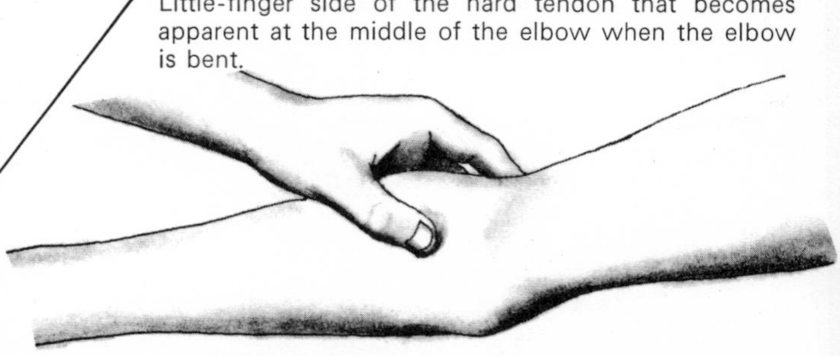

3. HT-7 (神門, *Shen-men*)
Innermost part of the inner surface of the wrist.

4. HC-7 (大陵, *Ta-ling*)
Point between the two large muscles in the middle of the inner side of the wrist.

5. LU-9 (太淵, *T'ai-yüan*)
When the fingers of the hand are outstretched to the maximum, a thick tendon becomes apparent at the base of the thumb. This tsubo is located on the thumb side of that tendon.

Fig. 2

6. TH-10 (天井, *T'ien-ching*)
On the back of the upper arm on the ulna about one sun from the elbow.

7. LI-11 (曲池, *Ch'ü-ch'ih*)
Thumb side of the bend of the elbow.

8. LI-5 (陽谿, *Yang-hsi*)
Point between the two hard tendons apparent on the back of the hand at the base of the thumb when the thumb is fully outstretched.

9. TH-4 (陽池, *Yang-ch'ih*)
When the palm is outstretched, on the back of the hand at the back of the wrist a hard, thick muscle becomes apparent. This tsubo is on the little-finger side of that muscle; that is, it is slightly to the little-finger side of the middle of the wrist.

10. SP-5 (商丘, *Shang-chiu*)
Inner ankle.

Fig. 3

11. KI-3 (太谿, *T'ai-hsi*)
Rear part of the inside of the ankle.

Fig. 4

12. ST-41 (解谿, *Chieh-hsi*)
Middle of the front part of the ankle.

13. BL-60 (崑崙, *K'un-lun*)
Immediately to the rear side of the outer ankle.

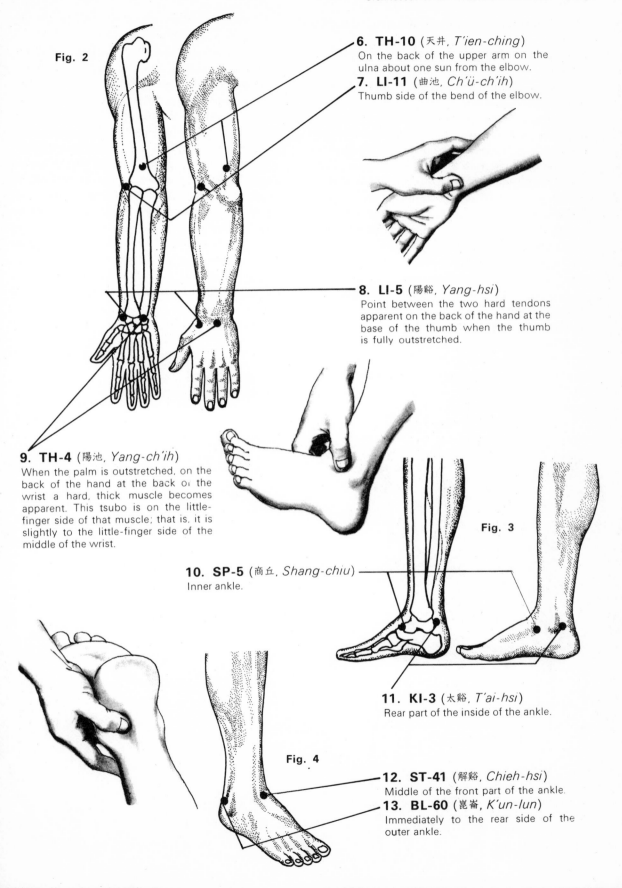

(2) Numbness in the Arms

During the mountain climbing season, people who are unaccustomed to carrying heavy loads on their backs complain of a kind of mild paralysis brought on by the packs that must be worn during long walks in mountainous terrain. The paralysis results from pressure applied by the pack and its harness to the nerves running from the base of the neck to the pit above the clavicles and through the armpits to the arms. Since this condition is rarely serious enough to cause permanent alteration in the nerves, it is not a source of worry. The paralysis can effect two zones: upper paralysis affecting the shoulders, shoulder blades, and muscles of the upper arms and lower paralysis affecting the elbows, hands, wrists, and fingers. As long as the situation is not serious, treatment with hot towels or a hair dryer will restore movement to the afflicted muscles.

After the hot packs have done their initial work, massage in the directions of the arrows on meridian ① on the rear of the neck and the extremities of the shoulders, meridian ② inside the shoulder blades, and meridian ③ below the projections of the shoulder blades (Fig. 5). Follow this with massage of these meridians: meridian ④ on the front of the base of the arms (Fig. 6), meridian ⑤ on the triceps muscle at the base of the arms, meridian ⑥ on the biceps muscle in the upper arm (Fig. 7), meridian ⑦ on the underside of the triceps muscle, meridian ⑧ running from the elbow to the thumb (Fig. 8), meridian ⑨ on the soft group of muscles on the thumb side of the front of the forearm (Fig. 7), and meridian ⑩ on the muscle group on the upper side forearm (Fig. 8). Perform this massage in stroking, rubbing, and squeezing motions with the palms. If this treatment does not cure the condition, damage may have been done to the nerves. In such cases, consult a physician.

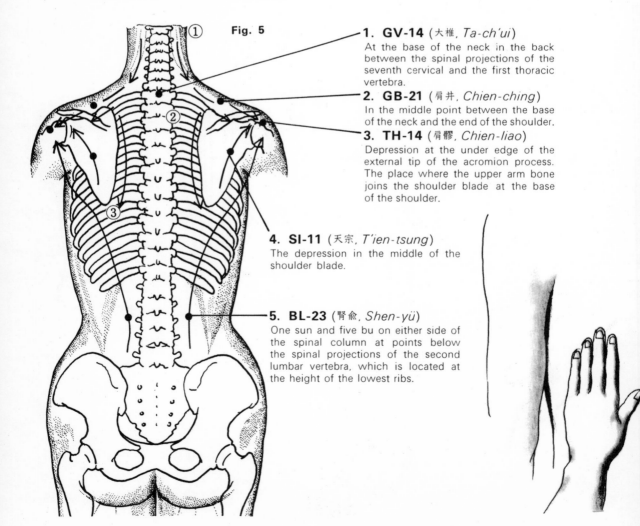

Fig. 5

1. GV-14 (大椎, *Ta-ch'ui*)
At the base of the neck in the back between the spinal projections of the seventh cervical and the first thoracic vertebra.

2. GB-21 (肩井, *Chien-ching*)
In the middle point between the base of the neck and the end of the shoulder.

3. TH-14 (肩髎, *Chien-liao*)
Depression at the under edge of the external tip of the acromion process. The place where the upper arm bone joins the shoulder blade at the base of the shoulder.

4. SI-11 (天宗, *T'ien-tsung*)
The depression in the middle of the shoulder blade.

5. BL-23 (腎兪, *Shen-yü*)
One sun and five bu on either side of the spinal column at points below the spinal projections of the second lumbar vertebra, which is located at the height of the lowest ribs.

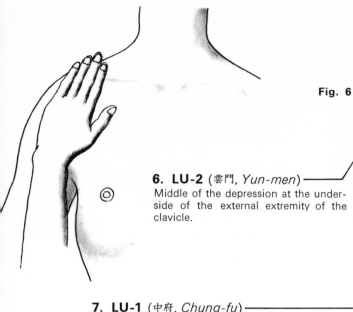

Fig. 6

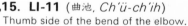

6. LU-2 (雲門, *Yun-men*)
Middle of the depression at the underside of the external extremity of the clavicle.

7. LU-1 (中府, *Chung-fu*)
Upper extremity of the exterior front chest wall at the second intercostal zone. Six sun on either side of the sternum.

8. LI-14 (臂臑, *Pi-nao*)
About seven sun above LI-11 on the thumb side of the upper arm; at the place in the upper arm where the triceps muscle gradually tapers to a tendon.

9. HT-3 (少海, *Shao-hai*)
Innermost point on the little-finger side of the large bone of the elbow joint.

10. LU-5 (尺沢, *Chi-tse*)
The hard tendon that is apparent in the inner side of the elbow when the wrist is bent.

11. HC-4 (郄門, *Hsi-men*)
Middle point of the inner side of the forearm at the midpoint between the elbow and the wrist.

12. HT-7 (神門, *Shen-men*)
Innermost part of the inner surface of the wrist.

15. LI-11 (曲池, *Ch'ü-ch'ih*)
Thumb side of the bend of the elbow.

16. LI-15 (陽谿, *Yang-hsi*)
Point between the two large tendons on the back of the hand at the base of the thumb when the thumb is fully outstretched.

17. TH-4 (陽池, *Yang-ch'ih*)
When the palm is outstretched, on the back of the hand at the back of the wrist a hard, thick muscles becomes apparent. This tsubo is on the little-finger side of that muscle; that is. it is slightly to the little-finger side of the middle of the wrist.

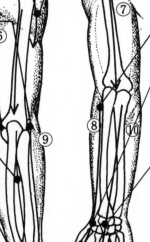

Fig. 7

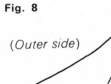

Fig. 8

(Outer side)

13. HC-7 (大陵, *Ta-ling*)
Point between the two large muscles in the middle of the inner side of the wrist.

(Inner side)

14. LU-9 (太淵, *T'ai-yüan*)
When the fingers of the hand are outstretched to the maximum, a thick tendon becomes apparent at the base of the thumb. This tsubo is located on the thumb side of that tendon.

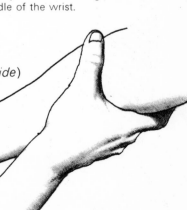

(3) Numbness in the Fingers

It is a common tendency to worry about numbness and discomfort in the fingers because such a condition is thought to presage an attack of a more serious nature. Undeniably, palsy and paralysis sometimes manifest this symptom in early stages; but, in general, numbness of the fingers can be accounted for by means of one of the following three causes. Slight deformation of a bone in the neck can apply pressure to the base of the nerves leading to the fingers and in this way cause numbness. Nerves branching from the first to eight cervical vertebra depart from the cervical region of the spinal cord. The ones branching from the fourth through the eighth cervical vertebra pass to the neck, arms, and hands. Obstruction—usually in vicinity of the vertebrae—in these nerves causes pain and numbness in the fingers. If the deformation or obstruction is at the fifth or sixth cervical vertebra, the thumbs will be affected; if at the sixth or seventh cervical vertebra, the middle fingers will be affected; and if at the seventh vertebra, the fourth and little fingers will be affected.

The second possible cause of numbness in the fingers is poor circulation caused by an obstruction in the sternomastoid artery, which runs from the heart to the hands. In these cases, the patient will experience severe stiffness in the scalenus muscle, which lies behind the sternomastoid muscle. The third possible cause—which resembles the second—is an anemic condition that adversely affects the circulation to the fingers. The symptoms of this condition are stiffness in the base of the neck and in the region from the neck to the shoulders, plus chilling of the fingers and low pulse at the wrist when the forearm is raised.

To treat the first condition, follow the therapy prescribed for ailments of the shoulders and the arms; in other words, use a hot pack on the cervical vertebrae on a level with the region from the nape of the neck to the tips of the shoulders (Fig. 9). Then gently massage both sides of the set of cervical vertebrae. For the second condition, treat the stiffness in the neck and shoulders with a hot pack or a heavy towel. Then, using the four fingers, massage LI-17, ST-12, HT-1, ST-11 (Fig. 10). At the same time, have the patient extend and contract his arm and swing it round and round. To treat numbness in the fingers caused by the third condition, it is necessary first to treat the anemia that is at the heart of the matter. Using the fingers of both hands, massage the meridians shown in Fig. 11, Then, thoroughly massage the area from the fingers to the wrists. Massage the arm to the base with the palms of the hands. Finally, stimulate circulation to the fingers by alternating hot and cold hand baths.

Fig. 9

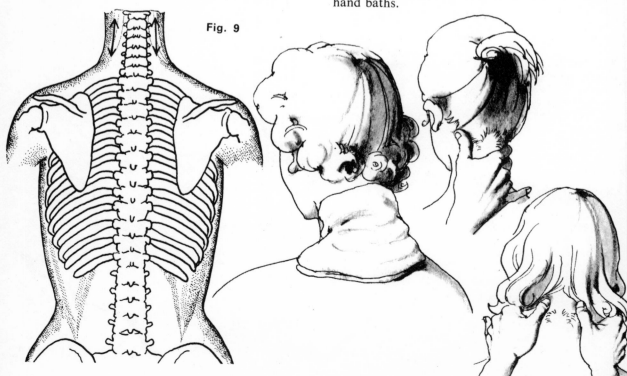

1. LI-17 (天鼎, *T'ien-ting*)
Near the peak of the triangular depression formed by the sternomastoid muscle (the muscle from the base of the neck to the ear; it becomes apparent when the neck is turned full to one side), the trapezius muscle (the large triangular muscle running from the neck to the shoulder tip), and the clavicles. Or three sun to the sides of the Adam's apple and one sun downward. Or the outer edge of the sternomastoid process.

Fig. 10

2. ST-12 (缺盆, *Chüeh-p'en*)
Immediately above the central point between the clavicles.

3. HT-1 (極泉, *Chi-ch'üan*)
Front part of the armpit at the arm joint.

4. ST-11 (気舎, *Ch'i-she*)
One sun and five bu on either side of the central point in the front of the neck. Inner tip of the clavicles and upper tip of the sternum.

Fig. 11

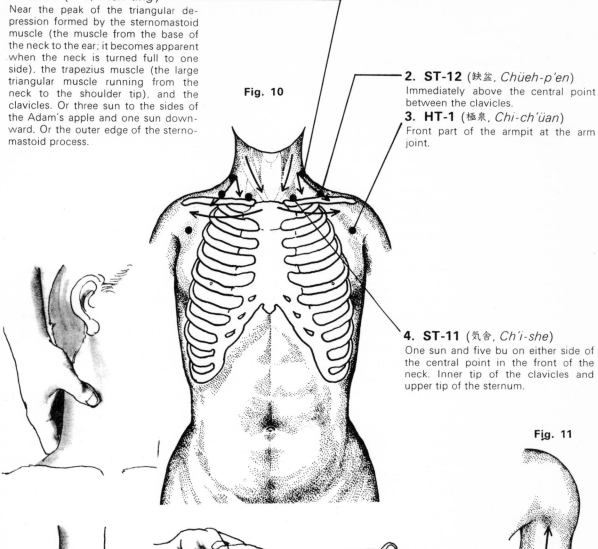
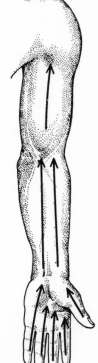

(4) Mild Pain in the Lower Back

Because he stands and walks on two instead of four limbs, man forces his lower back and pelvic region to bear the heavy load of the entire head, trunk, and upper limbs as well as that of the digestive and reproductive organs. It is not surprising, then, that these parts of the body should often become sites of pain and distress. Pain in the lower part of the back can result from many different causes. Sickness of the stomach, intestines, or urinary bladder may be the cause. Women suffering from female complaints often have backaches. Severe pain in this part of the body may be caused by hernia of the intervertebral discs (in such cases, lying on the side usually brings some relief). Suppurative spondylitis may be the cause of violent pain and fever in the back. Cancer produces pain in the back that is not relieved by lying down. Various symptoms of pain in the ischia of the pelvis produce pains in the back that extend all the way to the toes. When the intervertebral discs become deformed, they press on the nerves running to the feet and cause pain, numbness, and muscular contraction in the back and legs. Bone caries or destruction in the spinal column often forces old people to stand with sharply curved spines and shoulders. Sometimes the pain of backaches is very severe and localized at roughly the height of the belt or the upper protuberances of the pelvic bones. If there are no other remarkable symptoms, the patient may suffer from a condition affecting the fascia of the muscles of the back. This results usually from fatigue, cold, or some excessively energetic motion.

Even a physician has difficulty diagnosing the true causes of backaches of the kinds briefly mentioned above. If this is true, the amateur can hope to have little success in such an endeavor. Therefore, for the sake of tsubo therapy, I shall concentrate on bringing relief from the pain of backaches, which I classify into two types: mild and severe. In this section, I discuss treating the kind of mild ache in the back that plagues some people on arising in the morning yet that causes no physical manifestations traceable with X-ray photographs and no alterations in the rate of the patient's blood circulation. Bathing—especially in salt or sulfur mineral baths—brings relief from this condition; but, if such baths are impossible, a hot compress left in place for about twenty minutes followed by massage is equally effective. First, with both hands—right on bottom and left on top—press meridian ① (Fig. 12). Then, making circular motions with the palms of the hands, massage meridians ② and ③ (Fig. 13). Next, massage meridian ④ in the directions of the arrows and, finally, using the palms of the right and left hands at the same time and moving in the directions of the arrows, massage meridian ⑤, located on the buttocks. To strengthen the muscles of the abdomen, massage or apply shiatsu massage to the tsubo shown in Fig. 14. In addition, massage or shiatsu massage on the tsubo on the legs (Figs. 15 and 16) is very important.

Fig. 12

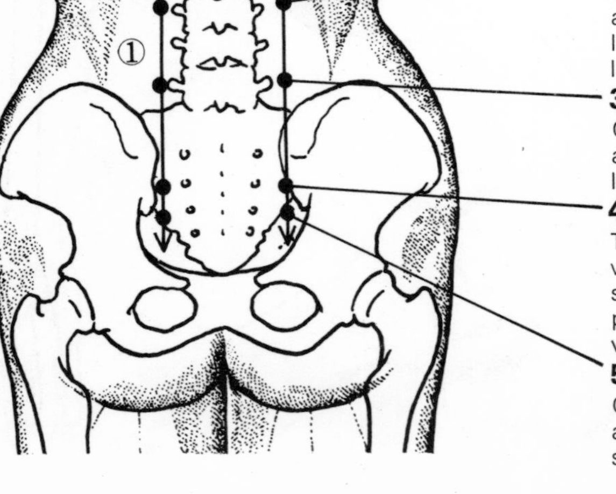

1. BL-22 (三焦兪, *San-chiao-yü*)
One sun and five bu on either side of the spinal column at points below the first lumbar vertebra.

2. BL-23 (腎兪, *Shen-yü*)
One sun and five bu on either side of the spinal column at points below the spinal projections of the second lumbar vertebra, which is located at the height of the lowest ribs.

3. BL-25 (大腸兪, *Ta-ch'ang-yü*)
One sun and five bu on either side of the spinal column at points below the spinal projections of the fourth lumbar vertebra.

4. BL-27 (小腸兪, *Hsiao-ch'ang-yü*)
The sacral vertebra are fused and formed into the rear wall of the pelvic cavity. These tsubo are located one sun and five bu on either side of the spinal column at points below the spinal projections of the first sacral vertebra.

5. BL-28 (膀胱兪, *P'ang-kuan-yü*)
One sun and five bu on either side of the spinal column at points below the spinal projections of the second sacral vertebra.

If you are using moxa, apply it to the tsubo on the lower part of the back when cold or chilling is thought to be the cause. Treat the tsubo shown in the chart if you think the cause is stomach or intestinal trouble or female complaints. Use medium-grade moxa from five to seven times on each tsubo once daily for three weeks.

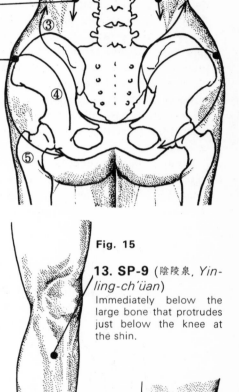

Fig. 13

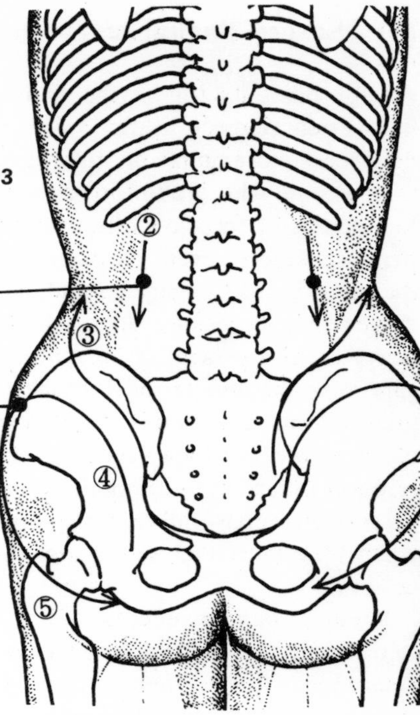

6. BL-47 (志室, *Chih-shih*)

Three sun on either side of the spinal column at points below the spinal projections of the second lumbar vertebra, on the outer sides of BL-23.

7. GB-29 (居髎, *Chü-liao*)

Eight sun and three bu below the extremities of the eleventh ribs. Exactly in the middle, but somewhat to the rear, of the hucklebone.

8. CV-12 (中脘, *Chung-wan*)

Four sun above the navel; midway between the navel and the diaphragm.

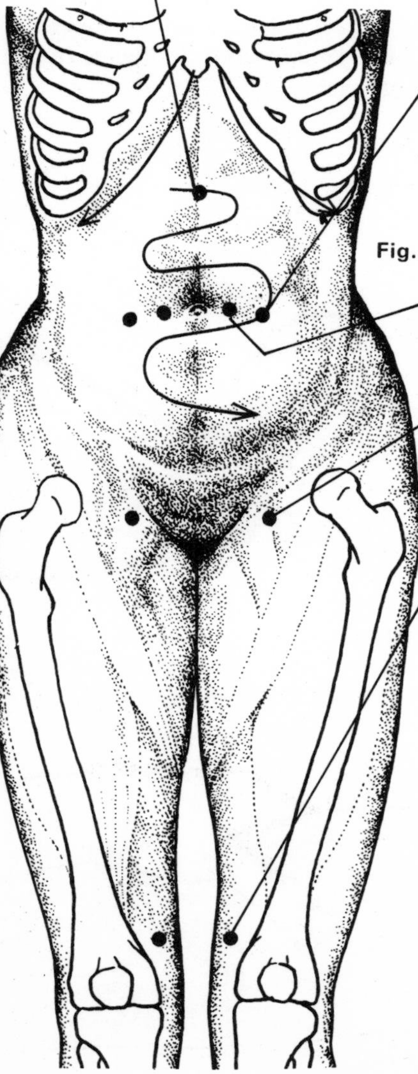

9. ST-25 (天枢, *T'ien-shu*)

Two sun on either side of the navel. Easily found by lining the thumb and index and middle fingers on either side of the navel.

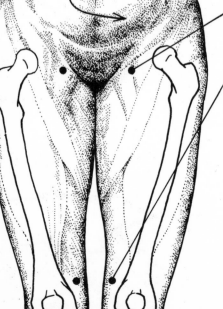

Fig. 14

10. KI-16 (肓俞, *Huang-yü*)

Points located five sun on either side of the navel.

11. LV-11 (陰廉, *Yin-lien*)

About two sun below the crotch on the inner side of the thigh.

12. SP-10 (血海, *Hsüeh-hai*)

Two sun and five bu above the kneecap on the inner side of the thigh.

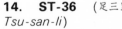

Fig. 15

13. SP-9 (陰陵泉, *Yin-ling-ch'üan*)

Immediately below the large bone that protrudes just below the knee at the shin.

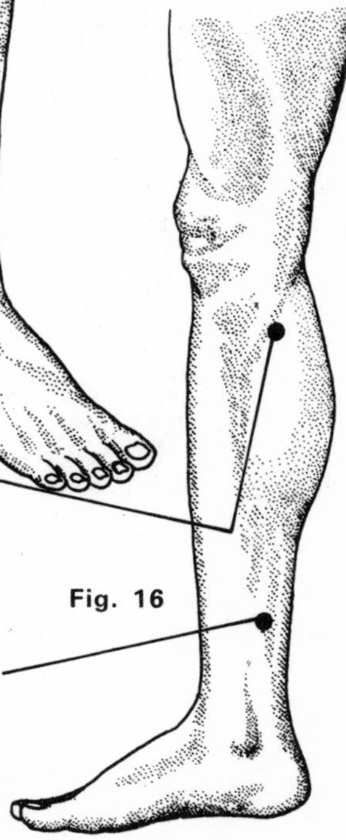

14. ST-36 (足三里, *Tsu-san-li*)

On the outer side of the calf three sun below the knee. Outer edge of the tibia or shin bone.

15. SP-6 (三陰交, *San-yin-chiao*)

Three sun upward on the side of the shin bone from the inner side of the ankle.

Fig. 16

(5) Severe Backache

As age takes its toll in the human body, the intervertebral discs in the spine may become deformed and angular or suffer a hernia condition. People who are unfortunate enough to be the victims of these conditions are likely to experience severe, even incapacitating, pains in the back if they engage in sudden or unusual movements, especially action involving lifting heavy articles. There are instances when actual sprains of the muscles of the back result. I have said that this condition is more prevalent among older people, but today even young people who rely too much on automobiles and thus fail to get enough exercise fall victim to severe backaches when they exert themselves more than is their custom.

Should a patient suffer an attack of this kind, immediately touch the aching part of the body to determine whether there is fever or swelling. If there is fever, apply a cold pack. If there is not,

apply a hot pack. And have the patient lie perfectly still for about twenty minutes. Then treat by massaging the tsubo on the feet (ST-41, Fig. 17). This must be done sharply with the thumbs of both hands at the same time. The patient must be lying with legs straight, feet together, and arms at sides. Then apply shiatsu massage to ST-36, BL-57 (Fig. 18), and ST-34 (Fig. 19).

When this treatment is over, have the patient lie on his stomach to enable you to massage the areas of the tsubo shown in Fig. 20: BL-22, BL-23, BL-25, BL-47, GB-29, BL-32, and BL-31. In other words, with the thumbs of both hands, apply shiatsu pressure to the back downward from the height of the elbows. Make arrow marks on the body at the ailing points where pressure brings relief. These points are the tsubo in this area. Continue treatment by applying fine-grade moxa to these tsubo from three to five times on each place for three days. Then increase the applications to seven times for each place daily. Acupuncture too helps relieve this kind of backache.

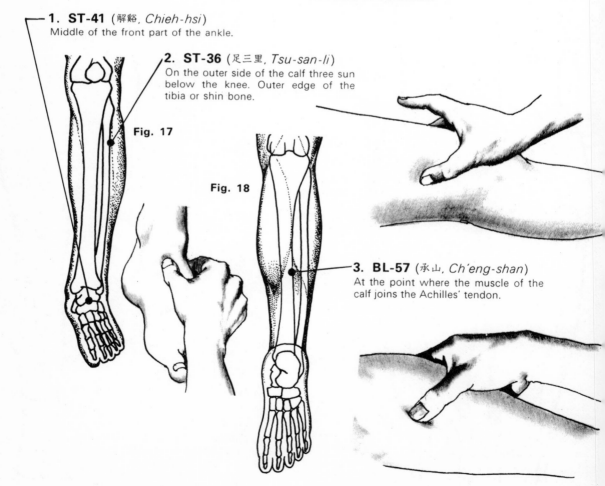

1. ST-41 (解谿, *Chieh-hsi*)
Middle of the front part of the ankle.

2. ST-36 (足三里, *Tsu-san-li*)
On the outer side of the calf three sun below the knee. Outer edge of the tibia or shin bone.

Fig. 17

Fig. 18

3. BL-57 (承山, *Ch'eng-shan*)
At the point where the muscle of the calf joins the Achilles' tendon.

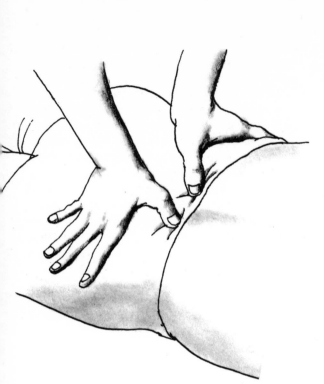

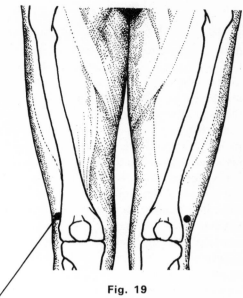

Fig. 19

4. ST-34 (梁丘, *Liang-chiu*)

Two sun above the upper edge of the kneecap. This can be easily located by fully extending the knee and finding the upper end of the groove formed on the outside of the kneecap.

Fig. 20

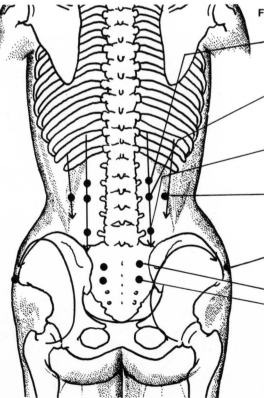

5. BL-22 (三焦兪, *San-chiao-yü*)

One sun and five bu on either side of the spinal column at points below the first lumbar vertebra.

6. BL-23 (腎兪, *Shen-yü*)

One sun and five bu on either side of the spinal column at points below the spinal projections of the second lumbar vertebra, which is located at the height of the lowest ribs.

7. BL-25 (大腸兪, *Ta-ch'ang-yü*)

One sun and five bu on either side of the spinal column at points below the spinal projections of the fourth lumbar vertebra.

8. BL-47 (志室, *Chih-shih*)

Three sun on either side of the spinal column at points below the spinal projections of the second lumbar vertebra; on the outer sides of BL-23.

9. GB-29 (居髎, *Chü-liao*)

Eight sun and three bu below the extremities of the eleventh ribs. Exactly in the middle, but somewhat to the rear, of the hucklebone.

10. BL-31 (上髎, *Shang-liao*)
11. BL-32 (次髎, *Tz'u-liao*)

Five sacral vertebra are fused to form a rear wall for the pelvic cavity. The four tsubo BL-31, BL-32, BL-33, and BL-34 are located beside the openings on either side of the projections of the top four of these vertebrae. The pair of tsubo designated BL-31 is on the level of the topmost of the sacral vertebrae, and the others proceed downward in ascending numerical order.

(6) Stiff Shoulders

The stiffness and pain in the shoulders that appear most frequently as a sign of aging are in fact a kind of inflammation of the shoulder joints and their peripheral areas. The condition usually begins with a dull heaviness or aching in the shoulders but proceeds to a more painful state. The pain is especially noticeable when the patient tries to bring his hand behind his back (as women do in combing their hair or unfastening a zipper in the back of a dress). Swinging the arms in any direction causes pain. There are cases in which the pain is so distressing that the patient finds it impossible to sleep at night. Gradually the discomfort decreases, though the shoulder may become thin and may develop places that are highly sensitive to any pressure at all. In a month or two, all pain may be gone, and the shoulder joint may return to completely normal functioning. It occasionally happens, however, that this condition disables the shoulder permanently. By bringing about mild inflammation in the muscles, ligaments, and tendons around the shoulder joint, aging causes this condition in older persons. In younger people it may result from external injury.

The following are some general rules of oriental medical therapy that may be applied in part to the case of stiff shoulders. If it is chilled, warm it. If it is feverish, cool it. If it is painful, press it with hands and fingers. If it is numb, stimulate it with moxa. When the shoulders are stiff, they are likely to be chilled. Consequently, in keeping with the rules just stated, oriental medical therapy prescribes a hot pack made from a heavy towel.

When the chilling has been successfully treated, using the four fingers of each hand, massage meridians ①, ②, and ③ in the directions of the arrows (Fig. 21). Then, having the patient lie on

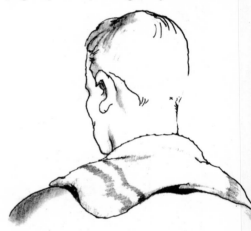

Fig. 21

1. LU-2 (雲門, *Yun-men*)
Middle of the depression at the underside of the external extremity of the clavicle.
2. LI-15 (肩髃, *Chien-yü*)
At the depression between the tip of the shoulder and the triceps muscle when the arm is held outstretched in a horizontal position. Thumb side of the upper arm at the tip of the acromion process.
3. LU-1 (中府, *Chung-fu*)
Upper extremity of the exterior front chest wall at the second intercostal zone. Six sun on either side of the sternum.

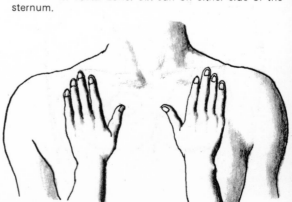

his stomach, massage meridians ④ through ⑨ (Fig. 22). Use light rubbing motions of the palms of the hands on meridians ④ through ⑦. When the pain has been relieved—as it will have been after the treatment described above—apply medium-grade moxa to the tsubo in Figs. 21 and 22.

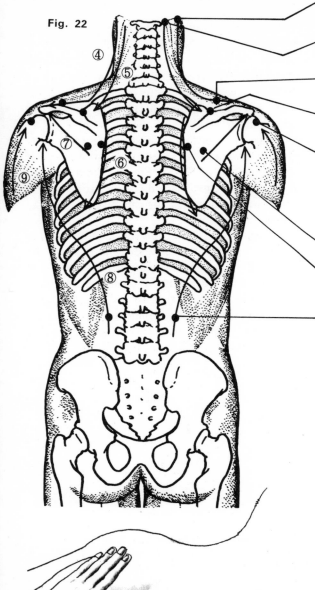

Fig. 22

4. GB-20 (風池, *Feng-ch'ih*)
Depressions on the right and left two sun below the central depression at the lower edge of the occiput.

5. BL-10 (天柱, *T'ien-chu*)
On the outer side of the two large muscles of the neck where they join the back of the head.

6. TH-15 (天髎, *T'ien-liao*)
The back, about one sun to the rear from the midpoint between the neck and tip of the shoulder.

7. SI-13 (曲垣, *Ch'ü-yüan*)
Inner side of the upper corner of the shoulder blade; or about one sun and five bu below TH-15.

8. TH-14 (肩髎, *Chien-liao*)
Depression at the under edge of the external tip of the acromion process. The place where the upper arm bone joins the shoulder blade at the base of the shoulder.

9. SI-11 (天宗, *T'ien-tsung*)
The depression in the middle of the shoulder blade.

10. BL-37 (魄戸, *P'o-hu*)
On the right and left, three sun below the third thoracic vertebra.

11. BL-23 (腎兪, *Shen-yü*)
One sun and five bu on either side of the spinal column at points below the spinal projections of the second lumbar vertebra, which is located at the height of the lowest ribs.

Moxa must be applied three times on each tsubo daily for at least three weeks. Acupuncture is effective in these cases as is the following iron exercise: have the patient hold an ordinary laundry iron in the hand on the side of the aching shoulder, bend forward slightly, and swing the iron forward and backward.

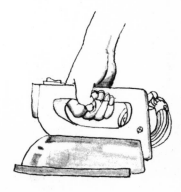

(7) Pains in the Knee

People—especially overweight women—in middle age or above frequently complain of the pain caused in their knees by rising, sitting, and climbing and descending stairs. The cause of this complaint is deformation in the joint. This deformation occurs with passing years. At first, the condition is mild; but, as it persists, it causes swelling, increasing sharp pain, and accumulation of liquid on the knee. In severe cases, the knee cap is obscured by this accumulation. The deformation often amounts to a sharpening and development of angles and edges in a joint that is naturally rounded. In light cases, a pain is felt on the inner side of the legs as the patient goes up and down steps. Since pain in the knees inevitably causes the patient to put an extra load on the back, thighs, and calves, these parts of the body may be put out of proper working order. The way to bring relief to the pain in them is to cure the aching in the knees by means of the following treatment. In short, relieving the pain and swelling in the knees will relieve similar related conditions in the back and legs.

The first step to take in treatment is to apply a hot compress made from a heavy towel. Leave the compress in place for twenty or thirty minutes or until the joint is thoroughly warmed. Next, conduct the following massage routine daily morning, noon, and evening for from five to six minutes a session.

Using the thumbs and fingers of one or both hands, massage meridians ①, ②, ③, and ④ (Figs. 23 and 24). Next, using the palm of the hand, massage meridian ⑤ on the calves. With a squeezing pressure of the palm of the hand, massage meridian ⑥ (Fig. 27). Follow this with shiatsu massage of the tsubo in Figs. 25 through 28. Continue this treatment regularly for two or three weeks. Fine-grade moxa applied to the vicinity of ST-35 (Fig. 28) from three to five times on each place daily for from two to three weeks increases the effectiveness of the treatment.

Even when the aching has subsided, the patient must be cautious, for undue motion of the joint will make the deformation permanent and will cause pain to resume. If it becomes necessary to move a great deal or to go up and down stairs often, the patient suffering from this condition must ensure adequate rest and must take care to see that the joint is kept warm.

Fig. 23

Fig. 24

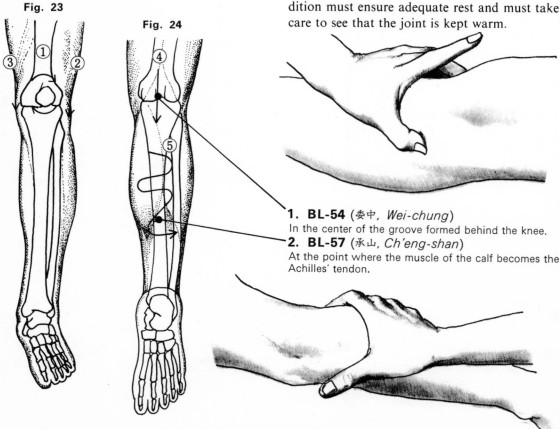

1. BL-54 (委中, *Wei-chung*)
In the center of the groove formed behind the knee.

2. BL-57 (承山, *Ch'eng-shan*)
At the point where the muscle of the calf becomes the Achilles' tendon.

3. LV-8 (曲泉, *Ch'ü-ch'üan*)

In the depression on the inner side of the knee joint. The extremity of the groove formed when the knee is bent.

4. BL-53 (委陽, *Wei-yang*)

Two sun to the outer sides of BL-54.

5. KI-1 (湧泉, *Yung-ch'üan*)

In the center of the arch of the foot immediately behind the bulge of the big toe.

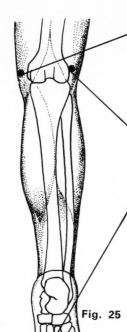

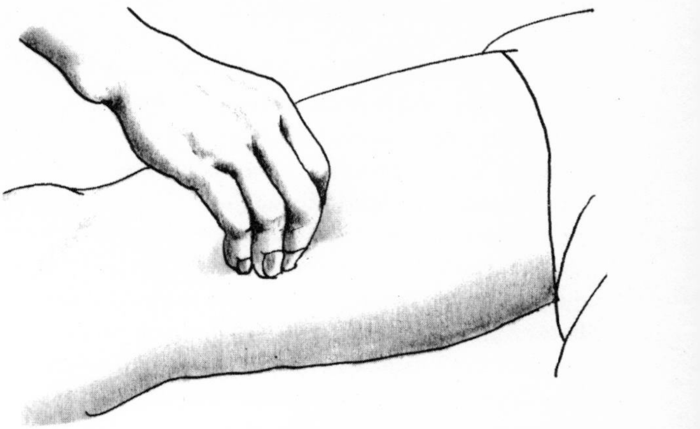

Fig. 25

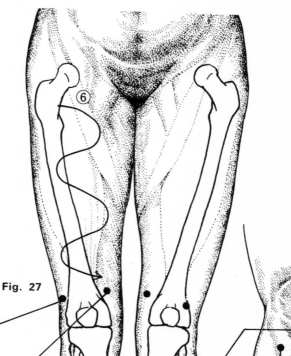

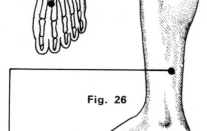

Fig. 26

6. SP-6 (三陰交, *San-yin-chiao*)

Three sun upward on the side of the shin bone from the inner side of the ankle.

7. ST-34 (梁丘, *Liang-chiu*)

Two sun above the upper edge of the kneecap. This can be easily located by fully extending the knee and finding the upper end of the groove formed on the outside of the kneecap.

8. SP-10 (血海, *Hsüeh-hai*)

Two sun and five bu above the kneecap on the inner side of the thigh. The place where a depression is formed two sun and five bu above the knee when the leg is outstretched.

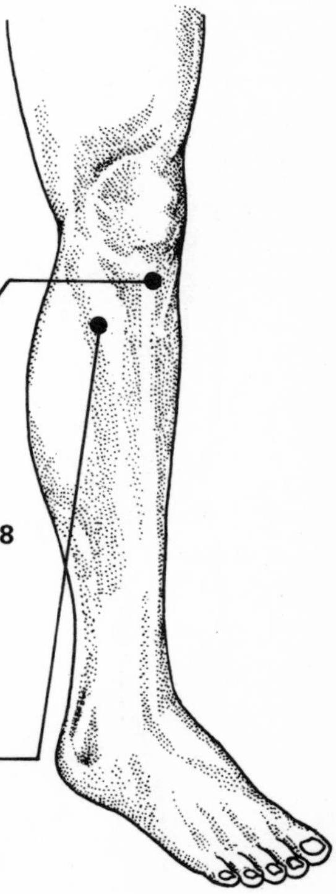

Fig. 27

9. ST-35 (犢鼻, *Tu-pi*)

The depression formed between the kneecap and the tubercle of the tibia when the knee is bent. The point in the exact middle of the zone between the kneecap and the tibia or shin bone.

10. ST-36 (足三里, *Tsu-san-li*)

On the outer side of the calf three sun below the knee. Outer edge of the tibia or shin bone.

Fig. 28

(8) Intercostal Neuralgia

Pains along the nerves running from the back, under the arms, along the ribs and to the sternum area can be excruciating. Caused by colds, excess fatigue, or overexertion, the condition sends spasms of sharp pain throughout the body at no more stimulus than speaking in a loud voice. Though exhalation is not painful, inhalation is difficult to bear when intercostal neuralgia strikes. It may affect either side, though it is more common for it to attack the center of the upper left part of the chest and the area around the left armpit. Points immediately to the side of the spine, the armpit, and the sternum area are hypersensitive to pressure in patients suffering from intercostal neuralgia. Slight bending even to the side that is not in pain is extremely distressing. Because caries, fracture of the ribs, and chest cancer can cause very similar symptoms, anyone experiencing this kind of pain must call on a specialist—a neurologist—at once. But if there is no fever and if X-ray photographs show no irregularities, intercostal neuralgia is a sound diagnosis. Since the eleventh and twelfth ribs are not attached to the sternum, strong pressure or twisting in their vicinities causes intercostal neuralgia. The patient must lie on his side—the side that is not in pain, of course—while a hot compress is applied to his ribs. Next, massage the meridians shown in Fig. 29 and use the four fingers of each hand to apply shiatsu pressure lightly in the directions of the ribs. Next, using four fingers, massage the meridians shown in Fig. 30 in the directions of the

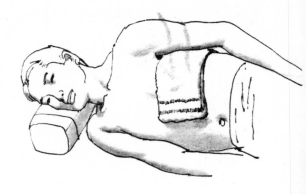

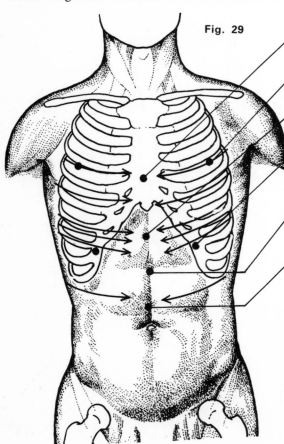

Fig. 29

1. CV-17 (膻中, *Shang-chung*)
Middle of the front of the sternum at the midpoint between the nipples.

2. HC-1 (天池, *T'ien-ch'ih*)
Front of the chest at the fourth intercostal zone, about one sun to the outside of the nipple line.

3. CV-14 (巨闕, *Chü-ch'üeh*)
Immediately below the diaphragm; two sun below the lower extremity of the sternum.

4. LV-14 (期門, *Ch'i-men*)
Extremities of the ninth ribs. Or a place located at the boundary between the rib and the abdomen directly below the nipple of the breast.

5. CV-12 (中脘, *Chung-wan*)
Four sun above the navel; midway between the navel and the diaphragm.

6. CV-9 (水分, *Shui-fen*)
One sun above the navel.

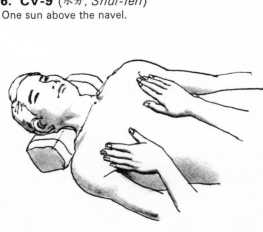

arrows. Then treat BL-15, BL-17, BL-18, BL-20, BL-22, and BL-23 (Fig. 30). Next treat CV-17, HC-1, CV-14, LV-14, CV-12, and CV-9 (Fig. 29). In this case, use the thumbs and fingers to exert about three kilograms of pressure.

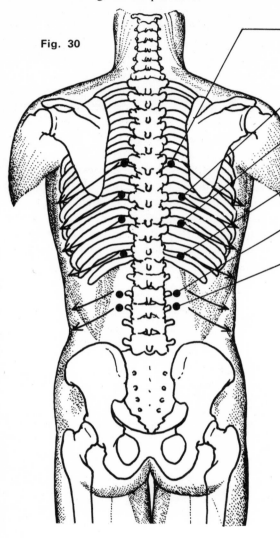

Fig. 30

7. BL-15 (心兪, *Hsin-yü*)
One sun and five bu on either side of the spinal column at points below the spinal projections of the fifth thoracic vertebra.

8. BL-17 (膈兪, *Ke-yü*)
One sun and five bu on either side of the spinal column at points below the seventh thoracic vertebra.

9. BL-18 (肝兪, *Kan-yü*)
One sun and five bu on either side of the spinal column at points below the spinal projections of the ninth thoracic vertebra.

10. BL-20 (脾兪, *P'i-yü*)
One sun and five bu on either side of the spinal column at points below the eleventh thoracic vertebra.

11. BL-22 (三焦兪, *San-chiao-yü*)
One sun and five bu on either side of the spinal column at points below the first lumbar vertebra.

12. BL-23 (腎兪, *Shen-yü*)
One sun and five bu on either side of the spinal column at points below the spinal projections of the second lumbar vertebra, which is located at the height of the lowest ribs.

Have the patient sit upright and, while breathing deeply, raise and lower his arms five or six times. In this way it is possible to stretch the intercostal nerves gently and thus bring relief from pain. Hot compresses or heat treatments with a hair dryer are sufficient to cure mild cases of this kind of neuralgia. Acupuncture and moxa, too, are effective on the tsubo listed above.

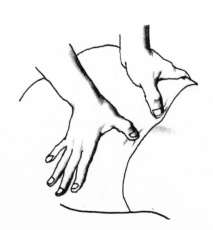

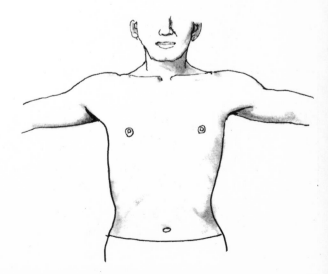

(9) Whiplash Syndrome

In automobile collisions, passengers sometimes have their heads and necks sharply snapped in a way resembling the action of the tip of a whip when it is cracked. As a consequence of this so-called whiplash, such people suffer a sprain of the cervical vertebrae, which later brings on headaches, stiff shoulders, ringing in the ears, numbness in the arms, sluggishness, and pains in the arms and legs. The sprain stretches the ligaments and small muscles in the neighborhood of the seven cervical vertebrae in the neck. Until these muscles and tendons return to normal, there is fever, swelling, and minor hemorrhage in the area. The headaches, stiff shoulders, ringing in the ears, sluggishness, and numbness in the arms subsequent to a whiplash experience result from the influence of the sprain on the nerves leading from the cervical vertebrae.

After a whiplash experience, the patient must remain quiet for four or five days until the fever has stopped and the swelling has gone down. Following this, apply a hot compress to the neck to relax the tendons and muscles. Then, with the thumbs, gently massage the back of the neck. Increase the effect of this treatment by combining it with massage on meridian ① and shiatsu on GV-14, GB-21, and LI-15 (Fig. 31). Next massage meridian ② (Fig. 32). Massaging meridians ③ and ④ (Figs. 33 and 34) relieves pain in the arms. Pain in the back of the neck and stiffness in the shoulder result from the effect of sprain on the first to fourth cervical vertebra. Pain in the arms, numbness in the fingers, and palpitations are caused by sprain in the fourth to the seventh cervical vertebra. For treatment of these conditions, see the entries in this book devoted to them. In all cases, shiatsu on the tsubo in Fig. 31 through Fig. 34 combined with massage increase the effect of the therapy. Moxa combustion is helpful when the symptoms of the whiplash condition seem to have become chronic.

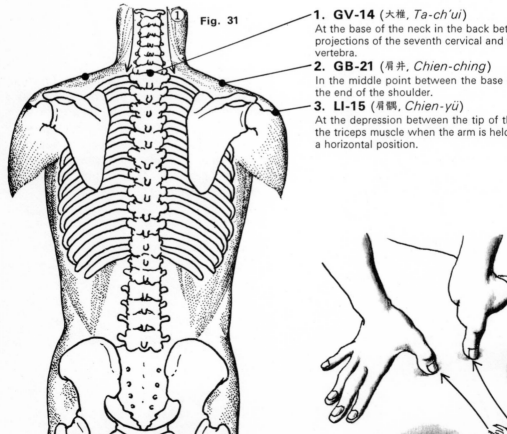

Fig. 31

1. GV-14 (大椎, *Ta-ch'ui*)
At the base of the neck in the back between the spinal projections of the seventh cervical and the first thoracic vertebra.

2. GB-21 (肩井, *Chien-ching*)
In the middle point between the base of the neck and the end of the shoulder.

3. LI-15 (肩髃, *Chien-yü*)
At the depression between the tip of the shoulder and the triceps muscle when the arm is held outstretched in a horizontal position.

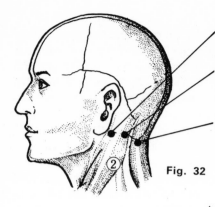

4. GB-12 (完骨, *Wan-ku*)
Depression in the back edge of the mastoid process behind the ear.

5. GB-20 (風池, *Feng-ch'ih*)
Depressions on the right and left two sun below the central depression at the lower edge of the occiput.

6. BL-10 (天柱, *T'ien-chu*)
On the outer side of the two large muscles of the neck where they join the back of the head.

Fig. 32

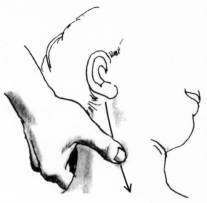

Fig. 33

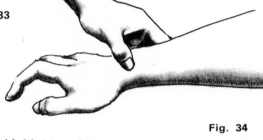

Fig. 34

7. LI-11 (曲池, *Ch'ü-ch'ih*)
Thumb side of the bend of the elbow.

8. LI-4 (合谷, *Ho-ku*)
The point exactly between the thumb and index finger on the back side of the hand.

9. HC-3 (曲沢, *Ch'ü-tse*)
Little-finger side of the hard tendon that becomes apparent at the middle of the elbow when the elbow is bent.

10. HT-3 (少海, *Shao-hai*)
Innermost point on the little-finger side of the large bone of the elbow joint.

11. HT-7 (神門, *Shen-men*)
Inner most part of the inner surface of the wrist.

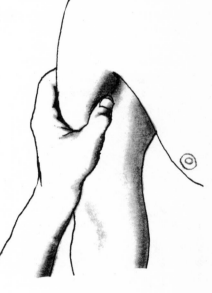

12. LU-5 (尺沢, *Chi-tse*)
The hard tendon that is apparent in the inner side of the elbow when the wrist is bent.

13. HC-4 (郄門, *Hsi-men*)
Middle point of the inner side of the forearm at the midpoint between the elbow and the wrist.

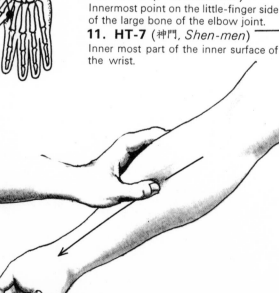

14. HC-7 (大陵, *Ta-ling*)
Point between the two large muscles in the middle of the inner side of the wrist.

(10) Sciatica

Sciatica is characterized by sharp pains in the backs of the hips, thighs, and calves and parts of the legs as low as the ankles. Though the patient may experience no discomfort under ordinary circumstances of bodily calm, coughing, sneezing, or bending of the body can bring on attacks. Sometimes the outer calves and the insteps are numb. Lying on the back and raising the legs (which remain outstretched) cause sharp pains in the backs of the thighs. The pain is the result of pressure on the sciatic nerves—the thickest in the body—which run from the hips to the thighs, legs, and feet. But, since disturbances in the spinal column, diabetes, sickness of the pelvic region, and cancer can be accompanied by the same symptoms, intensive physical examinations must be conducted before a certain diagnosis can be made. But if it is known that aging and deformation of the vertebrae, cold, chills, or dampness are the causes of neuralgic pains, which are only temporary, the following treatment brings relief.

First, heat the back well with a hot compress made from a thick towel. Allow the compress to remain in place for about twenty minutes. Then conduct the following massage. The patient must be lying on his stomach. First, using the palms of the hands, massage meridians ①, ②, and ③ (Fig. 35). Next, using the thumbs to apply from three to five kilograms of pressure for from three to five seconds for each place, treat each of the tsubo in Fig. 35 in the shiatsu fashion. Continue the same double treatment—massage with the palms followed by shiatsu with the thumbs—on meridians ④, ⑤, ⑥ and ⑦ (Fig. 36 and 37). Massage in the directions of the arrows.

When pain is slight and accompanied by a sensation of heaviness, use a hot-towel compress and a hair dryer. Acupuncture works well against sciatica, and moxa combustion is a good therapy for chronic cases. Three to five moxa applications on each of the tsubo shown above daily for three weeks will produce effects, but hair-dryer treatment works as well.

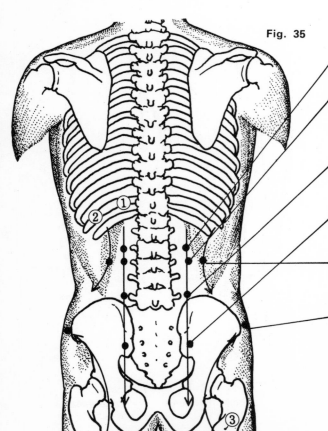

Fig. 35

1. BL-22 (三焦兪, *San-chiao-yü*)
One sun and five bu on either side of the spinal column at points below the first lumbar vertebra.

2. BL-23 (腎兪, *Shen-yü*)
One sun and five bu on either side of the spinal column at points below the spinal projections of the second lumbar vertebra, which is located at the height of the lowest ribs.

3. BL-25 (大腸兪, *Ta-ch'ang-yü*)
One sun and five bu on either side of the spinal column at points below the spinal projections of the fourth lumbar vertebra.

4. BL-28 (膀胱兪, *P'ang-kuan-yü*)
One sun and five bu on either side of the projections of the second sacral vertebra. The sacral vertebra form the rear wall of the pelvic cavity.

5. BL-47 (志室, *Chih-shih*)
Three sun on either side of the spinal column at points below the spinal projections of the second lumbar vertebra.

6. GB-29 (居髎, *Chü-liao*)
Eight sun and three bu below the extremities of the eleventh ribs. Exactly in the middle, but somewhat to the rear, of the hucklebone.

7. BL-50 (承扶, *Ch'eng-fu*)
In the centers of the grooves that form below the buttocks when the body is in military attention position.

8. BL-51 (殷門, *Yin-men*)
Exactly in the middle between BL-50 and BL-54; or in the middle of the rear part of the thigh.

9. BL-54 (委中, *Wei-chung*)
In the center of the groove formed behind the knee.

Fig. 36

10. BL-57 (承山, *Ch'eng-shan*)
At the point where the muscle of the calf doins the Achilles' tendon.

Fig. 37

11. GB-34 (陽陵泉, *Yang-ling-ch'üan*)
On the little-toe side of the calf about one sun below the knee. On the little-toe side directly below and in front of the head of the fibula.

12. GB-39 (懸鐘, *Hsüan-chung*)
Three sun above the outer ankle.

13. ST-36 (足三里, *Tsu-san-li*)
On the outer side of the calf three sun below the knee. Outer edge of the tibia or shin bone.

14. ST-41 (解谿, *Chieh-hsi*)
Middle of the front part of the ankle.

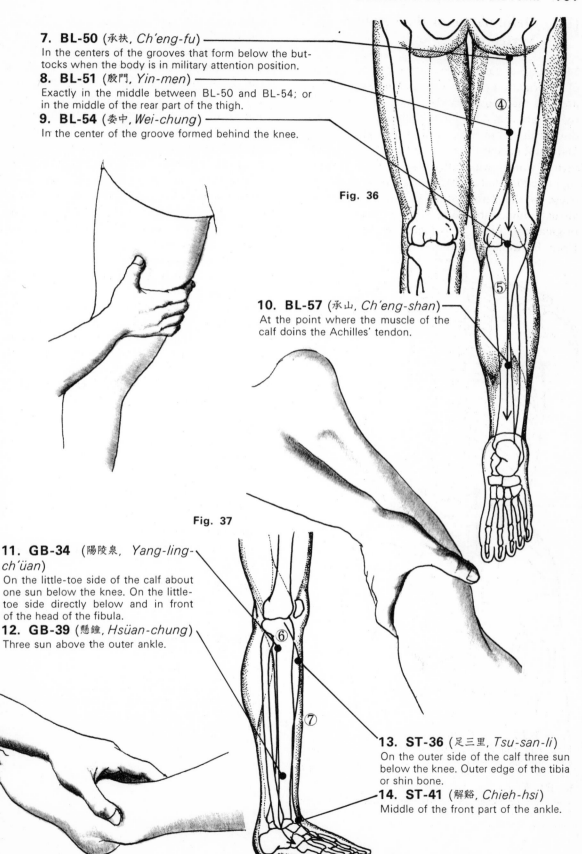

(11) **Deformation of the Lumbar Vertebrae**

Middle-aged women, the most numerous victims of deformation of the bones of the knee joints, are also the frequent victims of deformation of the vertebrae and the intervertebral cartilaginous discs. This malformation causes considerable pain and numbness in the back and legs. The percentage of women who suffer from this condition is said to equal that of men who go bald. Since the cause of the deformation is usually age, it is virtually impossible to return the bones to their original conditions. It is therefore important to treat this ailment at the first signs of pain or

numbness.

First apply a hot compress to the area between the first and third sacral vertebrae and the first and fifth lumber vertebrae in the regions of the tsubo shown in Fig. 38. After this, massage meridians ①, ②, and ③. Acupuncture and moxa combustion too are effective on these tsubo. Next, heat meridians ④, ⑤, ⑥, and ⑦ (Figs. 39 through 41) with a hair dryer; then massage them well in the directions of the arrows. In the cases of these tsubo as well, acupuncture and moxa combustion are effective. If the pain is severe in the vicinities of the knees, apply a hot pack and then massage the knees. Finally, have the patient sit on something high so that his legs hang free and his feet do not touch the floor. In this position, he must lightly bend and extend his knees. Most of the patients who visit my clinic because of this complaint are cured—even if they have been suffering for years—with from two to four months' treatment of three therapeutic sessions weekly. Even when the condition has been cured, however, the patient must be careful of chilling or excess fatigue, as such things can bring on a recurrence of the complaint.

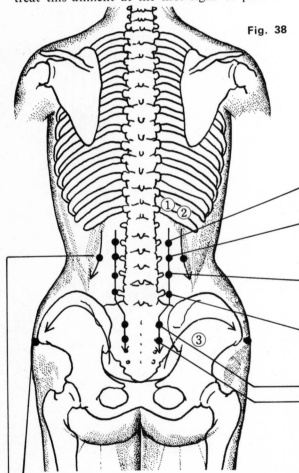

Fig. 38

1. BL-22 (三焦兪, *San-chiao-yü*)
One sun and five bu on either side of the spinal column at points below the first lumbar vertebra.

2. BL-23 (腎兪, *Shen-yü*)
One sun and five bu on either side of the spinal column at points below the spinal projections of the second lumbar vertebra, which is located at the height of the lowest ribs.

3. BL-24 (気海兪, *Ch'i-hai-yü*)
One sun and five bu on either side of the spinal column at points below the spinal projections of the third lumbar vertebra.

4. BL-25 (大腸兪, *Ta-ch'ang-yü*)
One sun and five bu on either side of the spinal column at points below the spinal projections of the fourth lumbar vertebra.

5. BL-31 (上髎, *Shang-liao*)
6. BL-32 (次髎, *Tz'u-liao*)
Five sacral vertebra are fused to form a rear wall for the pelvic cavity. The four tsubo BL-31, BL-32, BL-33, BL-34 are located beside the openings on either side of the projections of the top four of these vertebrae. The pair of tsubo designated BL-31 is on the level of the topmost vertebrae, and the others proceed downward in ascending numerical order.

7. GB-29 (居髎, *Chü-liao*)
Eight sun and three bu below the extremities of the eleventh ribs. Exactly in the middle, but somewhat to the rear, of the hucklebone.

8. BL-47 (志室, *Chih-shih*)
Three sun on either side of the spinal column at points below the spinal projections of the second lumbar vertebra; on the outer side of BL-23.

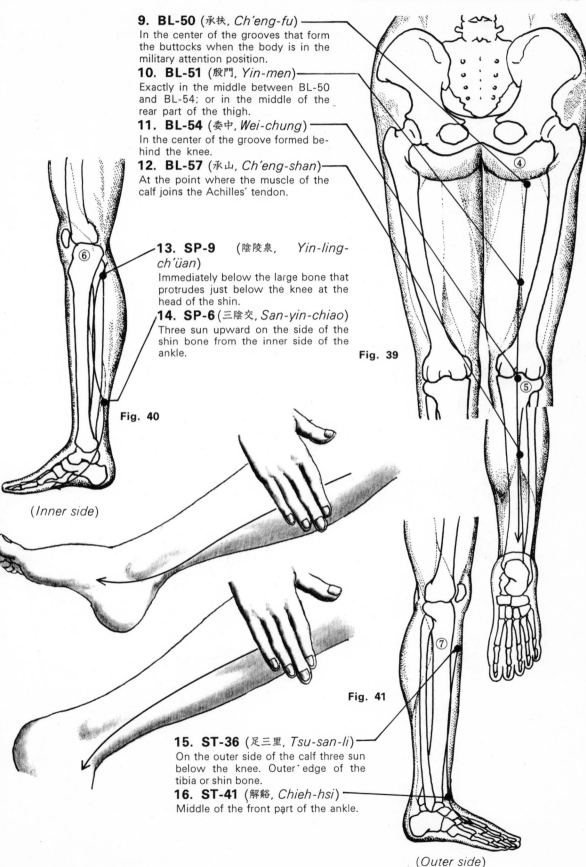

9. BL-50 (承扶, *Ch'eng-fu*)
In the center of the grooves that form the buttocks when the body is in the military attention position.

10. BL-51 (殷門, *Yin-men*)
Exactly in the middle between BL-50 and BL-54; or in the middle of the rear part of the thigh.

11. BL-54 (委中, *Wei-chung*)
In the center of the groove formed behind the knee.

12. BL-57 (承山, *Ch'eng-shan*)
At the point where the muscle of the calf joins the Achilles' tendon.

13. SP-9 (陰陵泉, *Yin-ling-ch'üan*)
Immediately below the large bone that protrudes just below the knee at the head of the shin.

14. SP-6 (三陰交, *San-yin-chiao*)
Three sun upward on the side of the shin bone from the inner side of the ankle.

Fig. 39

Fig. 40

(*Inner side*)

Fig. 41

15. ST-36 (足三里, *Tsu-san-li*)
On the outer side of the calf three sun below the knee. Outer edge of the tibia or shin bone.

16. ST-41 (解谿, *Chieh-hsi*)
Middle of the front part of the ankle.

(*Outer side*)

(12) Wryneck

Wryneck is a condition in which the neck and head are always tilted in one direction or another. It is an extreme inconvenience for the person afflicted. The causes are many. Wryneck can be congenital. It may be the result of shortening of the sternomastoid muscle brought on by some kind of violence during birth. It may be the outcome of paralysis or spasms in the nerves controlling the sternomastoid muscle. It can be the result of a prolonged habit of inclining the head in order to compensate for poor hearing or weak sight. Since the bones of infants are soft, mothers can inadvertently inflict wryneck on their children by allowing them to sleep always in the same position. This kind of wryneck, which is the most frequently encountered, is only temporary, but treatment for it is difficult. Consequently, mothers ought to take care to alter the infant's position during nursing and sleeping.

Muscular shortening in the sternomastoid muscle occurs when infants are pulled in birth, as they sometimes are when they are carried upside down in the mother's womb. Because this kind of thing is rarely made public, such babies are often thought to have congenital wryneck. If the condition is allowed to go untreated, the shortness of the muscle that causes wryneck can cause distortions in the shape of the face.

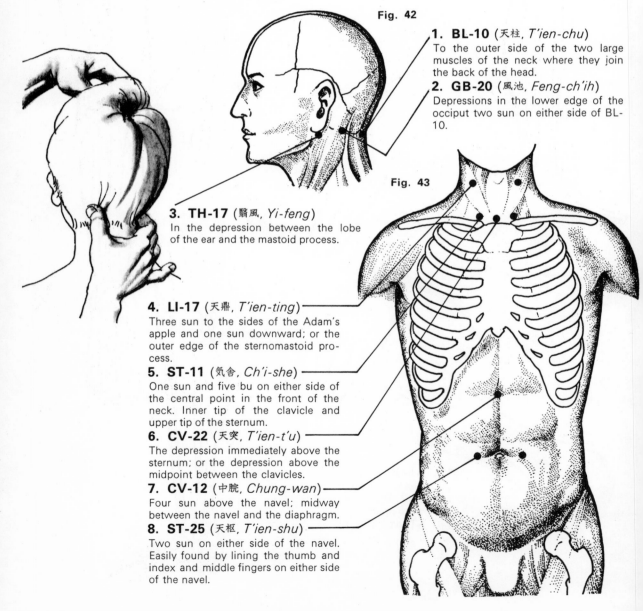

Fig. 42

1. BL-10 (天柱, *T'ien-chu*)
To the outer side of the two large muscles of the neck where they join the back of the head.
2. GB-20 (風池, *Feng-ch'ih*)
Depressions in the lower edge of the occiput two sun on either side of BL-10.

Fig. 43

3. TH-17 (翳風, *Yi-feng*)
In the depression between the lobe of the ear and the mastoid process.

4. LI-17 (天鼎, *T'ien-ting*)
Three sun to the sides of the Adam's apple and one sun downward; or the outer edge of the sternomastoid process.
5. ST-11 (気舎, *Ch'i-she*)
One sun and five bu on either side of the central point in the front of the neck. Inner tip of the clavicle and upper tip of the sternum.
6. CV-22 (天突, *T'ien-t'u*)
The depression immediately above the sternum; or the depression above the midpoint between the clavicles.
7. CV-12 (中脘, *Chung-wan*)
Four sun above the navel; midway between the navel and the diaphragm.
8. ST-25 (天枢, *T'ien-shu*)
Two sun on either side of the navel. Easily found by lining the thumb and index and middle fingers on either side of the navel.

Wryneck arising from nervous causes—pain, twistings of the head to compensate for poor sight and hearing, neuralgia, and so on—develop later than muscular wryneck and may be treated, though thorough medical examination must be conducted before home therapy can be initiated. Oriental tsubo therapy may be used to reinforce whatever treatment the doctor prescribes.

Massage or shiatasu in the vicinities of the tsubo in Figs. 42 through 44 assists in effecting a cure. In dealing with the tsubo on the face, massage only the ones on the side of the twist.

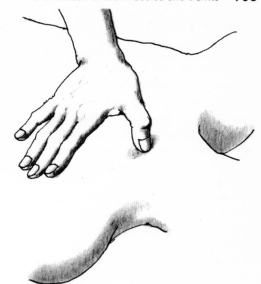

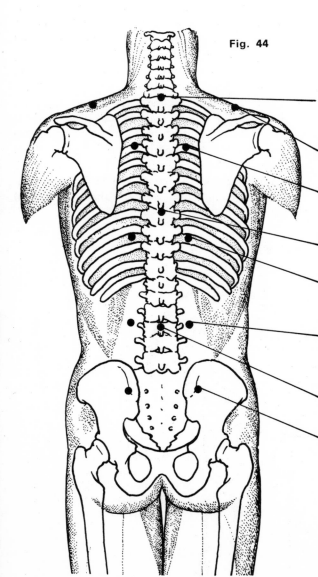

Fig. 44

9. GV-14 (大椎, *Ta-ch'ui*)
At the base of the neck in the back between the spinal projections of the seventh cervical and the first thoracic vertebra.

10. GB-21 (肩井, *Chien-ching*)
In the middle point between the base of the neck and the end of the shoulder.

11. BL-13 (肺俞, *Fei-yü*)
One sun and five bu on either side of the spinal column at points below the spinal projections of the third thoracic vertebra.

12. GV-9 (至陽, *Chih-yang*)
Below the spinal projections of the seventh thoracic vertebra.

13. BL-18 (肝俞, *Kan-yü*)
One sun and five bu on either side of the spinal column at points below the spinal projections of the ninth thoracic vertebra.

14. BL-23 (腎俞, *Shen-yü*)
One sun and five bu on either side of the spinal column at points below the spinal projections of the second lumbar vertebra, which is located at the height of the lowest ribs.

15. GV-4 (命門, *Ming-men*)
Below the spinal projections of the second lumbar vertebra.

16. BL-26 (関元俞, *Kuan-yüan-yü*)
One sun and five bu on either side of the spinal column at points below the spinal projections of the fifth lumbar vertebra.

(13) Bent Back

The several different malformations that can occur in the spinal column as a result of caries, tumors, and other pathological conditions alter the curve of the spine and, in this way, make it impossible for the back to bear the weight it is supposed to carry. This in turn puts an extra burden on the muscles, tendons, and soft tissues of the back. If the condition continues, it can greatly reduce the energy of the whole body. Surgery is the only way to correct some of the serious bends in the spinal column. When this is true, tsubo therapy can serve only as supplementary treatment.

When the cause of bent back is muscular and related to prolonged tension or overwork, tsubo therapy can effect cures. In Japan, where the traditional method of rice agriculture is wet paddies, until only recently, mechanization of labor in the fields has been considered difficult. Consequently, in the planting and harvesting seasons, Japanese farmers have been forced to spend long hours with their backs in bent positions, which, as aging proceeds, become pathological and cause pain and numbness. Sometimes this condition upsets the operation of the intes-

tines and stomach, makes breathing difficult, causes nausea, and even leads to constipation. To treat it, first place a large hot-towel compress and have the patient lie with it under his back. Next, lightly massage the tsubo shown in Fig. 45. Light acupuncture or shiatsu massage too is effective. Next, have him turn over on his stomach to permit you to treat the tsubo on the back (Fig. 46). If you use shiatsu, do not press directly on the spinal column. Making circular motions with the palms, continue to massage the meridians in the numerical order given. It is very important that the palms come into complete contact with the skin of the patient and that you move your shoulders and elbows as you move your hands.

Finally, have the patient limber his spinal column in the following way. He must place a fairly thick pillow or cushion under his back and lie on it with arms and legs outstretched. Then he must put the pillow under the base of his neck, lie on it for one or two minutes, then move it down slightly and lie on it again for one or two minutes. He must continue moving the cushion down until it reaches his hips. Treatment on the tsubo on the legs (Figs. 47 and 48) is good when used in conjunction with the therapy outlined above.

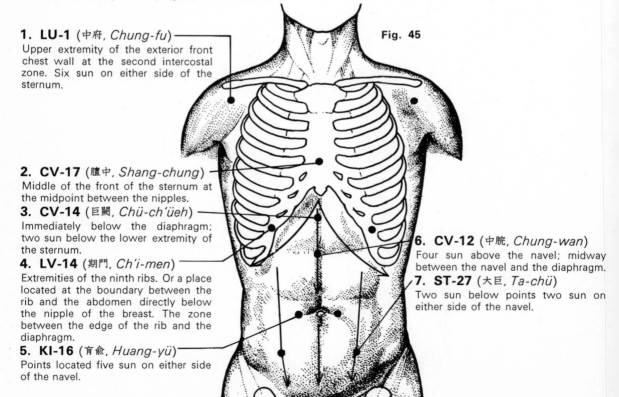

Fig. 45

1. LU-1 (中府, *Chung-fu*)
Upper extremity of the exterior front chest wall at the second intercostal zone. Six sun on either side of the sternum.

2. CV-17 (膻中, *Shang-chung*)
Middle of the front of the sternum at the midpoint between the nipples.

3. CV-14 (巨闕, *Chü-ch'üeh*)
Immediately below the diaphragm; two sun below the lower extremity of the sternum.

4. LV-14 (期門, *Ch'i-men*)
Extremities of the ninth ribs. Or a place located at the boundary between the rib and the abdomen directly below the nipple of the breast. The zone between the edge of the rib and the diaphragm.

5. KI-16 (肓兪, *Huang-yü*)
Points located five sun on either side of the navel.

6. CV-12 (中脘, *Chung-wan*)
Four sun above the navel; midway between the navel and the diaphragm.

7. ST-27 (大巨, *Ta-chü*)
Two sun below points two sun on either side of the navel.

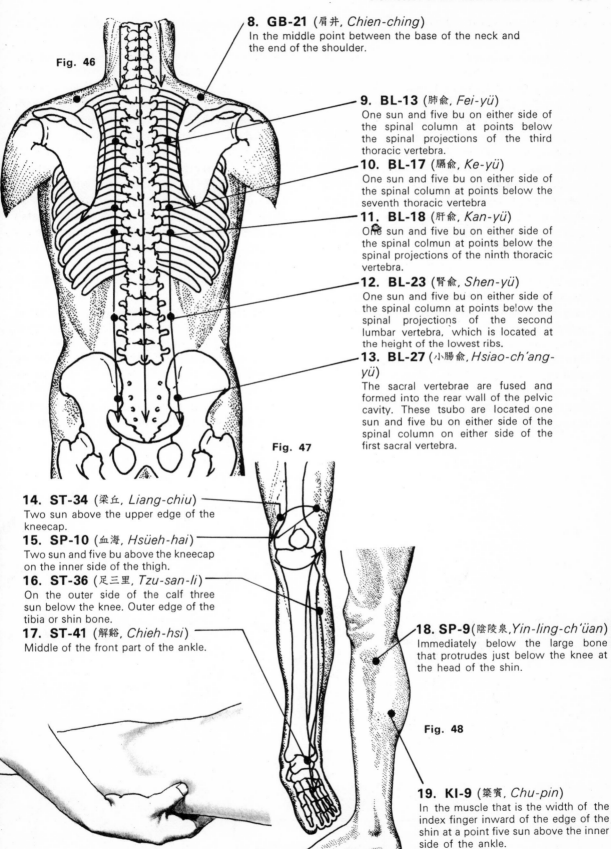

Fig. 46

8. GB-21 (肩井, *Chien-ching*)
In the middle point between the base of the neck and the end of the shoulder.

9. BL-13 (肺俞, *Fei-yü*)
One sun and five bu on either side of the spinal column at points below the spinal projections of the third thoracic vertebra.

10. BL-17 (膈俞, *Ke-yü*)
One sun and five bu on either side of the spinal column at points below the seventh thoracic vertebra

11. BL-18 (肝俞, *Kan-yü*)
One sun and five bu on either side of the spinal colmun at points below the spinal projections of the ninth thoracic vertebra.

12. BL-23 (腎俞, *Shen-yü*)
One sun and five bu on either side of the spinal column at points below the spinal projections of the second lumbar vertebra, which is located at the height of the lowest ribs.

13. BL-27 (小腸俞, *Hsiao-ch'ang-yü*)
The sacral vertebrae are fused and formed into the rear wall of the pelvic cavity. These tsubo are located one sun and five bu on either side of the spinal column on either side of the first sacral vertebra.

Fig. 47

14. ST-34 (梁丘, *Liang-chiu*)
Two sun above the upper edge of the kneecap.

15. SP-10 (血海, *Hsüeh-hai*)
Two sun and five bu above the kneecap on the inner side of the thigh.

16. ST-36 (足三里, *Tzu-san-li*)
On the outer side of the calf three sun below the knee. Outer edge of the tibia or shin bone.

17. ST-41 (解谿, *Chieh-hsi*)
Middle of the front part of the ankle.

18. SP-9 (陰陵泉, *Yin-ling-ch'üan*)
Immediately below the large bone that protrudes just below the knee at the head of the shin.

Fig. 48

19. KI-9 (築賓, *Chu-pin*)
In the muscle that is the width of the index finger inward of the edge of the shin at a point five sun above the inner side of the ankle.

Illnesses of the Urinary Tract and the Anus

(1) Hemorrhoids

Clotting in the many small blood vessels around the anus can obstruct circulation and cause blood-swelling and possible hemorrhage during defecation. This condition is called hemorrhoids. The bleeding usually stops after defecation; but, if the condition is allowed to go untreated, knots can form on the anus. In contrast to this condition, there is another kind of hemorrhoidal sickness in which cutlike wounds appear in the anal sphincter. Anal fistula is caused by different things and is usually suppurative. This condition —and, for that matter, all of the serious hemorrhoidal conditions—requires the attention of specialists. Tsubo therapy can be used to treat initial stages of hemorrhoids to prevent them from becoming serious.

The two major tsubo for treating hemorrhoids are GV-20, located on the top of the head, and GV-1, located on the coccyx bone. It may seem strange that the tsubo are so far apart and that one of them is on the head, but oriental medical tradition considers these two places to be closely related to each other and to this sickness because of the meridian on which they are both located. In addition, there is an old oriental medical belief that sicknesses affecting high parts of the body are to be treated on tsubo located low on the body, and vice versa.

Begin treatment with shiatsu pressure on GV-20 (Fig. 1) then use the same kind of massage on ST-25 (Fig. 2). Next, have the patient lie on his stomach as you apply shiatsu pressure to GV-14 (Fig. 3). Moxa combustion and shiatsu are effective on the following tsubo; but emphasis should be placed on massage, which is of maximum effectiveness: BL-21, BL-22, GV-1, BL-35 (Fig. 3), LU-6 (Fig. 4), LI-11 (Fig. 5), ST-36, (Fig. 6).

The patient should massage the tsubo on the lower back and hips himself each time he takes a hot bath. He should take care not to chill his hips or hands and feet. Sitz baths of hot water are effective in treating hemorrhoids. Finally, since constipation and hemorrhoids are closely related, treatment of the tsubo that cure constipation (p. 108) should be combined with treatment for hemorrhoids.

1. GV-20 (百会, *Pai-hui*)
At the point where a line directly upward from ear to ear crossing the top of the head and a line straight upward from the midpoint of the area between the shoulders to the top of the head intersect.

Fig. 1

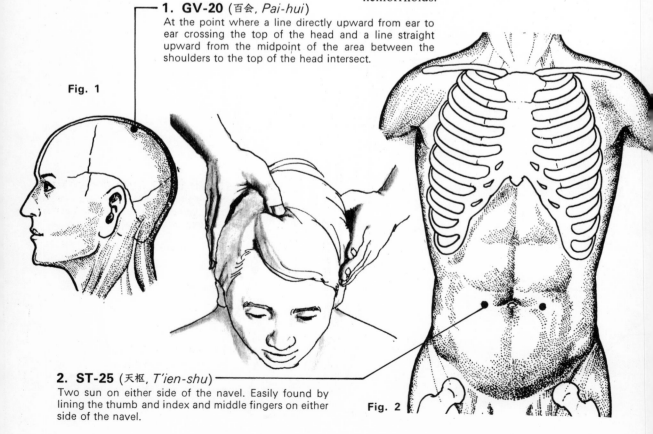

2. ST-25 (天枢, *T'ien-shu*)
Two sun on either side of the navel. Easily found by lining the thumb and index and middle fingers on either side of the navel.

Fig. 2

3. GV-14 (大椎, *Ta-ch'ui*)
At the base of the neck in the back between the spinal projections of the seventh cervical and the first thoracic vertebra.

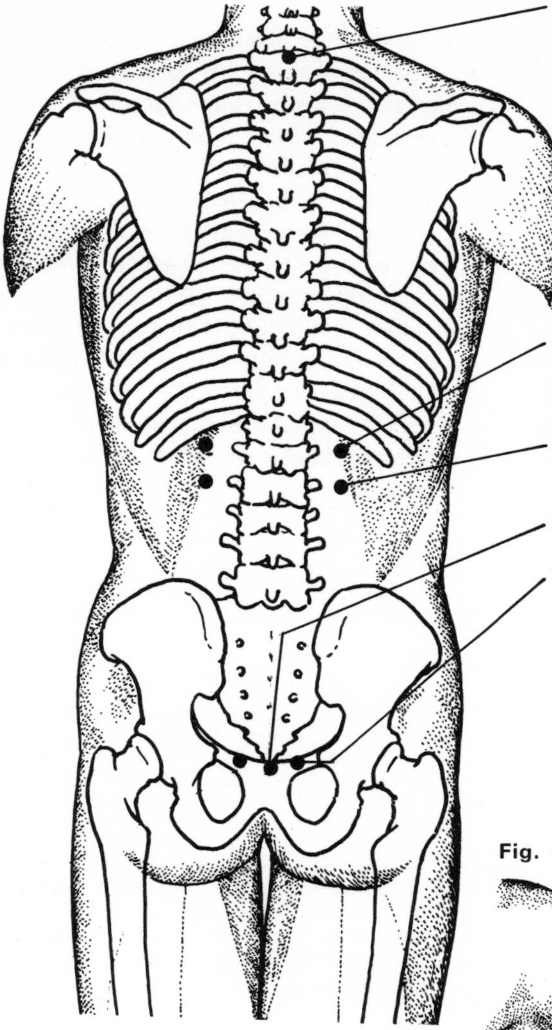

Fig. 3

4. BL-21 (胃兪, *Wei-yü*)
One sun and five bu on either side of the spinal column at points below the spinal projections of the twelfth thoracic vertebra.

5. BL-22 (三焦兪, *San-chiao-yü*)
One sun and five bu on either side of the spinal column at points below the first lumbar vertebra.

6. GV-1 (長強, *Chang-ch'iang*)
At the tip of the coccyx bone.

7. BL-35 (会陽, *Hui-yang*)
Immediately at the sides of GV-1.

Fig. 4

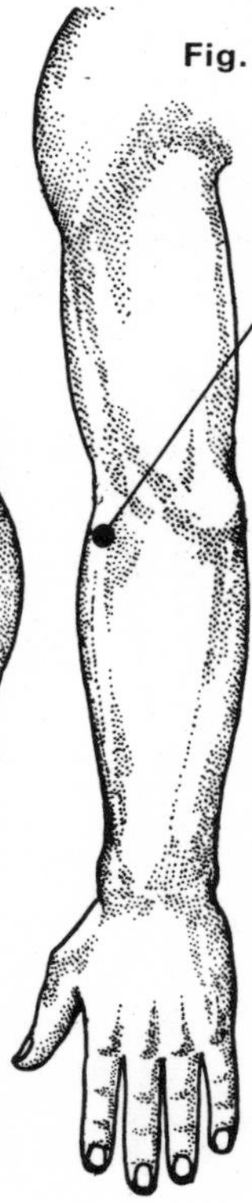

8. LU-6 (孔最, *K'ung-tsui*)
On the thumb side of the inner surface of the forearm at a point about one-third of the distance from the elbow to the wrist.

Fig. 5

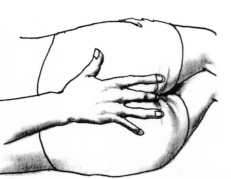

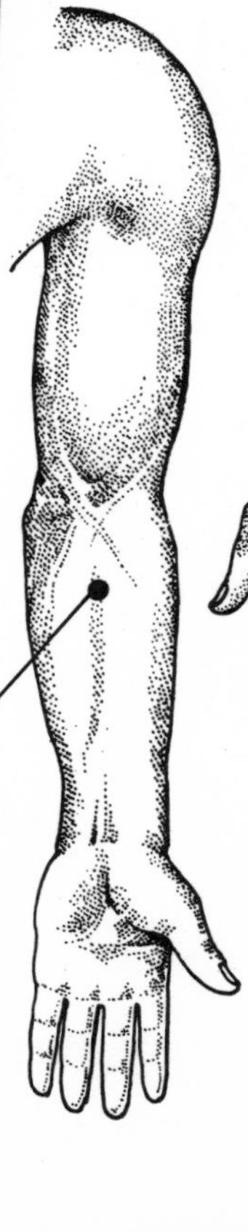

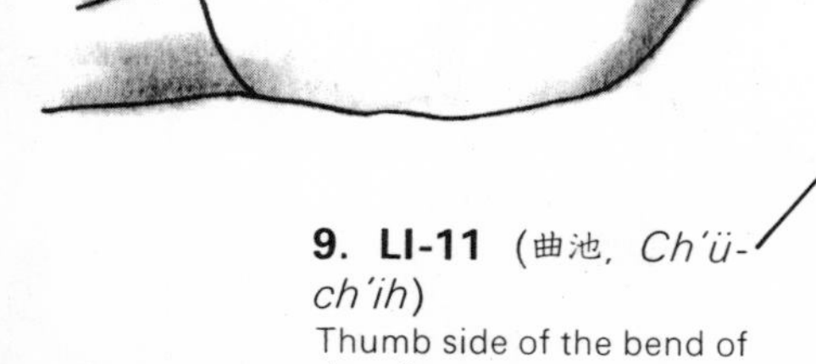

9. LI-11 (曲池, *Ch'ü-ch'ih*)
Thumb side of the bend of the elbow.

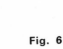

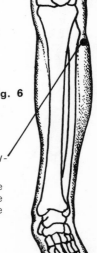

Fig. 6

10. ST-36 (足三里, *Tsu-san-li*)
On the outer side of the calf three sun below the knee. Outer edge of the tibia or shin bone.

(2) Enlargement of the Prostate Gland

In men of more than fifty years of age, often urges to urinate and inability to do so result from enlargement of the prostate gland. People suffering from this condition find that they wake several times in the middle of the night with the need to urinate. When they go to the toilet, however, they pass only very small amounts of urine. As the condition progresses, urination will take a long time to begin, the stream of urine will gradually become fine, and cessation of urination will be irregular and uneven. People with weak hearts too are often awakened in the night for urination, but they pass large amounts of waste at such times.

An enlargement—the reasons for which are unclear—occurring in the prostate gland, which is located between the urinary bladder and the urinary tract, presses on the urinary tract to cause the condition I have been describing. Examination, usually performed by inserting a finger into the anus and feeling the prostate gland, immediately reveals the presence of enlargement if there is any. In some cases, the gland itself enlarges; in others, the muscular fibers increase in number and cause swelling. In both instances, the symptoms are the same; and, as is always true, the oriental medical approach is to treat the symptoms. For surgical treatment of prostate-gland sicknesses, the attentions of a specialist are required.

Fig. 7

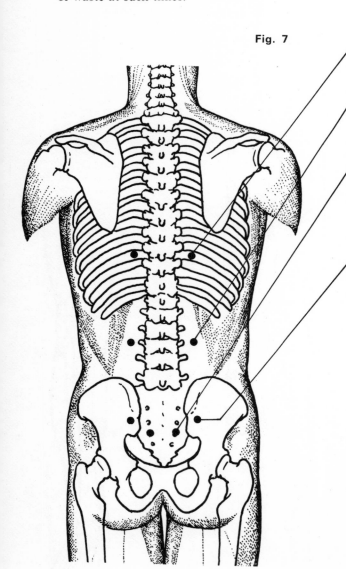

1. BL-18 (肝俞, *Kan-yü*)
One sun and five bu on either side of the spinal column at points below the spinal projections of the ninth thoracic vertebra.

2. BL-23 (腎俞, *Shen-yü*)
One sun and five bu on either side of the spinal column at points below the spinal projections of the second lumbar vertebra, which is located at the height of the lowest ribs.

3. BL-33 (中髎, *Chung-liao*)
Five sacral vertebrae are fused to form a rear wall for the pelvic cavity. The four tsubo BL-31, BL-32, BL-33, and BL-34 are located beside the openings on either side of the projections of the top four of these vertebrae. The pair of tsubo designated BL-31 is on the level of the topmost of the sacral vertebrae, and the others proceed downward in ascending numerical order.

4. BL-28 (膀胱俞, *P'ang-kuan-yü*)
One sun and five bu on either side of the projections of the second sacral vertebra.

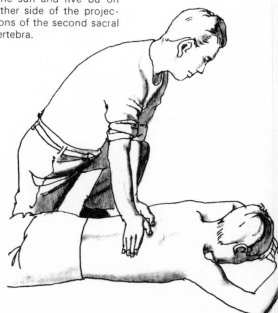

But, to treat the symptoms in the oriental fashion, have the patient lie on his stomach as you apply shiatsu pressure to BL-18, BL-23, BL-33, BL-28 (Fig. 7), CV-9, KL-16, CV-4, ST-28, CV-3 (Fig. 8), and KI-3 (Fig. 9). In massaging these tsubo, use both hands. Kneel on one knee and lean the upper part of your body forward to enable you to exert equal pressure with both arms. Use shiatsu pressure on CV-3 and BL-28. Press lightly on these two tsubo. If the patient experiences pain or if there is a depression in the location of the tsubo, the person is probably suffering from a disorder in the urinary bladder or urinary tract.

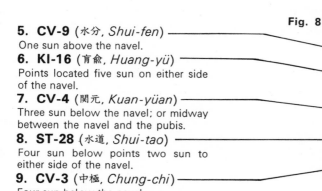

Fig. 8

5. CV-9 (水分, *Shui-fen*)
One sun above the navel.

6. KI-16 (肓兪, *Huang-yü*)
Points located five sun on either side of the navel.

7. CV-4 (関元, *Kuan-yüan*)
Three sun below the navel; or midway between the navel and the pubis.

8. ST-28 (水道, *Shui-tao*)
Four sun below points two sun to either side of the navel.

9. CV-3 (中極, *Chung-chi*)
Four sun below the navel.

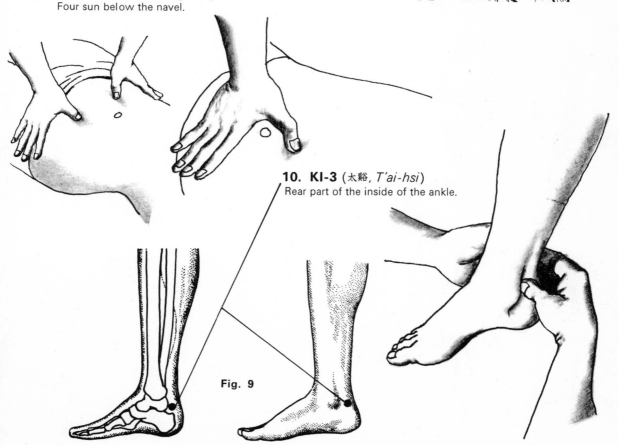

10. KI-3 (太谿, *T'ai-hsi*)
Rear part of the inside of the ankle.

Fig. 9

Illnesses of the Eyes, Ears, and Nose

(1) Tired Eyes

Television, glaring advertisements, dashing vehicles, and other visually taxing aspects of modern life cause almost everyone to experience occasional dizziness, pain behind the eyes, heaviness in the head, and other distressing symptoms of tired eyes. We must live in our society, of course, but we must not overtax our eyes, since they are irreplaceable. Furthermore, weariness and excess fatigue of the eyes can have an upsetting effect on the entire body. To refresh the eyes after long periods of close work or reading, I recommend simple massage or shiatsu massage. The person suffering from eye strain can perform this treatment for himself.

First, lying on your back and closing your eyes lightly, with your thumbs or with the four fingers of each hand, rub the rims of the eyes in the directions of the arrows (Fig. 1). Do not press directly on the eyeballs. The pressure of the thumbs or of the fingers must be directed toward the bone around the eye socket. Press gently at first and in a slanting direction.

Next, making circular motions with the four fingers of each hand, lightly massage the temples from the outer ends of the eyes to the fronts of the ears (Fig. 2). Then, leaving your eyes, closed, lightly press the eyelids with the fleshy balls of the four fingers of each hand. Press for from ten to fifteen seconds and then gently remove your fingers. With the fleshy tips of both thumbs, press the area from the nape of the neck to the backs of the ears (Fig. 3). Repeat this three or four times. Next, using either the thumbs or the palms of the hands, massage the area from the rear of the neck to the tips of the shoulders and to the scapulae in the directions of the arrows (Fig. 4). Moxa combustion on the tsubo shown in the charts is highly effective in resting the eyes.

Tsubo therapy can bring relief to eye complaints caused by weariness of the optical nerves, but it cannot cure faulty refraction in the lenses of the eyes. Such illnesses demand the attention of a specialist. Tsubo therapy improves conditions of blurring in the eyes; but treatment for this as well as for tired eye muscles, irregularities in the retina, low blood pressure, and weak stomach must be accompanied by treatment for these illnesses. Tsubo treatment cannot help conditions in which distant—but not near—vision is blurred, or vice versa, for this is the result of faulty refraction in the lens.

Fig. 1

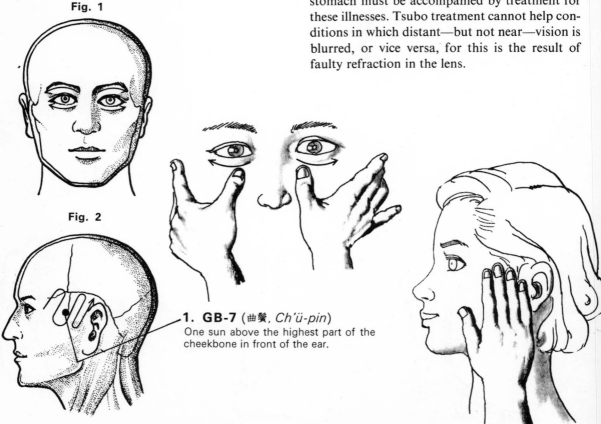

Fig. 2

1. GB-7 (曲鬢, *Ch'ü-pin*)
One sun above the highest part of the cheekbone in front of the ear.

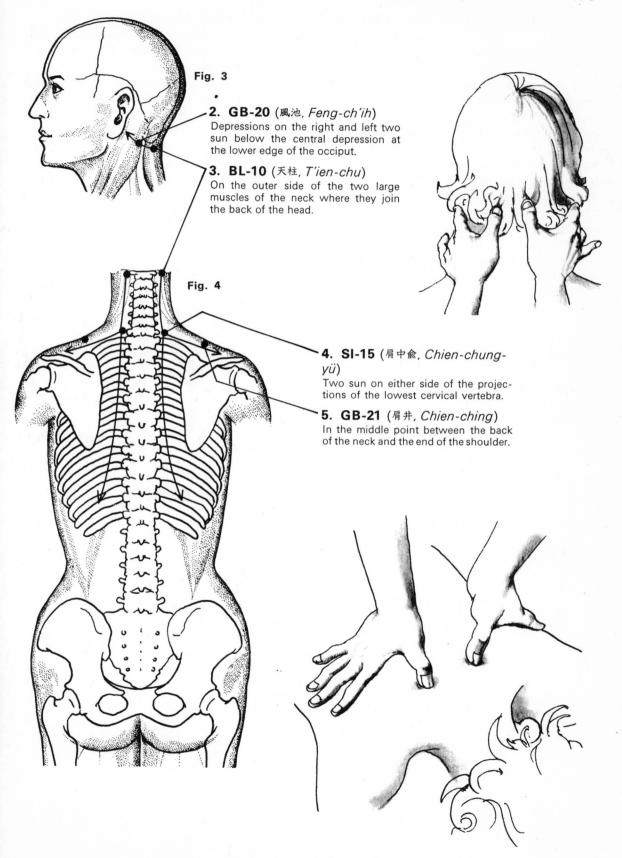

Fig. 3

2. GB-20 (風池, *Feng-ch'ih*)
Depressions on the right and left two sun below the central depression at the lower edge of the occiput.

3. BL-10 (天柱, *T'ien-chu*)
On the outer side of the two large muscles of the neck where they join the back of the head.

Fig. 4

4. SI-15 (肩中兪, *Chien-chung-yü*)
Two sun on either side of the projections of the lowest cervical vertebra.

5. GB-21 (肩井, *Chien-ching*)
In the middle point between the back of the neck and the end of the shoulder.

(2) Stuffy Nose

The simple condition of a stuffy nose, which leads people to gape and breathe through their mouths in an unattractive fashion and to snore in a roaring way when they sleep, can have more serious consequences. It can cause facial pains and can contribute to forgetfulness. It may be that a pathological condition is causing the stuffy nose. If so, consult a physician at once. Sometimes, however, colds, lack of sleep, allergies, and other minor things make the nose stuffy, cause it to run, or make it unnaturally dry. In such instances, try the following tsubo therapy.

The most important tsubo in this treatment are the ones located along the hairline at the back of the neck: BL-10 and GB-20 (Fig. 5). Firm pressure with the thumbs on these tsubo clears both the eyes and the nose. Stuffiness of the nose and nagging coughs are gradually reduced by shiatsu pressure on BL-4 and LI-20 (Fig. 6) and on BL-7 (Fig. 7).

Headaches and heaviness in the head often accompany stuffiness in the nose; these discomforts can be cured by means of shiatsu pressure on GV-20 and GV-21 (Fig. 7). Furthermore, shiatsu on the bladder meridian on the calves brings relief to these conditions. Consequently, I recommend shiatsu pressure on BL-58 and BL-60 (Fig. 8) to relieve the headaches and heaviness often experienced with stuffy nose. Moxa combustion on BL-10, GB-20, GV-20, GV-21, BL-7, and BL-60 is effective too.

Fig. 5

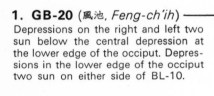

1. GB-20 (風池, *Feng-ch'ih*)
Depressions on the right and left two sun below the central depression at the lower edge of the occiput. Depressions in the lower edge of the occiput two sun on either side of BL-10.

2. BL-10 (天柱, *T'ien-chu*)
On the outer side of the two large muscles of the neck where they join the back of the head.

Fig. 6

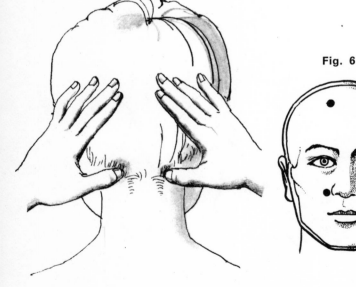

3. BL-4 (曲差, *Ch'ü-ch'a*)
One sun and five bu on either side of a point five bu above the hairline in the center of the forehead.

4. LI-20 (迎香, *Ying-hsiang*)
Either side of the flared part of the nostrils.

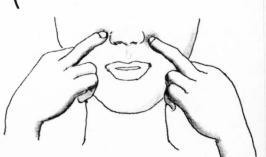

5. GV-21 (前頂, *Ch'ien-ting*)
One sun and five bu in front of GV-20.

6. GV-20 (百会, *Pai-hui*)
At the point where a line directly upward from ear to ear crossing the top of the head and a line straight upward from the midpoint of the area between the shoulders to the top of the head intersect.

Fig. 7

7. BL-7 (通天, *T'ung-t'ien*)
One sun and five bu from the very top of the head.

Fig. 8

8. BL-58 (飛陽, *Fei-yang*)
Rear side of the lower thigh seven sun above the outer side of the ankle.

9. BL-60 (崑崙, *K'un-lun*)
Immediately to the rear side of the outer ankle.

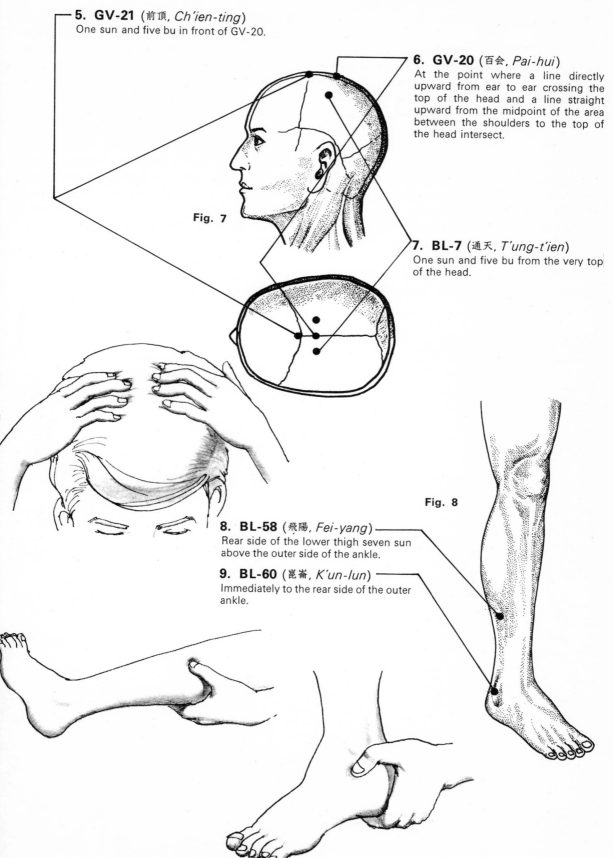

(3) Nosebleed

Wounds inflicted from the outside by such things as fingernails sometimes bring on nosebleed by damaging the nasal mucous membrane. But nosebleed is often related to the general condition of the body as well; and, in many instance, such things as the consumption of specially stimulating foods, leukemia, illness of the red blood corpuscles, arteriosclerosis, high blood pressure, and several others are the causes. In instances of this kind, it is imperative first to treat the basic sickness.

Not infrequently nosebleed occurs when no illness affects the patient and when he has suffered no exterior wound. Stress is the common cause of such nosebleed. The autonomic nervous system is put out of order for some reason, and the slightest stimulus causes the nose to bleed. The first thing a victim of this condition must do is to lie down and remain still. If the nosebleed recurs from time to time, it is wise to consult a physician.

But to cure the rare, apparently fortuitous nosebleed, try this therapy. Apply shiatsu massage to these tsubo: ST-3, BL-10 (Fig. 9), LI-7, LI-4 (Fig. 10), GV-14, and GV-12 (Fig. 11).

The patient must remain lying down or seated. Movement will cause the hemorrhage to recommence. The patient should keep his head as high as possible. Assist easy breathing by loosening neckties or collars. Insert a plug of sterile cotton in the nostril from which blood flows. If sterile cotton is unavailable, use something similar. The plugging matter, of course, must be clean. Cool the nose by means of an ice pack.

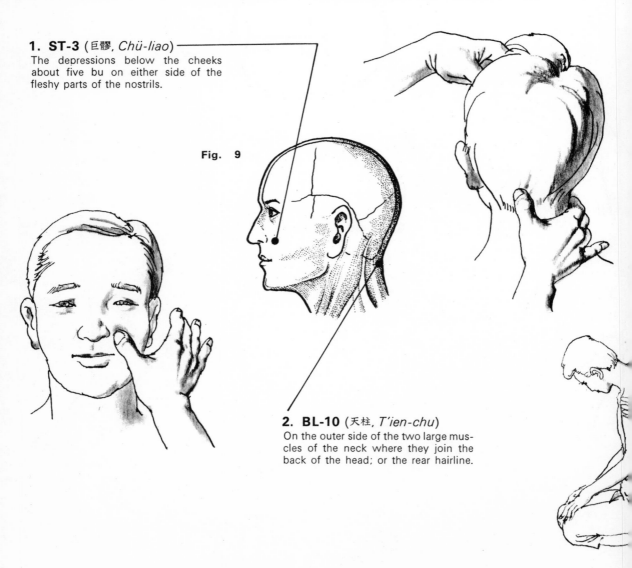

1. ST-3 (巨髎, *Chü-liao*)
The depressions below the cheeks about five bu on either side of the fleshy parts of the nostrils.

Fig. 9

2. BL-10 (天柱, *T'ien-chu*)
On the outer side of the two large muscles of the neck where they join the back of the head; or the rear hairline.

3. LI-7 (温溜, *Wen-liu*)

On the thumb side of the arm at a point half way between the wrist and the elbow.

Fig. 10

4. LI-4 (合谷, *Ho-ku*)

The point exactly between the thumb and index finger on the back side of the hand.

5. GV-14 (大椎, *Ta-ch'ui*)

At the base of the neck in the back between the spinal projections of the seventh cervical and the first thoracic vertebra.

6. GV-12 (身柱, *Shen-chu*)

Below the spinal projections of the third thoracic vertebra.

Fig. 11

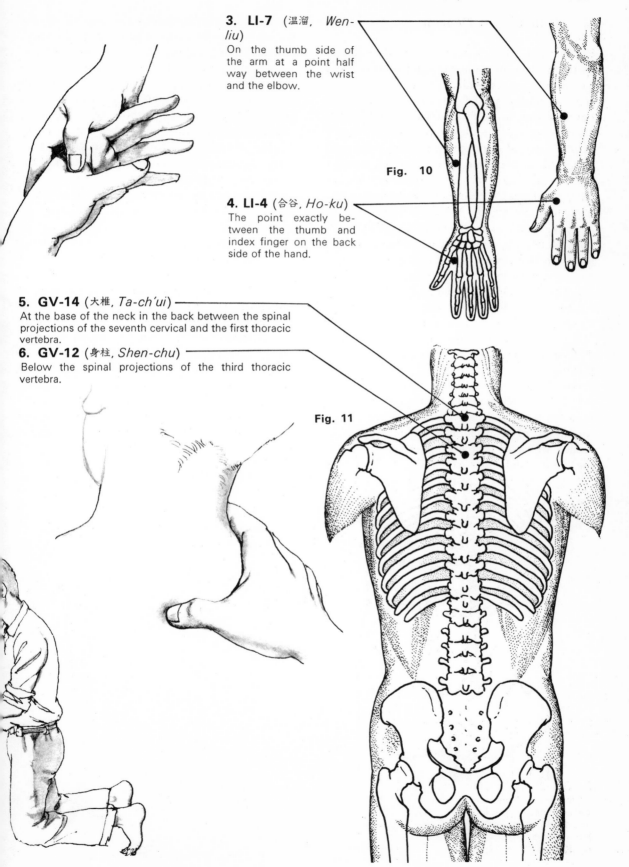

(4) Difficulty in Hearing

Hardness of hearing can range from the inability to hear very quiet sounds to total deafness. The condition may be divided into two major categories according to the part of the ear affected. Faulty transmission of sound is a condition affecting the outer and middle ear and caused by some kind of external stoppage or, possibly inflammation. The second kind of ear trouble involves loss of ability to perceive sounds and affects the inner ear. It may be caused by damage resulting from loud noises, by Ménière's syndrome, by hysteria, or by some illness affecting the entire body. Tsubo therapy, especially acupuncture, is most effective against hardness of hearing caused by hysteria, Ménière's syndrome, illness of the whole body, and perceptional difficulties that are largely psychological or nervous in cause. Among the difficulties caused by stoppage in the outer ear, those that involve the least organic damage are the ones that respond best to tsubo therapy.

Not all cases of hardness of hearing are of the simple kind. Some result from disturbances in both the inner and the outer ear. Whereas malformations or obstructions the outer ear usually reduce ability to hear low sounds and those in the middle and inner ear, ability to hear high sounds, there are cases of combined difficulty in which hearing of both sound ranges is impaired. To determine whether hardness of hearing in one of the patient's ears is related to transmission (outer ear) or to perception (inner and middle ears) perform this simple experiment. Strike a tuning fork and place it on the top of the patient's head. A person with normal hearing hears the sound of the fork with equal strength in both ears. A person suffering from obstruction of the outer ear hears it stronger with the affected ear, whereas a person suffering from a disturbance of the middle or inner ear hears the sound stronger with the well ear.

As the Chinese classics teach that the kidneys are related to hearing, tsubo therapy for ear troubles begin with an investigation of the kidney meridian. First, begin with shiatsu massage of BL-23, BL-47 (Fig. 12), GB-25, KI-16 (Fig. 13). All of these tsubo are very important. To cure the chilling of the feet that is common in people suffering from hearing difficulty, apply shiatsu massage to ST-41, BL-60 (Fig. 14), KI-3 (Fig. 15), CV-14, CV-12, CV-4, and ST-27 (Fig. 16). This treatment helps improve general body condition. Finally, direct treatment of the ear entails shiatsu massage on the following tsubo:

1. BL-23 (腎兪, *Shen-yü*)
One sun and five bu on either side of the spinal column at points below the spinal projections of the second lumbar vertebra, which is located at the height of the lowest ribs.

2. BL-47 (志室, *Chih-shih*)
Three sun on either side of the spinal column at points below the spinal projections of the second lumbar vertebra; on the outer side of BL-23.

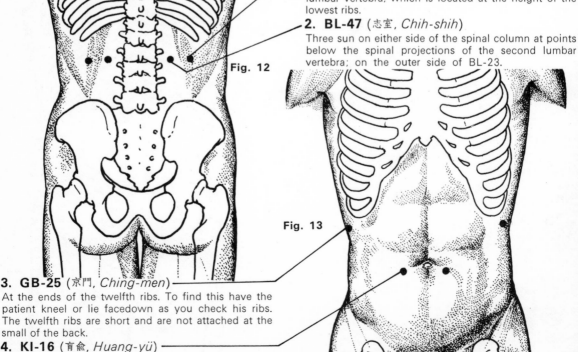

Fig. 12

Fig. 13

3. GB-25 (京門, *Ching-men*)
At the ends of the twelfth ribs. To find this have the patient kneel or lie facedown as you check his ribs. The twelfth ribs are short and are not attached at the small of the back.

4. KI-16 (肓兪, *Huang-yü*)
Points located five sun on either side of the navel.

TH-20, TH-21, TH-18, GB-11, GB-12, TH-17, SI-17. LI-17, and ST-11 (Fig. 17). If headaches accompany the hearing difficulty, apply shiatsu massage to GV-20, BL-10, and GB-20. Ordinary moxa combustion may be used in treating adults suffering from this condition, but moderate moxa is required for treatment of children.

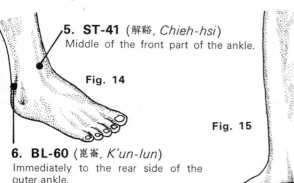

5. ST-41 (解谿, *Chieh-hsi*)
Middle of the front part of the ankle.

Fig. 14

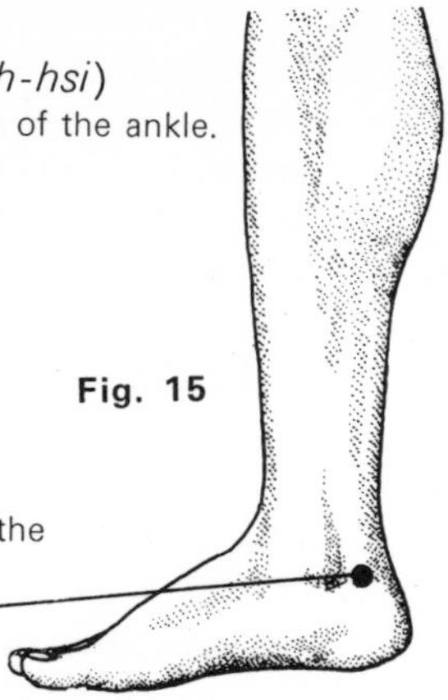

Fig. 15

Fig. 16

6. BL-60 (崑崙, *K'un-lun*)
Immediately to the rear side of the outer ankle.

7. KI-3 (太谿, *T'ai-hsi*)
Rear part of the inside of the ankle.

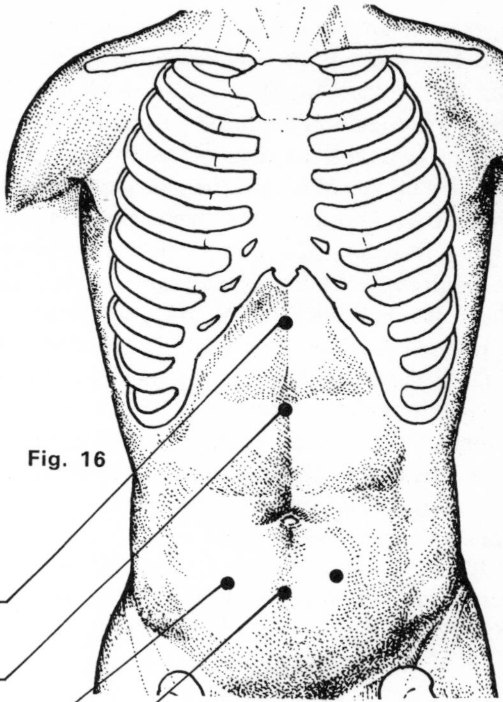

8. CV-14 (巨闕, *Ch'ü-ch'üeh*)
Immediately below the diaphragm; two sun below the lower extremity of the sternum.

9. CV-12 (中脘, *Chung-wan*)
Four sun above the navel; midway between the navel and the diaphragm.

10. ST-27 (大巨, *Ta-chü*)
Two sun below points two sun on either side of the navel.

11. CV-4 (関元, *Kuan-yüan*)
Three sun below the navel, midway between the navel and the pubis.

Fig. 17

12. GV-20 (百会, *Pai-hui*)
At the point where a line directly upward from ear to ear crossing the top of the head and a line straight upward from the midpoint of the area between the shoulders to the top of the head intersect.

13. TH-20 (角孫, *Chüeh-hsun*)
Immediately above the ear.

14. TH-21 (耳門, *Erh-men*)
Immediately in front of the ear hole.

15. TH-18 (瘈脈, *Chih-mei*)
The under part of the point of attachment of the earlobe moving from GB-11; or immediately below the lower extremity of the earlobe.

16. GB-11 (竅陰, *Ch'iao-yin*)
Point behind the ear directly opposite the ear hole.

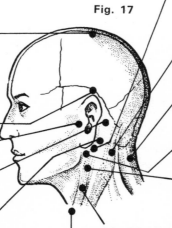

17. GB-12 (完骨, *Wan-ku*)
Depression in the back edge of the mastoid process behind the ear. In the depression that is located about the width of one finger above the mastoid process and four bu from the hairline.

18. GB-20 (風池, *Feng-ch'ih*)
Depressions in the lower edge of the occiput two sun on either side of BL-10.

19. BL-10 (天柱, *T'ien-chu*)
To the outer side of the two large muscles of the neck where they join the back of the head.

20. TH-17 (翳風, *Yi-feng*)
In the depression between the lobe of the ear and the mastoid process.

21. SI-17 (天容, *T'ien-jung*)
Below the ear at the corner of the lower jaw. Immediately in front of the sternomastoid muscle.

22. LI-17 (天鼎, *T'ien-ting*)
Near the peak of the triangular depression formed by the sternomastoid muscle (the muscle from the base of the neck to the ear; it becomes apparent when the neck is turned full to one side), the trapezius muscle (the large triangular muscle running from the neck to the shoulder tip), and the clavicle.

23. ST-11 (気舎, *Ch'i-she*)
One sun and five bu on either side of the central point in the front of the neck. Inner tip of the clavicle and upper tip of the sternum.

(5) Earache

Most of the earaches that patients complain of involve inflammation of the outer or middle ear and fall into one of two categories: acute and chronic inflammation. Acute inflammation strikes suddenly and can be so painful that the patient is unable to sleep. Infection caused by colds or other sickness in the passage connecting the throat and the ears bring this condition about. It occurs in adults but is more common in children, in whom the passages are short and thick. If it is not treated, it can recur often until it becomes chronic. Especially, when inflammation of the ear is toxic, the patient's condition greatly lower the resistance of the body, or the patient suffers from sickness of the throat or nose, earache is likely to be severe. If there is any suspicion of inflammation of the inner ear, consult a specialist at once.

If the earache begins mildly and gradually grows until chewing food causes pain, it is probably an inflammation of the outer ear. For patients of this condition, calm and quiet are essential. They must avoid all exercise and must refrain from bathing.

When there is no inflammation and no apparent organic cause for the pain, the earache is psychologically inspired, though it is nonetheless painful for the sufferer, who will have places around the ear that are sensitive to pressure. To apply oriental therapy to such patients, first use shiatsu massage on TH-20, GB-11, GB-20, TH-17, ST-6, and TH-21 (Fig. 18). The napply shiatsu massage to KI-16 (Fig. 19). BL-23 (Fig. 20) is an important tsubo for treatment of earache.

You must massage the patient with your body in the following position. Kneel on one knee with your weight forward and with both arms outstretched. Exert equal pressure with both hands. In addition to the ones listed, KI-7 and KI-3 (Fig. 21) are important tsubo in the treatment of headaches, earaches, and toothaches. Use shiatsu massage on them.

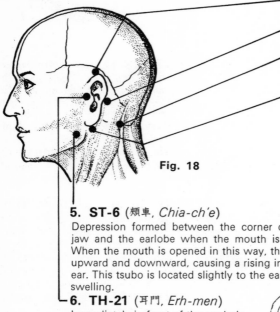

Fig. 18

1. TH-20 (角孫, *Chüeh-hsun*)
Immediately above the ear.
2. GB-11 (竅陰, *Ch'iao-yin*)
Point behind the ear directly opposite the ear hole.
3. GB-20 (風池, *Feng-ch'ih*)
Depressions on the right and left two sun below the central depression at the lower edge of the occiput.
4. TH-17 (翳風, *Yi-feng*)
In the depression between the lobe of the ear and the mastoid process.

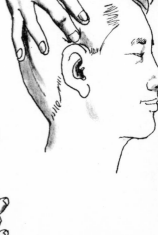

5. ST-6 (頬車, *Chia-ch'e*)
Depression formed between the corner of the lower jaw and the earlobe when the mouth is open wide. When the mouth is opened in this way, the jaws move upward and downward, causing a rising in front of the ear. This tsubo is located slightly to the ear side of that swelling.
6. TH-21 (耳門, *Erh-men*)
Immediately in front of the ear hole.

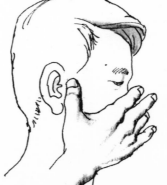

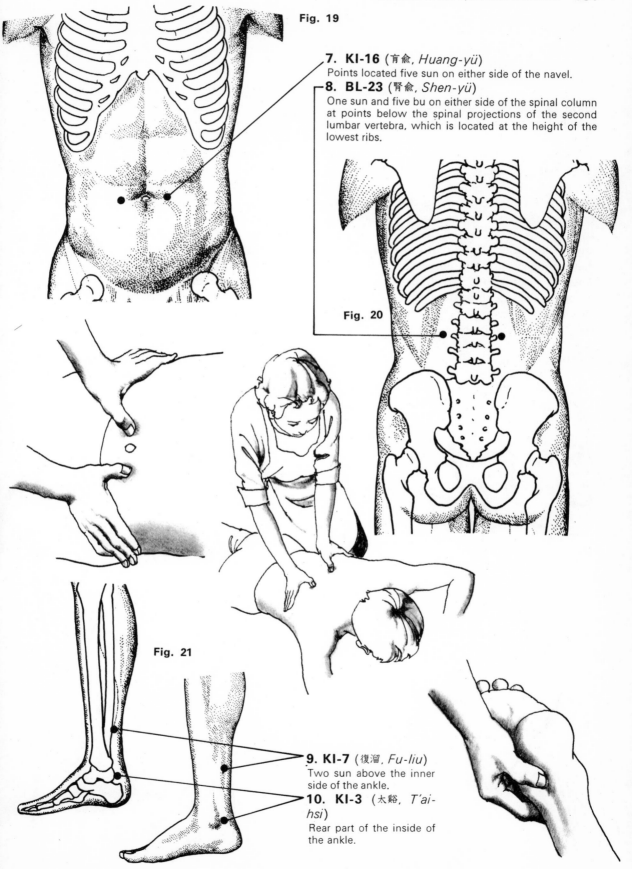

Fig. 19

7. KI-16 (肓兪, *Huang-yü*)
Points located five sun on either side of the navel.

8. BL-23 (腎兪, *Shen-yü*)
One sun and five bu on either side of the spinal column at points below the spinal projections of the second lumbar vertebra, which is located at the height of the lowest ribs.

Fig. 20

Fig. 21

9. KI-7 (復溜, *Fu-liu*)
Two sun above the inner side of the ankle.

10. KI-3 (太谿, *T'ai-hsi*)
Rear part of the inside of the ankle.

Illnesses of the Teeth and Mouth

(1) Oral Inflammation

The mouth is full of bacteria, but the action of saliva and mutual battling among the germs usually prevents any one kind from getting the upper hand and causing trouble. Sometimes, however, other things can bring about oral inflammation. Some of the causes are the bacteria themselves, virus infections, vitamin deficiencies, inadequacies of the blood, artificial dentures, tartar on the teeth, bits of bone from food, and so on. The term *oral inflammation* includes any inflammation of the oral membrane of the gums, tongue, lips, and corners of the mouth. Anemia, disorders of the autonomic nervous system, sicknesses of the stomach, and intestines, high fevers, menstrual periods, and pregnancy may bring the condition on. The basic symptoms may be divided into three categories: aphtous, catarrhal, and ulcerous. Aphthous inflammation

takes the form of round or oval, whitish or yellowish spots on the membrane. These spots are painful. If left untreated, they will usually be cured naturally, though they can sometimes become so serious that eating is highly uncomfortable. If they recur, they may develop into a troublesome condition.

Broad whitish areas or red and swollen areas and roughness in the oral cavity are symptoms of catarrhal oral inflammation. Swollen gums, malodorous breath, and burning discomfort in the mouth are the signs of ulcerous oral inflammation. The first thing to do in treating these conditions is to consult a physician, have him determine the cause, and permit him to cure the inflammation by curing the basic sickness that is bringing it on. But in many cases, the cause is not easy to pin down, though usually the stomach is involved. People who have developed oral inflammation must refrain from drinking alcohol, smoking, or eating or drinking anything that is highly stimulating.

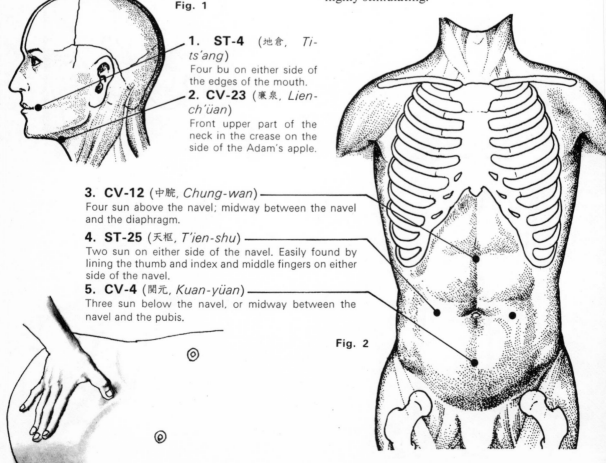

Fig. 1

1. ST-4 (地倉, *Ti-ts'ang*)
Four bu on either side of the edges of the mouth.

2. CV-23 (廉泉, *Lien-ch'üan*)
Front upper part of the neck in the crease on the side of the Adam's apple.

3. CV-12 (中脘, *Chung-wan*)
Four sun above the navel; midway between the navel and the diaphragm.

4. ST-25 (天枢, *T'ien-shu*)
Two sun on either side of the navel. Easily found by lining the thumb and index and middle fingers on either side of the navel.

5. CV-4 (関元, *Kuan-yüan*)
Three sun below the navel, or midway between the navel and the pubis.

Fig. 2

To apply oriental therapy, which treats the oral condition by striving to improve general bodily health, first perform shiatsu massage on ST-4, CV-23, CV-12, ST-25, and CV-4 (Figs. 1 and 2). Next perform shiatsu massage on GV-14, BL-18. BL-20, BL-23, LI-11, ST-36, and SP-6, (Figs. 3 through 6). In massaging the tsubo on the back, outstretch your arms and exert equal pressure with both hands.

6. GV-14 (大椎, *Ta-ch'ui*) ───────
At the base of the neck in the back between the spinal projections of the seventh cervical and the first thoracic vertebra.

7. BL-18 (肝兪, *Kan-yü*) ──────
One sun and five bu on either side of the spinal column at points below the spinal projections of the ninth thoracic vertebra.

8. BL-20 (脾兪, *P'i-yü*) ────────
One sun and five bu on either side of the spinal column at points below the eleventh thoracic vertebra.

9. BL-23 (腎兪, *Shen-yü*) ──────
One sun and five bu on either side of the spinal column at points below the spinal projections of the second lumbar vertebra; which is located at the height of the lowest ribs.

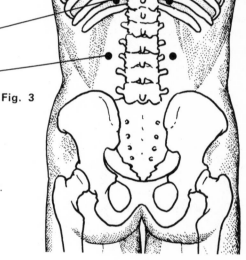

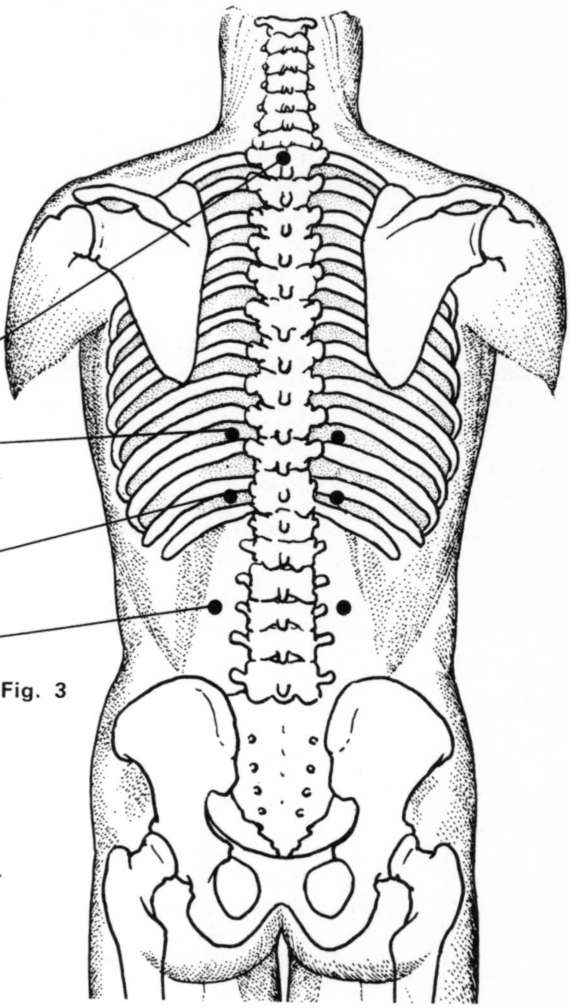

Fig. 3

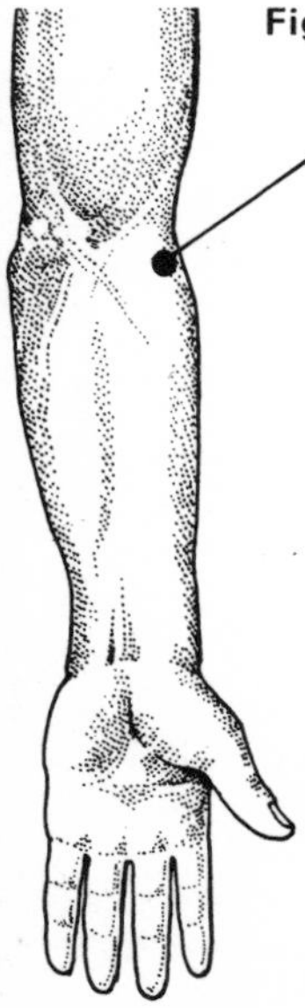

Fig. 4

10. LI-11 (曲池, *Ch'ü-ch'ih*)
Thumb side of the bend of the elbow.

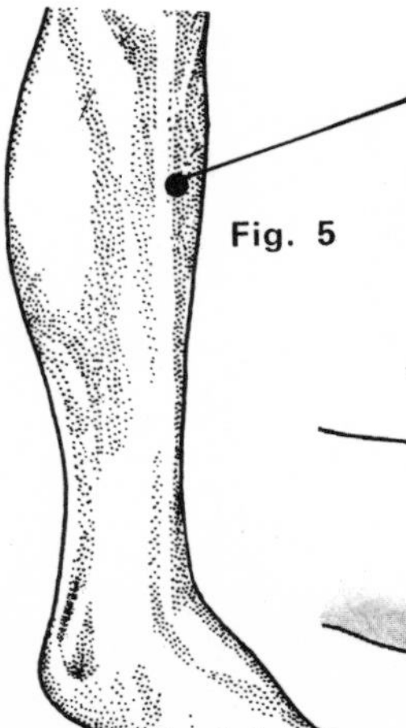

11. ST-36 (足三里, *Tsu-san-li*)
On the outer side of the calf three sun below the knee. Outer edge of the tibia or shin bone.

Fig. 5

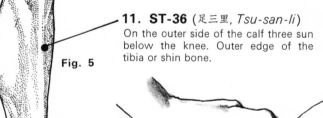

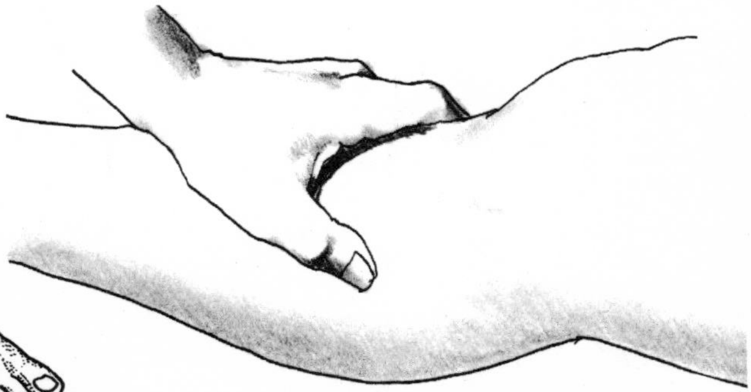

Fig. 6

12. SP-6 (三陰交, *San-yin-chiao*) ──────
Three sun upward on the side of the shin bone from the inner side of the ankle.

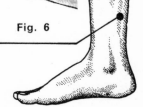

(2) Toothaches

The most common cause of toothache—one that has afflicted practically everyone at one time or another—is dental caries; that is, decay caused by bacteria. In addition to this, inflammation or infection of the gums can cause toothache, as can incorrect eruption or impacting of such teeth as the wisdom teeth, especially those of the lower jaw.

Furthermore, pain in the dental region can result from the extraction of teeth, inflammation of the alveolar bone or of dental pulp, spreading to the periodontium and giving rise to suppuration. Cancer or ulcers, of course, can cause severe dental pain. Furthermore, general bodily debility sometimes aggravates latent inflammation, which then becomes acute and creates great pain in the dental regions. This is often accompanied by trigeminal facial neuralgia (see p. 124).

Obviously, for dental caries or any of the strictly organic conditions described above, consult a dentist at once and have him treat the cause of the trouble. For the kind of psychological toothache that strikes together with trigeminal facial neuralgia, use the following oriental tsubo therapy. For toothache in the lower jaw, shiatsu on ST-3 and ST-5 (Fig. 7) is effective.

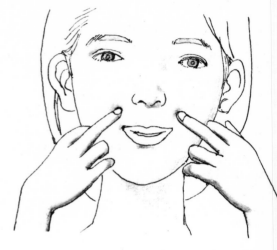

Fig. 7

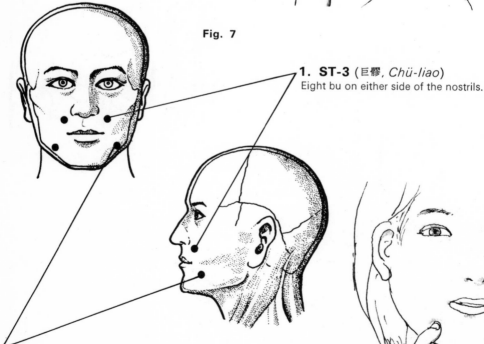

1. ST-3 (巨髎, *Chü-liao*)
Eight bu on either side of the nostrils.

2. ST-5 (大迎, *Ta-ying*)
Depression in the lower jaw one sun and five bu from its corner; or the depression in the bone at a point located diagonally downward from the ends of the mouth.

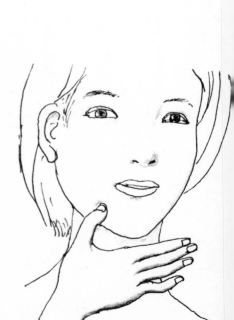

Often toothache in the lower jaw results from lack of sleep and headaches; shiatsu on ST-5 is effective in such cases. To treat toothaches in the upper jaw, use shiatsu massage on ST-2 (Fig. 8). Shiatsu with the thumbs on ST-6 too is effective, as is treatment of ST-7. For further details on treating toothaches related to trigeminal facial neuralgia. Remember that this treatment has no effect on toothaches caused by dental caries. Moxa, because of its very nature as a material to be burned, is scarcely recommendable for use on the face, although mild moxa on ST-6 on the forehead helps cure toothaches.

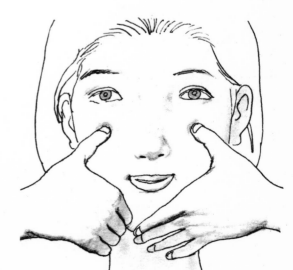

3. ST-2 (四白, *Szu-pai*)
Directly to the side of the nose about one sun lower than the edge of the bone at the bottom of the eye.

Fig. 8

5. ST-6 (頬車, *Chia-ch'e*)
Depression formed between the corner of the lower jaw and the earlobe when the mouth is open wide. When the mouth is opened in this way, the jaws move upward and downward, causing a rising in front of the ear. This tsubo is located slightly to the ear side of that swelling.

4. ST-7 (下関, *Hsia-kuan*)
The depression in front of the part of the lower jaw that passes in front of the ear hole. Lower edge of the zygomatic arch. Depression under the cheek bone (zygomatic arch) opposite the nostrils.

(3) Pyorrhea

Bad breath and a slimy feeling in the mouth are two of the earliest signs of pyorrhea. Since this disease is not usually accompanied by the kind of severe pain associated with toothaches, many people tend to allow it to go unchecked. But this is dangerous since pyorrhea affects the organisms around the teeth—gums, periodontium, alveolar bone, cement—and, if allowed to reach advanced stages, can cause the teeth to fall out. Pyorrhea is rarely seen in small children, but it strikes people after they reach the age of fourteen or fifteen. In older people there is little sex-related difference in the frequencies of people suffering from pyorrhea, although in younger people the condition seems to strike women more often than men.

The following factors play a role in the generation of the disease. (1) The tissues and organs around the teeth are susceptible to pyorrhea. (2) Exterior elements have a bad influence on the gums; for instance, dental tartar, remains of food, extremes of cold and heat, or bacterial infection may cause the disease. (3) The condition may be caused by an inner disturbance in the body: diabetes or some other sickness related to the metabolism, irregularities in the secretions of the thyroid glands, vitamin deficiency, irregularities in the autonomic nervous system, allergies, and so on. There are many unexplained things related to possible internal causes of pyorrhea.

When the condition has attacked, immediately consult a dentist to have him examine the patient and prescribe ways to prevent the pyorrhea from getting out of hand. Following his advice, regularly massage or give shiatsu massage to the tsubo listed below to reinforce dental therapy. The combined treatment will cure the disease and prevent its recurrence.

First, treat LI-20, LI-19, ST-5, CV-24, and BL-10 (Fig. 9). Then treat CV-12, KI-16 (Fig. 10), in the shiatsu fashion. Massage and shiatsu on BL-18, BL-23, LI-11, and LI-10 (Figs. 11 and 12) are effective. The symptoms of pyorrhea are stubborn and seem to resist treatment. Consequently, carry out the treatment outlined here regularly and daily.

Fig. 9

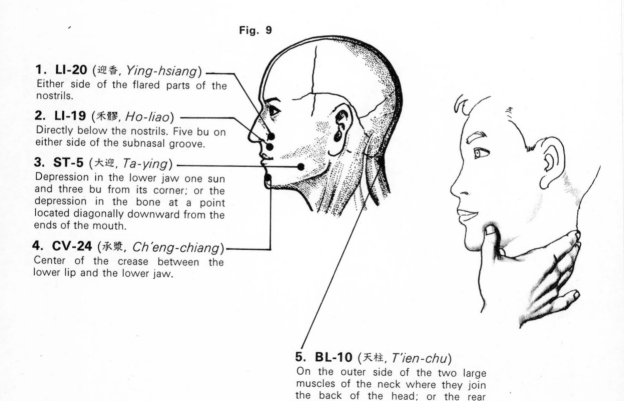

1. LI-20 (迎香, *Ying-hsiang*)
Either side of the flared parts of the nostrils.

2. LI-19 (禾髎, *Ho-liao*)
Directly below the nostrils. Five bu on either side of the subnasal groove.

3. ST-5 (大迎, *Ta-ying*)
Depression in the lower jaw one sun and three bu from its corner; or the depression in the bone at a point located diagonally downward from the ends of the mouth.

4. CV-24 (承漿, *Ch'eng-chiang*)
Center of the crease between the lower lip and the lower jaw.

5. BL-10 (天柱, *T'ien-chu*)
On the outer side of the two large muscles of the neck where they join the back of the head; or the rear hairline.

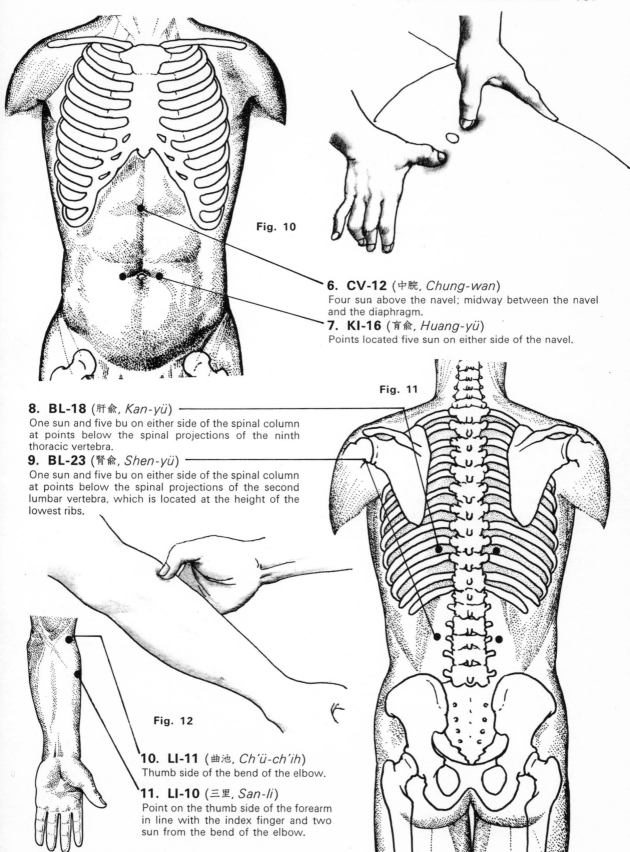

Fig. 10

6. CV-12 (中脘, *Chung-wan*)
Four sun above the navel; midway between the navel and the diaphragm.

7. KI-16 (肓俞, *Huang-yü*)
Points located five sun on either side of the navel.

Fig. 11

8. BL-18 (肝俞, *Kan-yü*)
One sun and five bu on either side of the spinal column at points below the spinal projections of the ninth thoracic vertebra.

9. BL-23 (腎俞, *Shen-yü*)
One sun and five bu on either side of the spinal column at points below the spinal projections of the second lumbar vertebra, which is located at the height of the lowest ribs.

Fig. 12

10. LI-11 (曲池, *Ch'ü-ch'ih*)
Thumb side of the bend of the elbow.

11. LI-10 (三里, *San-li*)
Point on the thumb side of the forearm in line with the index finger and two sun from the bend of the elbow.

(4) Eruptions around the Mouth

When a person has roughness at the ends of the mouth and when his face is marked with eruptions, it is usual for him to experience heaviness in the region of the diaphragm, lack appetite, belch frequently, and feel generally rundown. This is because the roughness of the skin and the eruptions are a sign of gastric disorder. The important thing to do is to stimulate the areas in which the eruptions develop: massage ST-4 and CV-24 (Fig. 13). Oriental medicine has long held that the location of ST-4 is intimately related to the condition of the stomach and that, for this reason, it is the place where eruptions of the kind under discussion are most likely to occur. Perform thorough shiatsu massage on ST-4 and CV-24. Next, to put the digestive organs back in good working order, massage (shiatsu) with the thumbs the following tsubo: BL-18, BL-20, and BL-21 (Fig. 14) in the directions of the arrows.

Supplement this treatment with massage of CV-14, ST-19, LV-14, CV-12, and ST-25 (Fig. 15). Using the four fingers of each hand, massage in the directions of the arrows; then perform shiatsu massage on the same places. This will greatly increase the effectiveness of treatment. Finally, perform shiatsu massage on ST-36 (Fig. 16).

Many people tend to think that commercial salves and ointments are sufficient to cure pimples and facial eruptions, but this is not true in the case of disfigurements of the kind caused by gastric disorders. To clear up the skin in such instances, it is necessary first to put the stomach and digestive tract in good condition.

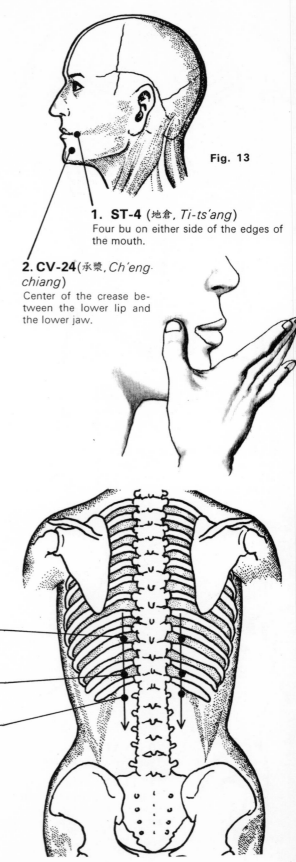

Fig. 13

1. ST-4 (地倉, *Ti-ts'ang*)
Four bu on either side of the edges of the mouth.

2. CV-24 (承漿, *Ch'eng-chiang*)
Center of the crease between the lower lip and the lower jaw.

Fig. 14

3. BL-18 (肝兪, *Kan-yü*) ——————
One sun and five bu on either side of the spinal column at points below the spinal projections of the ninth thoracic vertebra.
4. BL-20 (脾兪, *P'i-yü*) ——————
One sun and five bu on either side of the spinal column at points below the eleventh thoracic vertebra.
5. BL-21 (胃兪, *Wei-yü*) ——————
One sun and five bu on either side of the spinal column at points below the spinal projections of the twelfth thoracic vertebra.

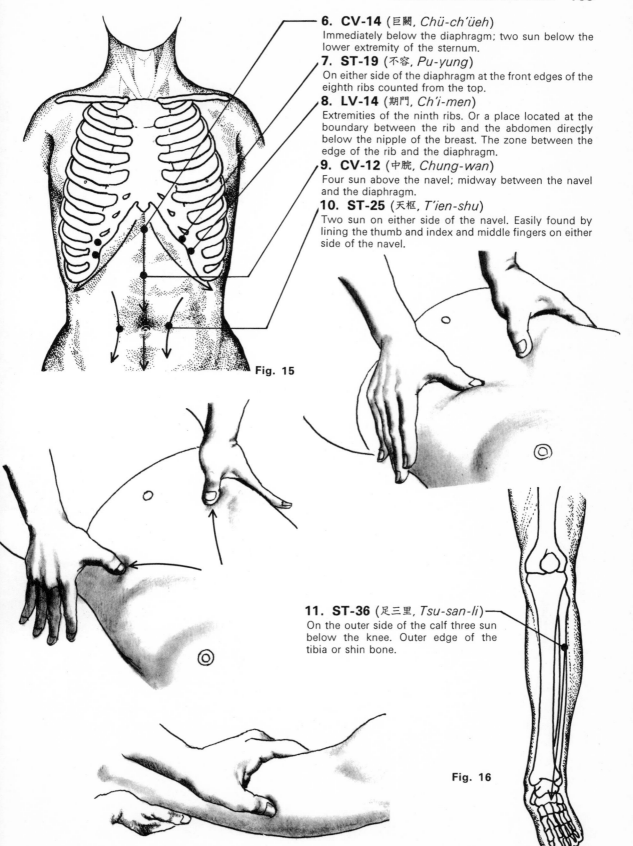

6. CV-14 (巨闕, *Chü-ch'üeh*)
Immediately below the diaphragm; two sun below the lower extremity of the sternum.

7. ST-19 (不容, *Pu-yung*)
On either side of the diaphragm at the front edges of the eighth ribs counted from the top.

8. LV-14 (期門, *Ch'i-men*)
Extremities of the ninth ribs. Or a place located at the boundary between the rib and the abdomen directly below the nipple of the breast. The zone between the edge of the rib and the diaphragm.

9. CV-12 (中脘, *Chung-wan*)
Four sun above the navel; midway between the navel and the diaphragm.

10. ST-25 (天樞, *T'ien-shu*)
Two sun on either side of the navel. Easily found by lining the thumb and index and middle fingers on either side of the navel.

Fig. 15

11. ST-36 (足三里, *Tsu-san-li*)
On the outer side of the calf three sun below the knee. Outer edge of the tibia or shin bone.

Fig. 16

10. Skin Diseases

(1) Eczema

Victims of eczema complain of a total-body itchiness that keeps them awake at night. They lose appetite and suffer from constipation. Their skin is often marked with bloody wounds that they have inflicted on themselves by scratching. The skin all over their bodies is rough and dark. The area from the neck to the tips of the shoulders is stiff because of muscular contraction. The lymph glands in their necks are usually swollen. The causes of eczema are uncertain. It can occur on any part of the body; and, in its acute form, it is almost invariably characterized by itching, redness, and the formation of blisters or scales of skin. It can be topical, and it can spread by contact. In its chronic form, eczema displays less drastic symptoms; but the skin becomes thick, and the wrinkles in it are clearly apparent.

Since it is deeply related to overall bodily condition, eczema can only be cured by putting the entire body into a state of sound health. To help do this, perform the following treatment. Using commercially available, fine-grade moxa, apply moxa combustion from three to five times on each of the following tsubo: CV-14, LV-14, CV-12, KI-16, ST-27, ST-25, and CV-4 (Fig. 1). Then massage on the meridians shown in Fig. 1; massage in the directions of the arrows.

You may increase the effectiveness of treatment by supplementing it with moxa combustion on the following: GB-21, BL-13, BL-22, BL-23, BL-25, BL-31, BL-32, BL-33, and BL-34 (Fig. 2). Once again, massage must center on these tsubo and must follow the directions of the arrows. When itching and skin roughness are severe, moxa combustion on the affected places—whether they are the locations of tsubo or not—brings relief.

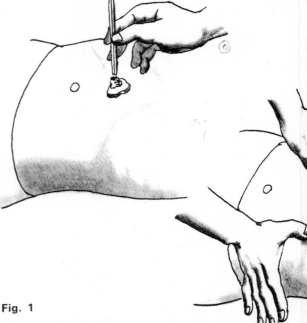

Fig. 1

1. CV-14 (巨闕, *Chü-ch'üeh*)
Immediately below the diaphragm; two sun below the lower extremity of the sternum.

2. LV-14 (期門, *Ch'i-men*)
Extremities of the ninth ribs. Or a place located at the boundary between the rib and the abdomen directly below the nipple of the breast. The zone between the edge of the rib and the diaphragm.

3. CV-12 (中脘, *Chung-wan*)
Four sun above the navel; midway between the navel and the diaphragm.

4. KI-16 (肓兪, *Huang-yü*)
Points located five sun on either side of the navel.

5. ST-25 (天枢, *T'ien-shu*)
Two sun on either side of the navel. Easily found by lining the thumb and index and middle fingers on either side of the navel.

6. ST-27 (大巨, *Ta-chü*)
Two sun below the points two sun on either side of the navel; that is, two sun below ST-25.

7. CV-4 (関元, *Kuan-yüan*)
Three sun below the navel, or midway between the navel and the pubis.

Regular, protracted tsubo therapy geared to improve the total body condition is the best way to approach chronic eczema and to do away with the thick skin and other conditions it produces. Recently, medical science has been employing the adrenal cortical hormone to treat eczema, which remains, however, a difficult disease to cure. Nonetheless, patient perseverance in tsubo therapy has cured many cases in the past. When tsubo therapy begins taking effect—as it will if performed faithfully—the swelling in the lymph glands in the neck will subside, and the patient will become surprisingly healthy and vigorous.

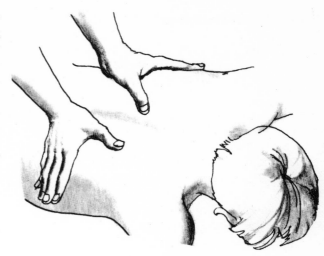

8. GB-21 (肩井, *Chien-ching*)
In the middle point between the base of the neck and the end of the shoulder.

9. BL-13 (肺兪, *Fei-yü*)
One sun and five bu on either side of the spinal column at points below the spinal projections of the third thoracic vertebra.

10. BL-22 (三焦兪, *San-chiao-shu*)
One sun and five bu on either side of the spinal column at points below the first lumbar vertebra.

Fig. 2

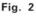

11. BL-23 (腎兪, *Shen-yü*)
One sun and five bu on either side of the spinal column at points below the spinal projections of the second lumbar vertebra, which is located at the height of the lowest ribs.

12. BL-25 (大腸兪, *Ta-ch'ang-yü*)
One sun and five bu on either side of the spinal column at points below the spinal projections of the fourth lumbar vertebra.

13. BL-31 (上髎, *Shang-liao*)
14. BL-32 (次髎, *Tz'u-liao*)
15. BL-33 (中髎, *Chung-liao*)
16. BL-34 (下髎, *Hsia-liao*)
Five sacral vertebrae are fused to form a rear wall for the pelvic cavity. The four tsubo BL-31, BL-32, BL-33, and BL-34 are located beside the openings on either side of the projections of the top four of these vertebrae. The pair of tsubo designated BL-31 is on the level of the topmost of the sacral vertebrae, and the others proceed downward in ascending numerical order.

(2) Urticaria (Hives)

The condition known as hives is characterized by an intolerable itching all over the body and an outbreaking of red risings, which gradually expand. Acute hives may last only a few minutes hours, or days; chronic hives can occurs over a period of months or even years. When the hives subside, the skin returns to its normal condition. The cause of hives depends largely on the person experiencing them and may range from such external factors as friction, cold, heat, and the use of chemicals or drugs on the skin to such internal matters as foods, medicines, injections, organic or metabolic sicknesses, nervous conditions, or hysteria. Although stomach or intestinal problems can cause hives, in most cases they are brought on by allergies that make the person hypersensitive to some condition or material. When the allergy manifests itself in the subdermal tissues, the eyes fail to function properly, the person tires easily and may fall victim to nose colds or stomach and intestinal ailments. If the allergy manifests itself in the muscles surrounding the internal organs, cramps and bronchial asthma may result. Curing the manifestations of the sickness is achieved only by curing the allergy.

Characteristically, people who suffer from allergies have stains, blotches, or rough skin in the areas from the base of the neck to the tips of the shoulders. Pressure on the base of the neck at the location of the seventh cervical vertebra causes severe pain in such people. Moxa combustion on points right and left and top and bottom of GV-14 (Fig. 3) will greatly reduce the frequency of attacks of the hives. Treat further by massaging or applying shiatsu massage on the following tsubo: GV-14, BL-13, BL-18, BL-23, BL-25 (Fig. 3), CV-17, CV-12, CV-4, and TH-4 (Figs. 4 and 5). Follow this with thorough shiatsu pressure on KI-3 (Fig. 6). This treatment decidedly has effect, though the reasons for its benefits are uncertain. In conjunction with massage on these tsubo, moxa combustion on the back, abdomen, and TH-4 increases the effectiveness of the therapy. Using fine- or medium-grade moxa, burn it from three to five times on the tsubo. Use mild moxa for children. Without fail, continue this therapy for three weeks. If the treatment agrees with the bodily constitution of the patient, it will have amazing effect. It can be advantageously combined with acupuncture or with the use of magnetized metal balls with adhesive tape.

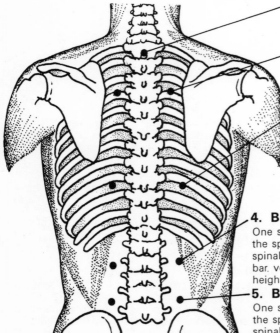

Fig. 3

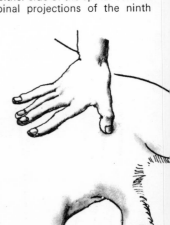

1. GV-14 (大椎, *Ta-ch'ui*)
At the base of the neck in the back between the spinal projections of the seventh cervical and the first thoracic vertebra.

2. BL-13 (肺俞, *Fei-yü*)
One sun and five bu on either side of the spinal column at points below the spinal projections of the third thoracic vertebra.

3. BL-18 (肝俞, *Kan-yü*)
One sun and five bu on either side of the spinal column at points below the spinal projections of the ninth thoracic vertebra.

4. BL-23 (腎俞, *Shen-yü*)
One sun and five bu on either side of the spinal column at points below the spinal projections of the second lumbar. vertebra, which is located at the height of the lowest ribs.

5. BL-25 (大腸俞, *Ta-ch'ang-yü*)
One sun and five bu on either side of the spinal column at points below the spinal projections of the fourth lumbar vertebra.

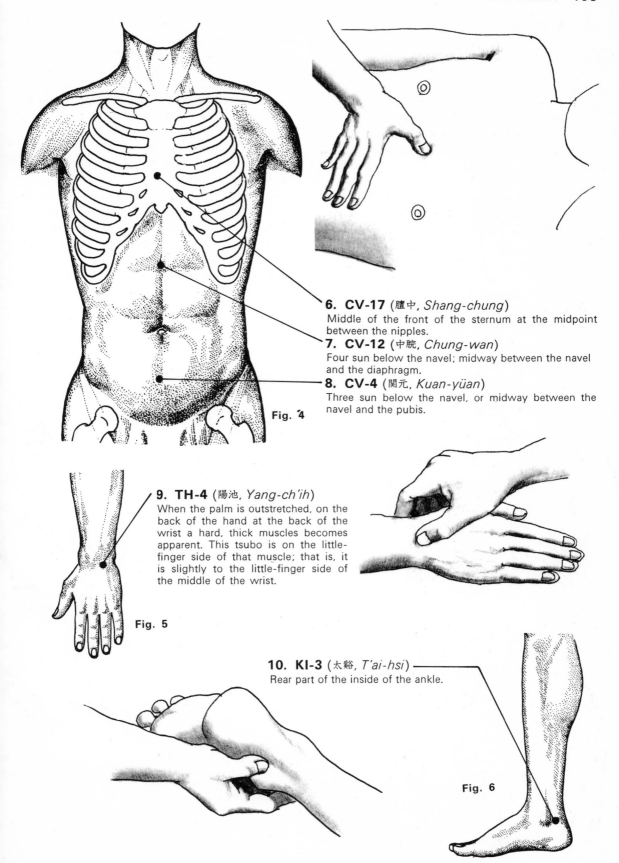

Fig. 4

6. CV-17 (膻中, *Shang-chung*)
Middle of the front of the sternum at the midpoint between the nipples.

7. CV-12 (中脘, *Chung-wan*)
Four sun below the navel; midway between the navel and the diaphragm.

8. CV-4 (関元, *Kuan-yüan*)
Three sun below the navel, or midway between the navel and the pubis.

9. TH-4 (陽池, *Yang-ch'ih*)
When the palm is outstretched, on the back of the hand at the back of the wrist a hard, thick muscles becomes apparent. This tsubo is on the little-finger side of that muscle; that is, it is slightly to the little-finger side of the middle of the wrist.

Fig. 5

10. KI-3 (太谿, *T'ai-hsi*)
Rear part of the inside of the ankle.

Fig. 6

(3) Chilblains

This condition, characterized by painful swellings and discolorations on the hands or feet, is directly caused by exposure to cold; but its true cause is poor circulation of the blood. In our clinic, we place great emphasis on the circulation and, in prescribing treatment, always measure the temperatures of the patient's forehead, hands, and feet. In normal people, body temperature ranges from twenty-six to thirty degrees centigrade, whereas in people with poor circulation it is generally much lower. Cold and chills cause the capillaries of the circulation system to become sluggish, thus bringing about anemia or congestion in the feet and hands. And this is the source of the blackish swellings typical of chilblains.

The tsubo therapy for curing this sickness is to return the entire body to good health and to improve the circulation of the blood. To effect this, treatment of the following tsubo is very important: BL-14, BL-15 (Fig. 7), CV-17, CV-14, and SP-12 (Fig. 8). Massage meridians ①, ②, and ③ and then perform thorough shiatsu on tsubo BL-23 and BL-25, which are central to the meridians designated for massage. To improve circulation in the hands, treat TH-4, LI-4 (Fig. 9), and HT-7 (Fig. 10). To improve circulation in the feet, massage ST-36 (Fig. 11), SP-9, SP-6, and KI-1 (Figs. 12 and 13). Concentrate on the circulatory organs in meridians ④, ⑤, ⑥, and ⑦. Shiatsu massage and ordinary massage performed as prescribed here from late autumn will prevent chilblains. Certainly it is better to prevent the condition in people susceptible to it than to try to treat it once it strikes. Amazingly, when oriental therapy has removed the danger of chilblains, the entire physical condition of the patient improves greatly.

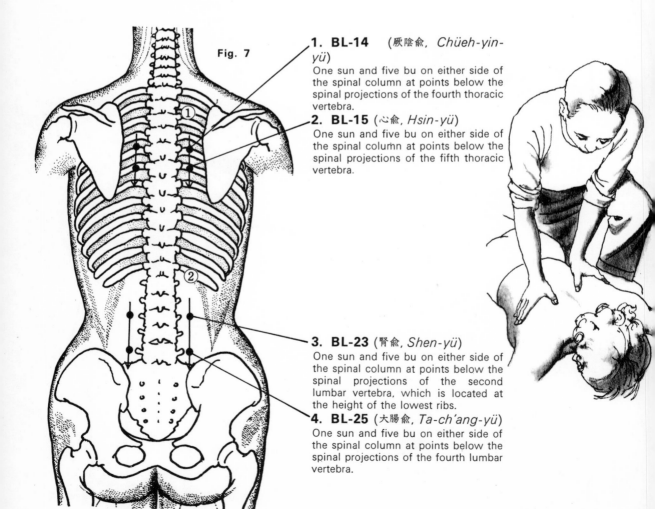

Fig. 7

1. BL-14 (厥陰兪, *Chüeh-yin-yü*)
One sun and five bu on either side of the spinal column at points below the spinal projections of the fourth thoracic vertebra.

2. BL-15 (心兪, *Hsin-yü*)
One sun and five bu on either side of the spinal column at points below the spinal projections of the fifth thoracic vertebra.

3. BL-23 (腎兪, *Shen-yü*)
One sun and five bu on either side of the spinal column at points below the spinal projections of the second lumbar vertebra, which is located at the height of the lowest ribs.

4. BL-25 (大腸兪, *Ta-ch'ang-yü*)
One sun and five bu on either side of the spinal column at points below the spinal projections of the fourth lumbar vertebra.

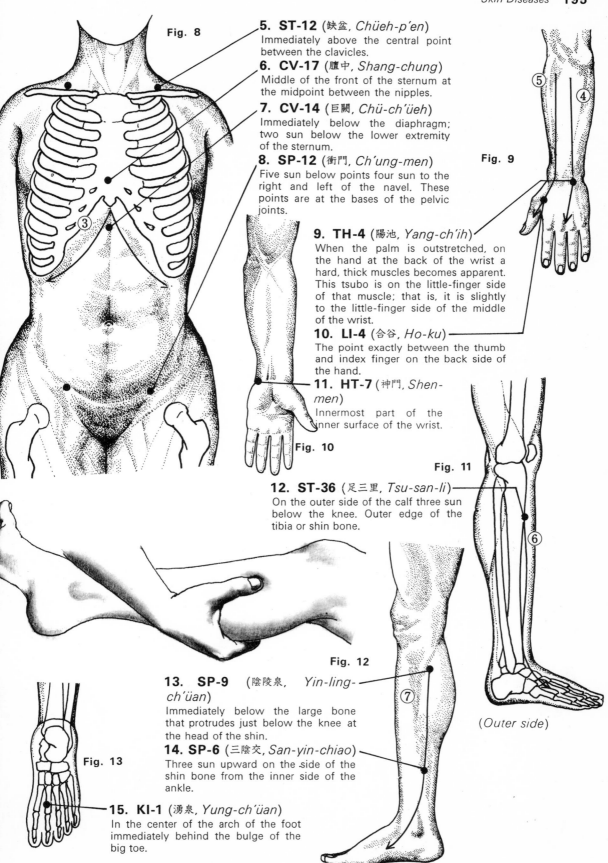

Fig. 8

5. ST-12 (缺盆, *Chüeh-p'en*)
Immediately above the central point between the clavicles.

6. CV-17 (膻中, *Shang-chung*)
Middle of the front of the sternum at the midpoint between the nipples.

7. CV-14 (巨闕, *Chü-ch'üeh*)
Immediately below the diaphragm; two sun below the lower extremity of the sternum.

8. SP-12 (衝門, *Ch'ung-men*)
Five sun below points four sun to the right and left of the navel. These points are at the bases of the pelvic joints.

9. TH-4 (陽池, *Yang-ch'ih*)
When the palm is outstretched, on the hand at the back of the wrist a hard, thick muscles becomes apparent. This tsubo is on the little-finger side of that muscle; that is, it is slightly to the little-finger side of the middle of the wrist.

10. LI-4 (合谷, *Ho-ku*)
The point exactly between the thumb and index finger on the back side of the hand.

11. HT-7 (神門, *Shen-men*)
Innermost part of the inner surface of the wrist.

Fig. 9

Fig. 10

Fig. 11

12. ST-36 (足三里, *Tsu-san-li*)
On the outer side of the calf three sun below the knee. Outer edge of the tibia or shin bone.

Fig. 12

13. SP-9 (陰陵泉, *Yin-ling-ch'üan*)
Immediately below the large bone that protrudes just below the knee at the head of the shin.

14. SP-6 (三陰交, *San-yin-chiao*)
Three sun upward on the side of the shin bone from the inner side of the ankle.

(Outer side)

Fig. 13

15. KI-1 (湧泉, *Yung-ch'üan*)
In the center of the arch of the foot immediately behind the bulge of the big toe.

(4) Falling Hair

There are many different kinds of baldness, all brought on by different reasons. The most common is hereditary, pattern baldness that afflicts men in middle years. Another is the distressing round-spot baldness (*alopecia areata*) that sometimes strikes young people. If slight, the condition will clear up naturally, and hair will grow again on the bald spot or spots that have developed. Secondary syphilis causes the hair to fall out in undefined patches. Cold-wave permanents sometimes cause falling hair in women, as do coiffures that involve extensive pulling and tying of the hair. For all of these kinds of baldness, either consult a physician or stop doing whatever is causing the trouble. In one kind of baldness, however, oriental tsubo therapy can be of help; this is the baldness caused by psychological stress. To prevent this condition, use massage, shiatsu, acupuncture, or moxa combustion on the tsubo shown in Figs. 14 through 18. Incidentally, our clinic has success in treating *alopecia areata* by means of moxa therapy on GV-20, BL-10, BL-23, CV-12, CV-4, and LI-4.

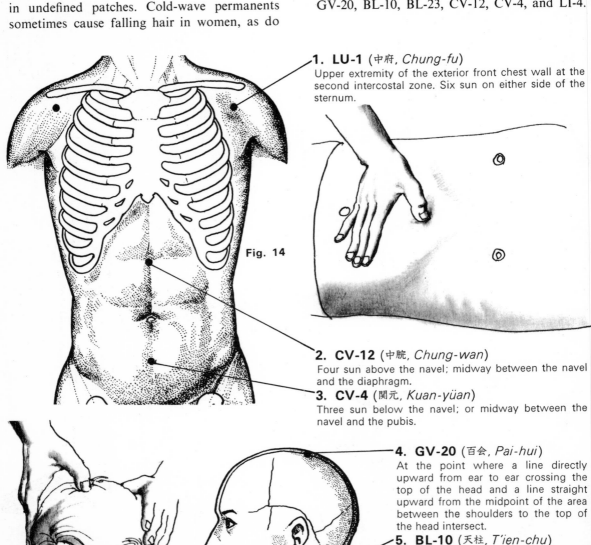

1. LU-1 (中府, *Chung-fu*)
Upper extremity of the exterior front chest wall at the second intercostal zone. Six sun on either side of the sternum.

Fig. 14

2. CV-12 (中脘, *Chung-wan*)
Four sun above the navel; midway between the navel and the diaphragm.

3. CV-4 (関元, *Kuan-yüan*)
Three sun below the navel; or midway between the navel and the pubis.

4. GV-20 (百会, *Pai-hui*)
At the point where a line directly upward from ear to ear crossing the top of the head and a line straight upward from the midpoint of the area between the shoulders to the top of the head intersect.

5. BL-10 (天柱, *T'ien-chu*)
On the outer side of the two large muscles of the neck where they join the back of the head; or the rear hairline.

6. GB-20 (風池, *Feng-ch'ih*)
Depressions in the lower edge of the occiput two sun on either side of BL-10.

Fig. 15

7. GV-14 (大椎, *Ta-ch'ui*)
At the base of the neck in the back between the spinal projections of the seventh cervical and the first thoracic vertebra.

8. GV-12 (身柱, *Shen-chu*)
Below the spinal projections of the third thoracic vertebra.

9. BL-13 (肺俞, *Fei-yü*)
One sun and five bu on either side of the spinal column at points below the spinal projections of the third thoracic vertebra.

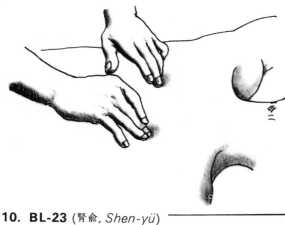

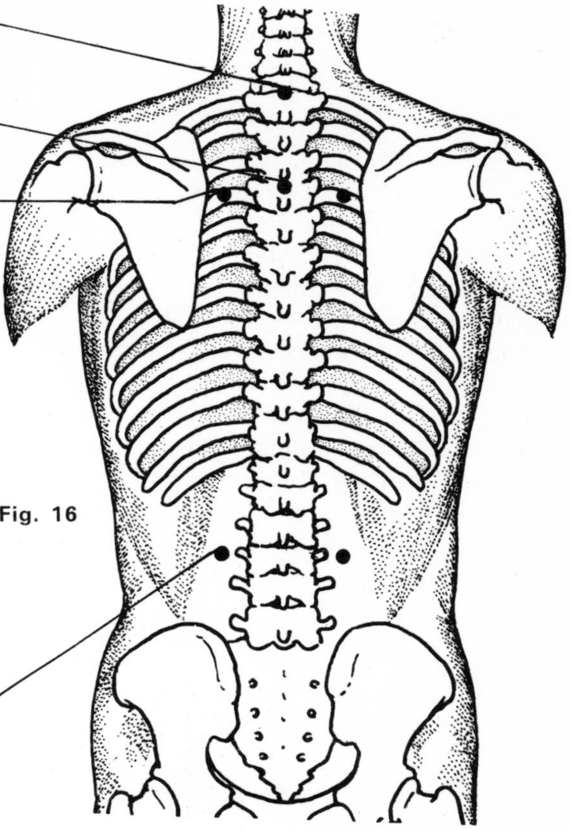

Fig. 16

10. BL-23 (腎俞, *Shen-yü*)
One sun and five bu on either side of the spinal column at points below the spinal projections of the second lumbar vertebra, which is located at the height of the lowest ribs.

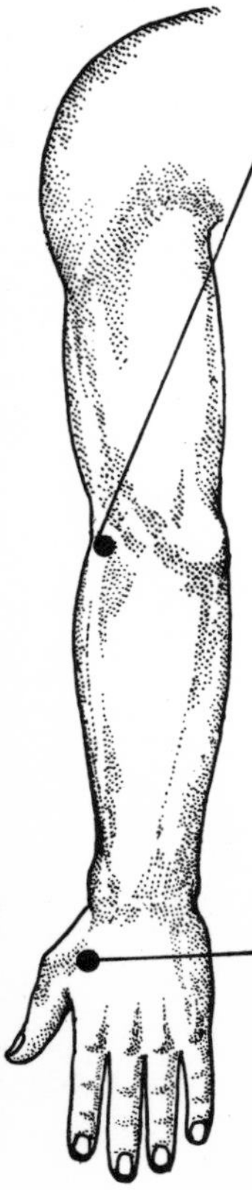

11. LI-11 (曲池, *Ch'ü-ch'ih*)
Thumb side of the bend of the elbow.

Fig. 17

13. LU-6 (孔最, *K'ung-tsui*)
On the thumb side of the inner surface of the forearm at a point about one-third of the distance from the elbow to the wrist.

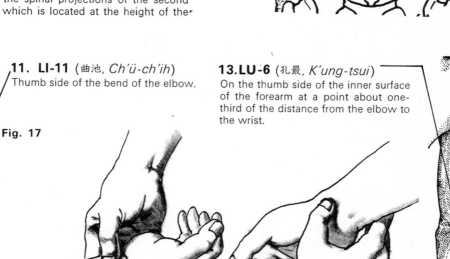

Fig. 18

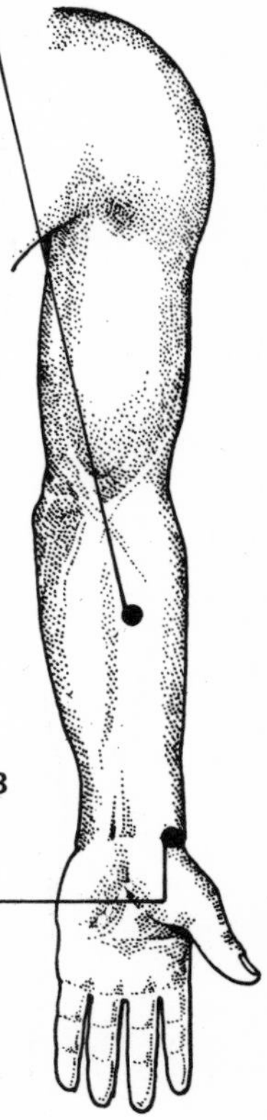

12. LI-4 (合谷, *Ho-ku*)
The point exactly between the thumb and index finger on the back side of the hand.

14. LU-9 (太淵, *T'ai-yüan*)
When the fingers of the hand are outstretched to the maximum, a thick tendon becomes apparent at the base of the thumb. This tsubo is located on the thumb side of that tendon.

Juvenile Sicknesses

(1) Irritability

Some small children are prone to a juvenile neurosis that causes them to cry excessively, throw temper tantrums, and behave in erratic and upsetting ways. Manifestations of this state include thumb sucking beyond infancy and, later, biting of the fingernails. Oriental medical therapy has long prescribed acupuncture for this condition. And, in our clinic, we use a special metal device devised for children. But you do not require special equipment to perform successful treatment in the home. Using something like the blunt end of a toothpick, you can safely and effectively stimulate an infant's sensitive skin and produce an effect as strong as the

acutal insertion of an acupuncture needle produces in an adult. After lightly tapping the areas around the tsubo listed below with the blunt end of a toothpick, massage or perform shiatsu treatment on them: GV-14, GV-12, and BL-18 (Fig. 1).

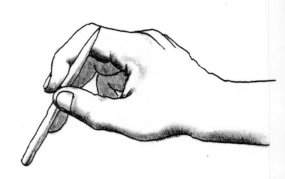

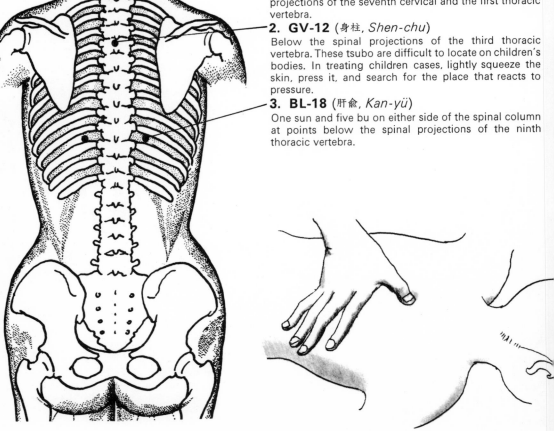

Fig. 1

1. GV-14 (大椎, *Ta-ch'ui*)
At the base of the neck in the back between the spinal projections of the seventh cervical and the first thoracic vertebra.

2. GV-12 (身柱, *Shen-chu*)
Below the spinal projections of the third thoracic vertebra. These tsubo are difficult to locate on children's bodies. In treating children cases, lightly squeeze the skin, press it, and search for the place that reacts to pressure.

3. BL-18 (肝兪, *Kan-yü*)
One sun and five bu on either side of the spinal column at points below the spinal projections of the ninth thoracic vertebra.

Perform the same kind of treatment on CV-15, CV-12, and CV-7 (Fig. 2). The important thing to bear in mind in using the toothpick is to tap the skin lightly and quickly. For infants, shiatsu must be performed lightly.

The treatment outlined here, if performed regularly, will calm the infant's hypersensitive nerves, improve his digestion, and relieve whatever intestinal troubles he may suffer from.

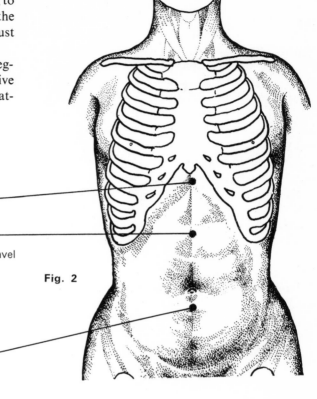

4. CV-15 (鳩尾, *Chiu-wei*)
At the diaphragm.
5. CV-12 (中脘, *Chung-wan*)
Four sun above the navel; midway between the navel and the diaphragm.

Fig. 2

6. CV-7 (陰交, *Yin-chiao*)
One sun below the navel.

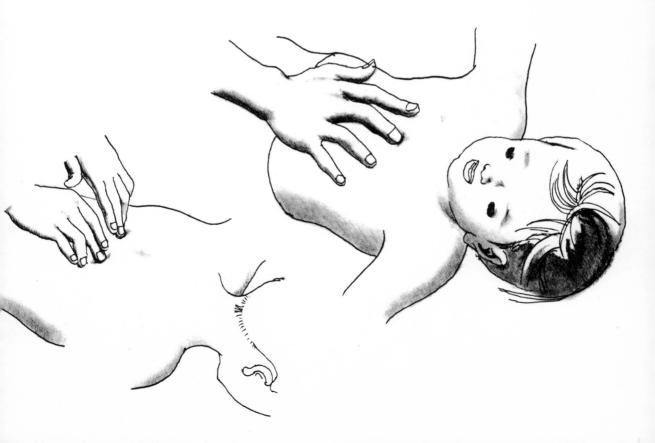

(2) **Bedwetting**

Although the speed at which the habit is developed varies with the child and with his upbringing, most infants learn to control urination before the age of three. Children who frequently wet their clothes or their beds after this age have something wrong with them. In modern cities, many children develop bronchial asthma, which has the side effect of causing bedwetting. In addition to this sickness, kidney, bladder, and urinary-tract disturbances can make a child lose control of his urine. If such seems to be the case, consult a physician at once. But there are other things that lead children to wet themselves. For instance, a child who has been perfectly well behaved in this connection before, may begin to wet his bed shortly after the birth of a little brother or sister. The reason is psychological and relates to a sudden and serious change in the child's way of life. Chilling can cause bedwetting; indeed, most children who are prone to this bad habit are chilly to the touch in the buttocks and legs. To cure the chills and the bedwetting at the same time, shiatsu massage, ordinary massage, and moxa combustion on CV-4 and CV-3 (Fig. 3) are highly effective. In addition, BL-23, BL-47, BL-28 (Fig. 4), ST-36, SP-6, and KI-3 (Figs. 5 and 6) require treatment.

Traditionally, LV-1, located beside the nail on the big toes, has been considered an excellent tsubo for moxa combustion for the prevention of bedwetting. This is not surprising, since the tsubo is connected with the control of the liver, which generates heat. In short, the moxa burned on these tsubo relieves the chills that cause loss of control of urination. Instead of scolding and punishing, cure children of bedwetting by means of moxa combustion, as our clinic did with five of thirty such cases from a large Tokyo children's institution. If ordinary moxa is too uncomfortable for children, use mild moxa.

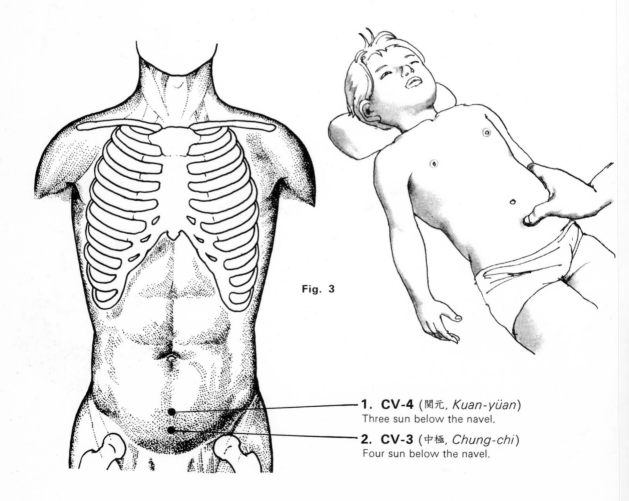

Fig. 3

1. CV-4 (関元, *Kuan-yüan*)
Three sun below the navel.

2. CV-3 (中極, *Chung-chi*)
Four sun below the navel.

Fig. 4

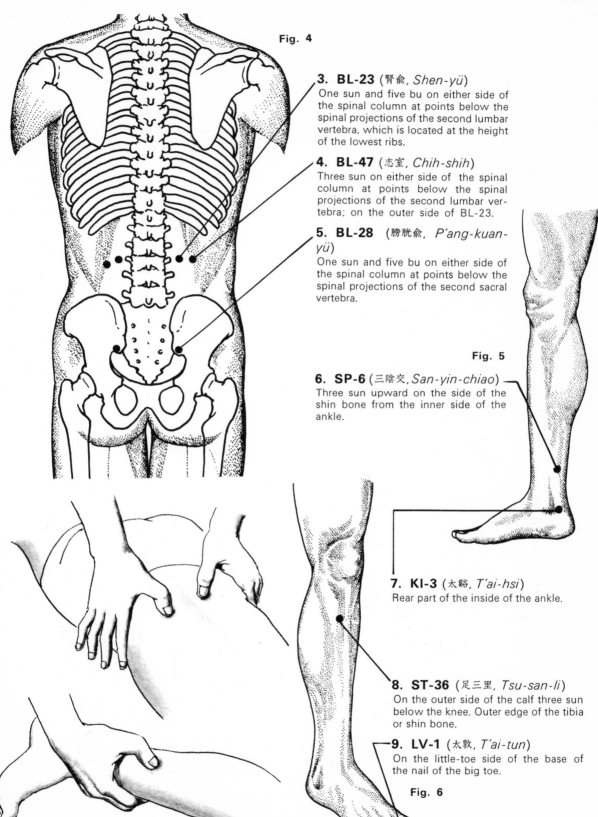

3. BL-23 (腎兪, *Shen-yü*)
One sun and five bu on either side of the spinal column at points below the spinal projections of the second lumbar vertebra, which is located at the height of the lowest ribs.

4. BL-47 (志室, *Chih-shih*)
Three sun on either side of the spinal column at points below the spinal projections of the second lumbar vertebra; on the outer side of BL-23.

5. BL-28 (膀胱兪, *P'ang-kuan-yü*)
One sun and five bu on either side of the spinal column at points below the spinal projections of the second sacral vertebra.

Fig. 5

6. SP-6 (三陰交, *San-yin-chiao*)
Three sun upward on the side of the shin bone from the inner side of the ankle.

7. KI-3 (太谿, *T'ai-hsi*)
Rear part of the inside of the ankle.

8. ST-36 (足三里, *Tsu-san-li*)
On the outer side of the calf three sun below the knee. Outer edge of the tibia or shin bone.

9. LV-1 (太敦, *T'ai-tun*)
On the little-toe side of the base of the nail of the big toe.

Fig. 6

(3) Poliomyelitis

Poliomyelitis, an acute, highly infectious disease caused by a virus that invades the gray matter of the spinal cord, was formerly very much dreaded, though, fortunately, thanks to the development of the Salk vaccine, it is no longer as feared as it once was. About 90 percent of cases of the sickness, which strikes most often in summer and early autumn, are subclinical. This means that, after two or three days of fever, headaches, and diarrhea, the disease is cured. In more serious cases, after these primary symptoms have disappeared, the patient becomes paralyzed in his

Fig. 7

hands or legs because virus inflammation in the spinal cord obstructs the passage of impulses from the brain. Since the immobilized parts of the bodies of polio victims are very cold, they should be treated with hot compresses before massage. When the flesh is quite warm, massage along the meridians shown in the chart. Pay special attention to massage of the buttocks and the shoulder blades in order to strengthen the muscles in these areas.

Using the four fingers and the thumbs of each hand, massage along the sternomastoid muscle and clavicles in the directions of the arrows in Fig. 7. Massage along the ribs, abdomen, knees, and legs in a similar way (Fig. 8). Continue by rubbing the meridians on the back (Fig. 9) and those on both arms and both legs (Figs. 10 through 12). The following tsubo must be the major points of concern in massage: GV-14, SI-14, BL-25, LI-14, LI-11, LI-10, LU-9, and LI-4. In addition, the follow tsubo are effective in treating spinal infantile paralysis: BL-22, BL-23, ST-34, and ST-36. While performing the massage, do not allow the child to lie still. Instead, keep him moving as much as possible.

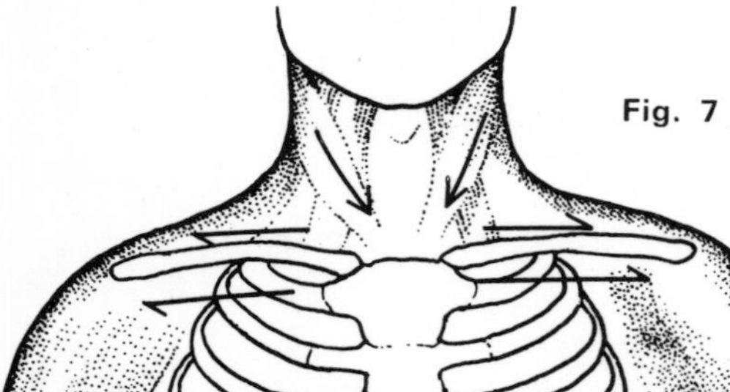

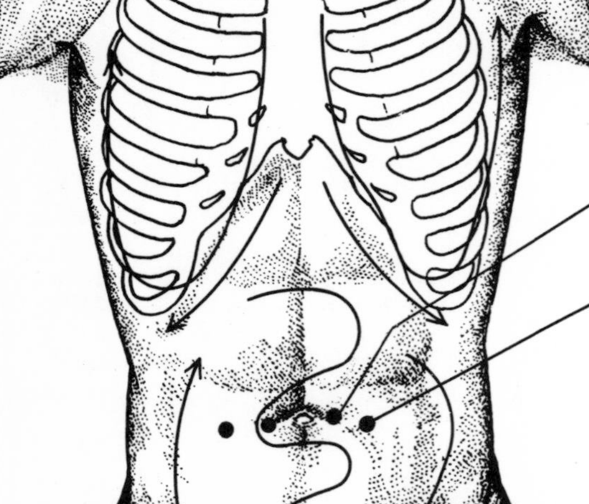

1. ST-25 (天枢, *T'ien-shu*)
Two sun on either side of the navel. Easily found by lining the thumb and index and middle fingers on either side of the navel.

2. KI-16 (肓俞, *Huang-yü*)
Points located five sun on either side of the navel.

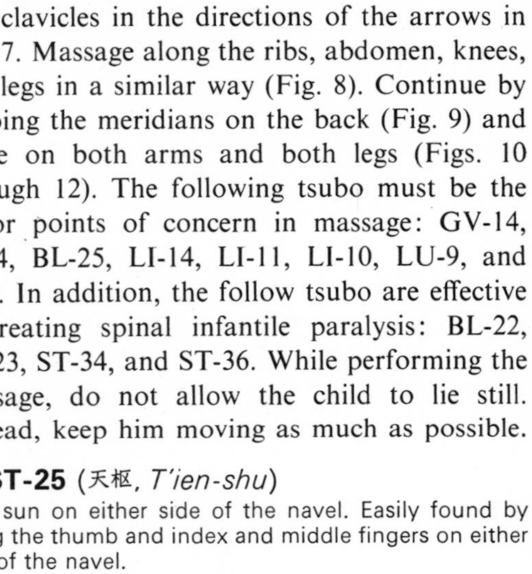

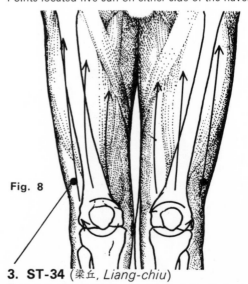

Fig. 8

3. ST-34 (梁丘, *Liang-chiu*)
Two sun above the upper edge of the kneecap. This can be easily located by fully extending the knee and finding the upper end of the groove formed on the outside of the kneecap. In other words, it is on the front of the thigh, two sun above the upper outer edge of the kneecap.

4. GV-14 (大椎, *Ta-ch'ui*)
At the base of the neck in the back between the spinal projections of the seventh cervical and the first thoracic vertebra.

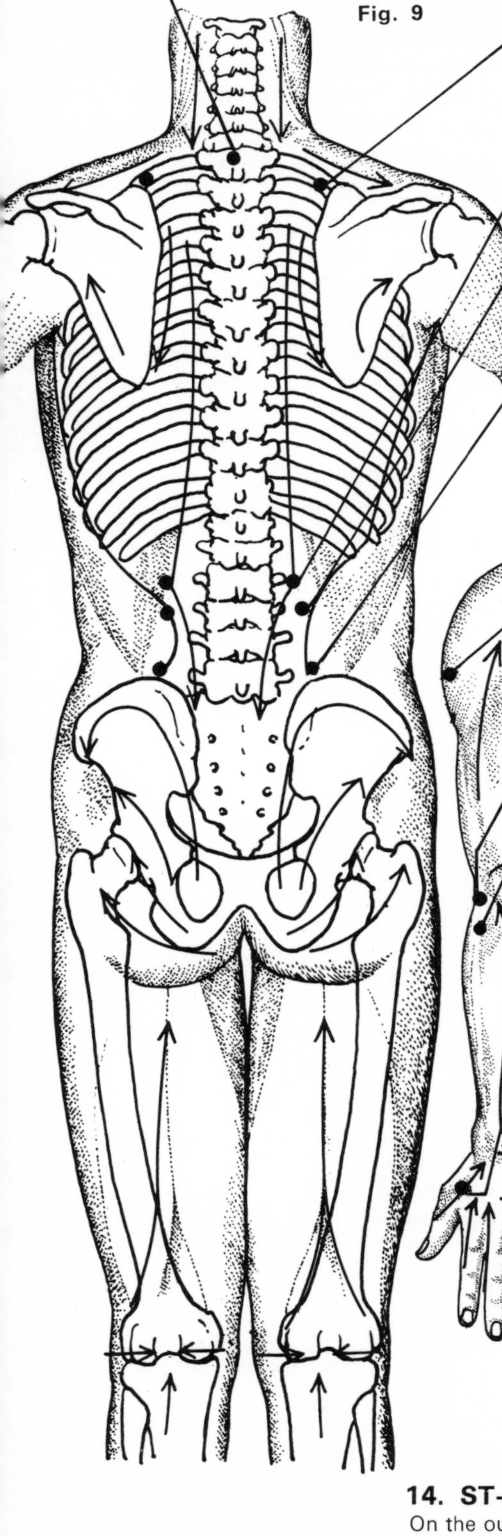

Fig. 9

5. SI-14 (肩外俞, *Chien-wai-yü*)
Below the first thoracic vertebra. About two sun on either side of the spinal column at the upper corner of the inner side of the shoulder blades.

6. BL-22 (三焦俞, *San-chiao-yü*)
One sun and five bu on either side of the spinal column at points below the first lumbar vertebra.

7. BL-23 (腎俞, *Shen-yü*)
One sun and five bu on either side of the spinal column at points below the spinal projections of the second lumbar vertebra, which is located at the height of the lowest ribs.

8. BL-25 (大腸俞, *Ta-ch'ang-yü*)
One sun and five bu on either side of the spinal column at points below the spinal projections of the fourth lumbar vertebra.

9. LU-9 (太淵, *T'ai-yüan*)
When the fingers of the hand are outstretched to the maximum, a thick tendon becomes apparent at the base of the thumb. This tsubo is located on the thumb side of that tendon.

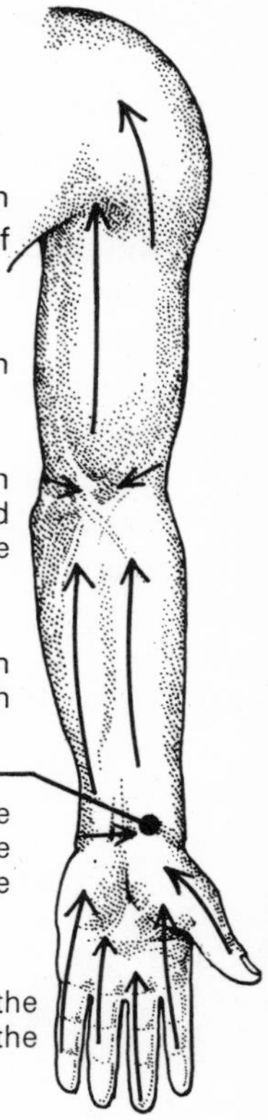

10. LI-14 (臂臑, *Pi-nao*)
About seven sun above LI-11 on the thumb side of the upper arm; at the place in the upper arm where the triceps muscle gradually tapers to a tendon.

11. LI-11 (曲池, *Ch'ü-ch'ih*)
Thumb side of the bend of the elbow.

12. LI-10 (三里, *San-li*)
Point on the thumb side of the forearm in line with the index finger and two sun from the bend of the elbow.

13. LI-4 (合谷, *Ho-ku*)
The point exactly between the thumb and index finger on the back side of the hand.

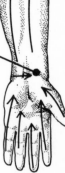

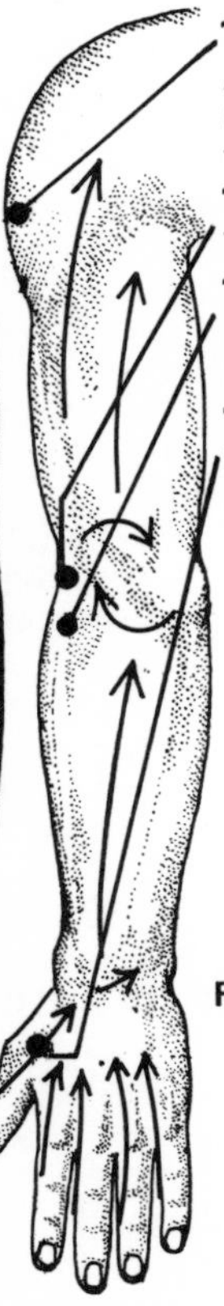

Fig. 10

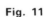

Fig. 11

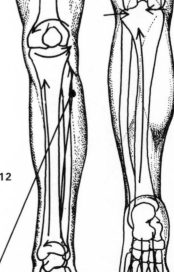

Fig. 12

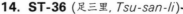

14. ST-36 (足三里, *Tsu-san-li*)
On the outer side of the calf three sun below the knee. Outer edge of the tibia or shin bone.

(4) Cerebral Palsy

In contrast to infantile paralysis, which attacks after birth and can be prevented by means of vaccines, cerebral palsy is either hereditary or caused by viruses attacking the prenatal fetus or the infant at birth. There is no known cure for it; and, in may parts of the world today, facilities to treat and care for the victims, who cannot control their muscular movements and are sometimes mentally retarded, are far from adequate. Although it cannot cure cerebral palsy, tsubo therapy, if performed regularly and over a long period of time, can lessen spasms and rigidity in the limbs of patients.

Treatment is performed on the head, arms, abdomen, back, and legs as shown in the charts.

Since the trouble arises in the head, begin by treating GV-20 and BL-10 (Fig. 13). Continue by performing massage or shiatsu massage on the following tsubo: GV-14, LI-15, BL-17, BL-21, BL-23, BL-25 (Fig. 14), LI-11 (Fig. 15), CV-15, CV-14, LV-14, CV-12, ST-25, CV-4, LV-11, LV-9 (Fig. 16), SP-9, and SP-6 (Fig. 17).

Massage and shiatsu as well as moderate and regular moxa combustion on these tsubo are certain to produce results as long as they are used regularly and for a long time. In conjunction with these treatments, have the patient join his hands behind his head and execute situps. He should then try relaxing exercises to relieve bodily tension and he should sit cross-legged on the floor and practice holding his head in a straight position.

Fig. 13

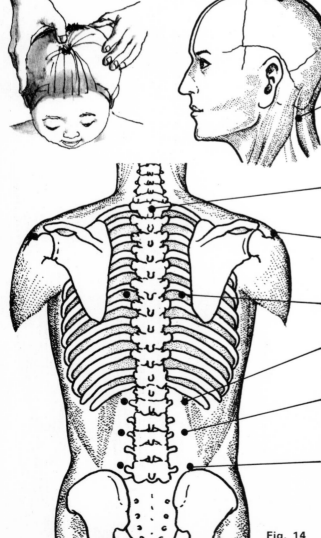

1. GV-20 (百会, *Pai-hui*)
At the point where a line directly upward from ear to ear crossing the top of the head and a line straight upward from the midpoint of the area between the shoulders to the top of the head intersect.

2. BL-10 (天柱, *T'ien-chu*)
On the outer side of the two large muscles of the neck where they join the back of the head.

3. GV-14 (大椎, *Ta-ch'ui*)
At the base of the neck in the back between the spinal projections of the seventh cervical and the first thoracic vertebra.

4. LI-15 (肩髃, *Chien-yü*)
At the depression between the tip of the shoulder and the triceps muscle when the arm is held outstretched in a horizontal position. Thumb-side of the upper arm at the tip of the acromion process.

5. BL-17 (膈俞, *Ke-yü*)
One sun and five bu on either side of the spinal column at points below the seventh thoracic vertebra.

6. BL-21 (胃俞, *Wei-yü*)
One sun and five bu on either side of the spinal column at points below the spinal projections of the twelfth thoracic vertebra.

7. BL-23 (腎俞, *Shen-yü*)
One sun and five bu on either side of the spinal column at points below the spinal projections of the second lumbar vertebra, which is located at the height of the lowest ribs.

8. BL-25 (大腸俞, *Ta-ch'ang-yü*)
One sun and five bu on either side of the spinal column at points below the spinal projections of the fourth lumbar vertebra.

Fig. 14

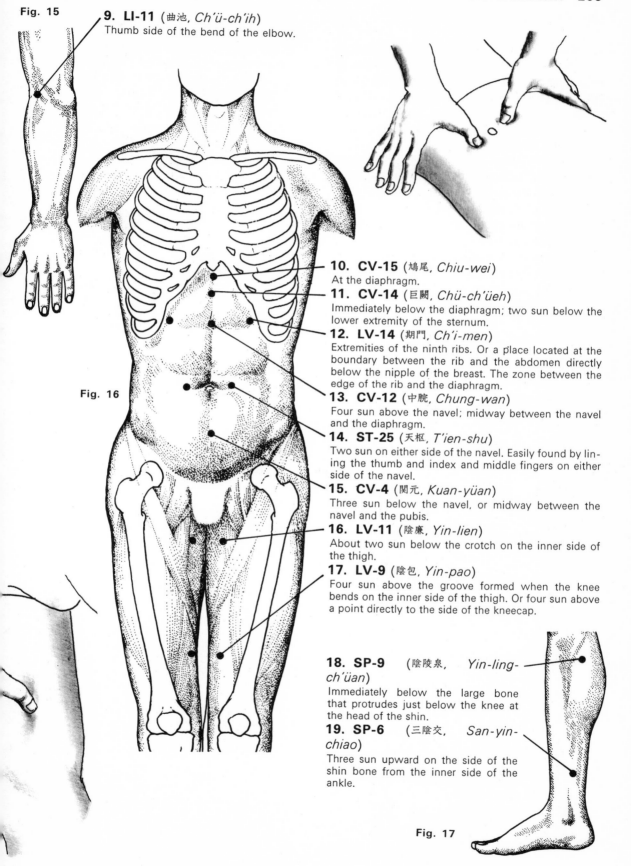

Fig. 15

9. LI-11 (曲池, *Ch'ü-ch'ih*)
Thumb side of the bend of the elbow.

Fig. 16

10. CV-15 (鳩尾, *Chiu-wei*)
At the diaphragm.

11. CV-14 (巨闕, *Chü-ch'üeh*)
Immediately below the diaphragm; two sun below the lower extremity of the sternum.

12. LV-14 (期門, *Ch'i-men*)
Extremities of the ninth ribs. Or a place located at the boundary between the rib and the abdomen directly below the nipple of the breast. The zone between the edge of the rib and the diaphragm.

13. CV-12 (中脘, *Chung-wan*)
Four sun above the navel; midway between the navel and the diaphragm.

14. ST-25 (天枢, *T'ien-shu*)
Two sun on either side of the navel. Easily found by lining the thumb and index and middle fingers on either side of the navel.

15. CV-4 (関元, *Kuan-yüan*)
Three sun below the navel, or midway between the navel and the pubis.

16. LV-11 (陰廉, *Yin-lien*)
About two sun below the crotch on the inner side of the thigh.

17. LV-9 (陰包, *Yin-pao*)
Four sun above the groove formed when the knee bends on the inner side of the thigh. Or four sun above a point directly to the side of the kneecap.

18. SP-9 (陰陵泉, *Yin-ling-ch'üan*)
Immediately below the large bone that protrudes just below the knee at the head of the shin.

19. SP-6 (三陰交, *San-yin-chiao*)
Three sun upward on the side of the shin bone from the inner side of the ankle.

Fig. 17

(5) Night Crying

To calm a baby who is crying at night, disturbing his mother and father and conceivably keeping awake the people in the next house, massage GV-12 (Fig. 18). The bodies of infants are small enough to make the locating of some of the tsubo difficult. Find this one by lightly massaging from the hairline on the rear of the neck toward the shoulders. When pressure is applied to the point where GV-12 is located, the baby will sharply move his body or react in some other way. Traditionally, in the Orient, moxa—very mild— is burned on this point. But more advisable for home therapy is massage or shiatsu centering on GV-12 and including BL-18 and BL-23. Massage lightly and slowly with the tips of the thumbs. Pressure must be light (no more than from 500 grams to 1 kilogram).

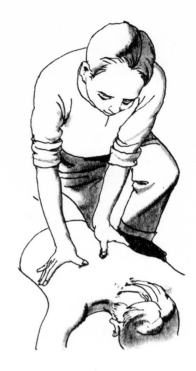

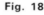

1. GV-12 (身柱, *Shen-chu*)
Below the spinal projections of the third thoracic vertebra.

Fig. 18

2. BL-18 (肝兪, *Kan-yü*)
One sun and five bu on either side of the spinal column at points below the spinal projections of the ninth thoracic vertebra.

3. BL-23 (腎兪, *Shen-yü*)
One sun and five bu on either side of the spinal column at points below the spinal projections of the second lumbar vertebra, which is located at the height of the lowest ribs.

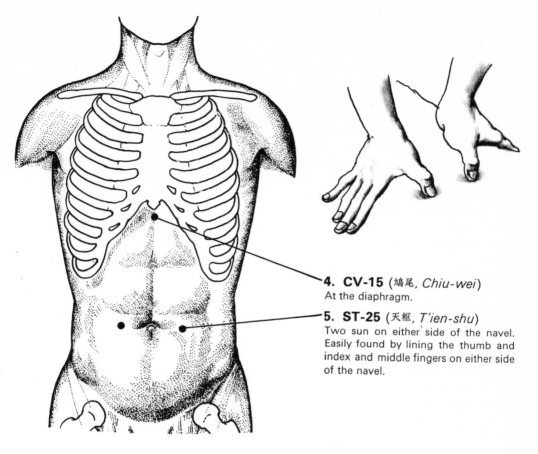

4. CV-15 (鳩尾, *Chiu-wei*)
At the diaphragm.

5. ST-25 (天枢, *T'ien-shu*)
Two sun on either side of the navel.
Easily found by lining the thumb and
index and middle fingers on either side
of the navel.

Fig. 19

Continue by massaging CV-15 and ST-25 (Fig.
19). Magnetized metal balls and adhesive tape
too may be used to produce a calming effect on a
crying baby.

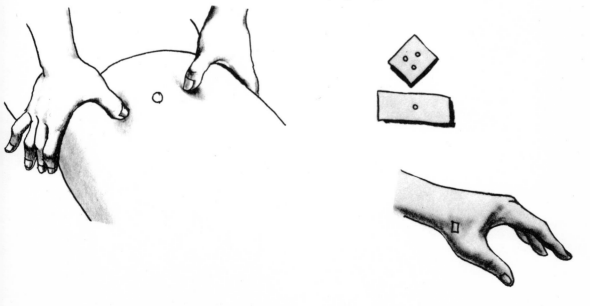

Female Complaints

(1) Menstrual Pains

Some women never experience menstrual pains, some have them in mild degrees, and some suffer so severely that they must take medicines and go to bed in order to bear up under the attack. In a few cases, the pains are mild at first and grow worse, whereas the reverse is frequently true. About half of all women experience tolerable pains on the first day of the menstrual period. Some have pains in the lower abdominal region for from two to three days before the beginning of the menstrual period. The pains may last for from two to three days longer than the period and may force the woman to go to bed. Frequently, women experience headaches, pains in the breast, and anxiety a week before the menstrual period begins. The pains are caused by contractions of muscles in the uterus in the effort to force out the menstrual flux. If the muscles of the uterus are strong, severe pains result; if the mouth of the uterus is wide, pain does not occur. In most cases, the pain is

no greater than the woman can bear; consequently, putting up with the situation becomes a matter of monthly habit. For such people, I recommend massage and shiatsu performed on the tsubo listed below for alleviation of the unpleasantness of this unavoidable condition.

Begin with massage or shiatsu on BL-22, BL-23, BL-31, BL-33, BL-34, and BL-48 (Fig. 1). Continue with similar treatment on CV-12, CV-6, CV-4, ST-27, KI-12, and CV-3 (Fig. 3). Treatment is made more effective if you massage LI-4, KI-9, SP-6, and KI-3 (Figs. 2 and 4). If menstrual pains are prolonged or rendered severe by tumors in the uterine muscles or by serious uterine metrectopy, consult a physician.

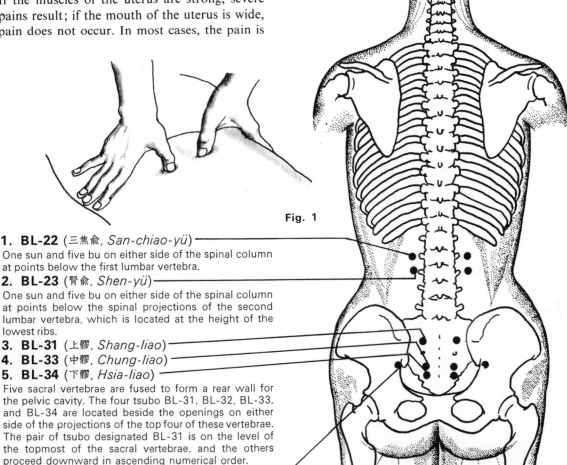

Fig. 1

1. BL-22 (三焦俞, *San-chiao-yü*)
One sun and five bu on either side of the spinal column at points below the first lumbar vertebra.

2. BL-23 (腎俞, *Shen-yü*)
One sun and five bu on either side of the spinal column at points below the spinal projections of the second lumbar vertebra, which is located at the height of the lowest ribs.

3. BL-31 (上髎, *Shang-liao*)
4. BL-33 (中髎, *Chung-liao*)
5. BL-34 (下髎, *Hsia-liao*)
Five sacral vertebrae are fused to form a rear wall for the pelvic cavity. The four tsubo BL-31, BL-32, BL-33, and BL-34 are located beside the openings on either side of the projections of the top four of these vertebrae. The pair of tsubo designated BL-31 is on the level of the topmost of the sacral vertebrae, and the others proceed downward in ascending numerical order.

6. BL-48 (胞肓, *Pao-huang*)
Three sun on either side of the spinal column at points below the second sacral vertebra.

7. LI-4 (合谷, *Ho-ku*)
The point exactly between the thumb and index finger on the back side of the hand.

Fig. 2

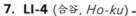

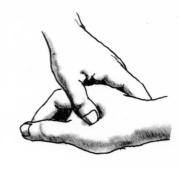

8. CV-12 (中脘, *Chung-wan*)
Four sun above the navel; midway between the navel and the diaphragm.
9. CV-6 (気海, *Ch'i-hai*)
One sun and five bu below the navel.
10. CV-4 (関元, *Kuan-yüan*)
Three sun below the navel.
11. ST-27 (大巨, *Ta-chü*)
Two sun below points two sun on either side of the navel.

Fig. 3

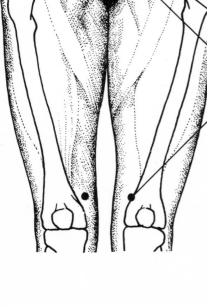

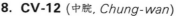

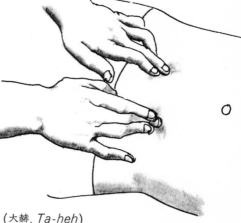

12. KI-12 (大赫, *Ta-heh*)
Four sun below points five bu on either side of the navel.
13. CV-3 (中極, *Chung-chi*)
Four sun below the navel.
14. SP-10 (血海, *Hsüeh-hai*)
Two sun and five bu above the kneecap on the inner side of the thigh.

15. KI-9 (築賓, *Chu-pin*)
In the muscle that is the width of the index finger inward from the edge of the shin at a point five sun above the inner side of the ankle.
16. SP-6 (三陰交, *San-yin-chiao*)
Three sun upward on the side of the shin bone from the inner side of the ankle.
17. KI-3 (太谿, *T'ai-hsi*)
Rear part of the inside of the ankle.

Fig. 4

(2) **Menstrual Irregularity**

Emotional disturbances, sudden shocks, weather, insufficient nourishment or sleep, overwork, and many other conditions can influence a woman's menstrual period and make her irregular. The diencephalon—the interbrain between the right and left lobes of the brain—controls human emotions and the secretion of the hormone produced by the anterior lobe of the hypophysis of the pituitary gland. It is this hormone that regulates ovulation. Consequently, since emotional upsets influence the diencephalon, they simultaneously influence ovulation regularity.

Ordinarily, the menstrual period occurs roughly once in four weeks; that is, two weeks after the development of the ovum. Irregularities in the production of the pituitary hormone make it impossible to predict menstrual periods with any certainty. Sometimes menstruation occurs at intervals of less than twenty days. Sometimes it occurs only once in two or three months. There are some cases in which it does not take place for as long as six months and others in which the periods of ovulation and nonovulation become confused. To put ovulation and the menstrual cycle back on a regular schedule, the production of the hormone of the pituitary gland must be returned to normal. To do this, lead a regular life with adequate nourishing food and sleep, strive to remain emotionally stable, and practice the shiatsu and massage outlined below.

Perform massage or shiatsu massage on GV-4 and BL-23. BL-23 is traditionally believed to control the energy with which the body is congenitally endowed. BL-22 controls the energy the body receives after birth. Continue treatment by massaging BL-22, BL-47, BL-31, BL-32, BL-33, and BL-34 (Fig. 5). Next, press CV-6, CV-4, ST-27, and SP-10 (Fig. 7). Treatment of GV-20, GV-19, GV-21, BL-10, and GB-20 (Fig. 6) relieves the headaches and heaviness in the head that often accompany menstrual irregularity. For chills in the feet, perform shiatsu massage on KI-9, KI-7, and KI-3 (Fig. 7). All of the tsubo listed here are traditonally considered excellent places for moxa combustion in connection with curing menstrual irregularity. Women who are prone to this complaint must take care to keep their feet warm. They would be well-advised to wear stockings while sleeping.

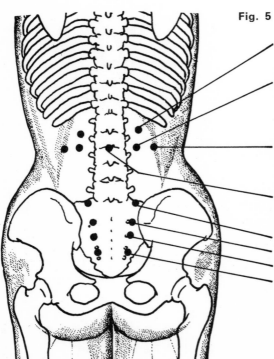

Fig. 5

1. BL-22 (三焦兪, *San-chiao-yü*)
One sun and five bu on either side of the spinal column at points below the first lumbar vertebra.

2. BL-23 (腎兪, *Shen-yü*)
One sun and five bu on either side of the spinal column at points below the spinal projections of the second lumbar vertebra, which is located at the height of the lowest ribs.

3. BL-47 (志室, *Chih-shih*)
Three sun on either side of the spinal column at points below the spinal projections of the second lumbar vertebra; on the outer sides of BL-23.

4. GV-4 (命門, *Ming-men*)
Between BL-23 and below the spinal projections of the second lumbar vertebra.

5. BL-31 (上髎, *Shang-liao*)
6. BL-32 (次髎, *Tz'u-liao*)
7. BL-33 (中髎, *Chung-liao*)
8. BL-34 (下髎, *Hsia-liao*)
These four sets of tsubo are located adjacent to the sacral hiatuses of the four fused sacral vertebra.

Fig. 6

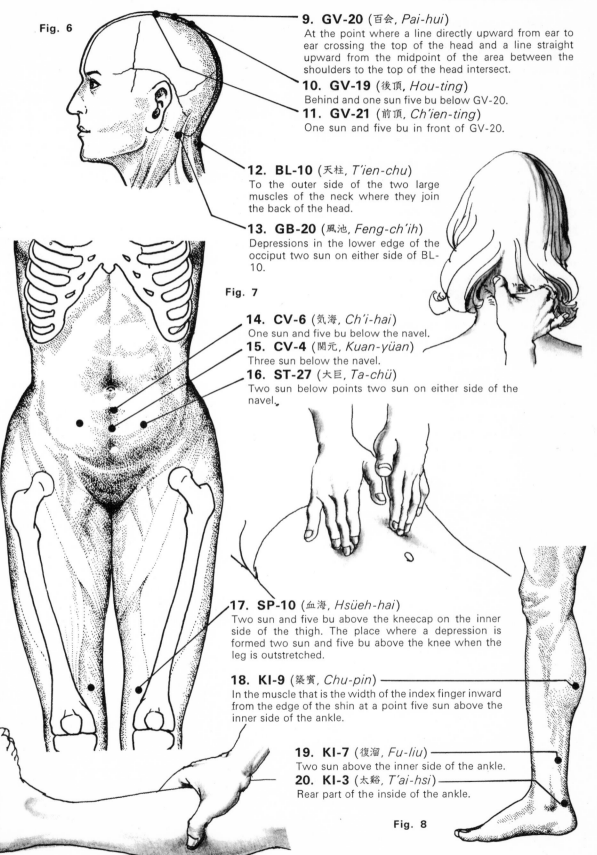

9. GV-20 (百会, *Pai-hui*)
At the point where a line directly upward from ear to ear crossing the top of the head and a line straight upward from the midpoint of the area between the shoulders to the top of the head intersect.

10. GV-19 (後頂, *Hou-ting*)
Behind and one sun five bu below GV-20.

11. GV-21 (前頂, *Ch'ien-ting*)
One sun and five bu in front of GV-20.

12. BL-10 (天柱, *T'ien-chu*)
To the outer side of the two large muscles of the neck where they join the back of the head.

13. GB-20 (風池, *Feng-ch'ih*)
Depressions in the lower edge of the occiput two sun on either side of BL-10.

Fig. 7

14. CV-6 (気海, *Ch'i-hai*)
One sun and five bu below the navel.

15. CV-4 (関元, *Kuan-yüan*)
Three sun below the navel.

16. ST-27 (大巨, *Ta-chü*)
Two sun below points two sun on either side of the navel.

17. SP-10 (血海, *Hsüeh-hai*)
Two sun and five bu above the kneecap on the inner side of the thigh. The place where a depression is formed two sun and five bu above the knee when the leg is outstretched.

18. KI-9 (築賓, *Chu-pin*)
In the muscle that is the width of the index finger inward from the edge of the shin at a point five sun above the inner side of the ankle.

19. KI-7 (復溜, *Fu-liu*)
Two sun above the inner side of the ankle.

20. KI-3 (太谿, *T'ai-hsi*)
Rear part of the inside of the ankle.

Fig. 8

(3) Insufficient Lactation

Breast feeding is the ideal nourishment for infants; consequently, mothers ought to feel responsible for eating proper, wholesome foods that enable them to produce the kind of milk their babies require to grow strong. In addition, women must avoid artificial food preservatives and chemical additives that, in the modern world of environmental pollution, can cause harm to mother and baby alike. But there are women who, even though carefully controlling their own diets, find that they fail to lactate sufficiently.

In each breast are mammary glands, each composed of from fifteen to twenty lobes. Each lobe carries a vessel connecting it to the nipple of the breast. Fat is packed among the lobes of the mammary glands, and it is this fat that gives the breasts their tactile texture and their size and shape.

A number of reasons can be advanced for poor lactation. First the mammary glands themselves may be underdeveloped and may fail to produce milk, even after the child has been born. Sometimes, on the other hand, milk congests in the breast. This state of affairs causes inflammation which, in turn, reduces the flow of lactation. When this happens, the entire breast becomes red, feverish, and sore. Lumps in the breast may reduce lactation. Breast cancer is the most feared cause of such lumps. But not all cases of this abnormality can be traced to cancer, for in some instances fat among the lobes of the mammary glands hardens and produces knotty structures. By compressing the vessels connecting the glands and the nipple, these lumps of fat reduce lactation. This condition is frequent with first births. In a number of instances, the way the baby sucks the nipple weakens the flow. This too has adverse effects on the amounts of milk produced by the mammary glands.

Although, because it directly stimulates the breasts, massage is an excellent treatment for insufficient lactation, it can have harmful effects if cancer or inflammation of the mammary membrane is involved. Therefore, careful diagnosis of the case must be made before treatment is begun.

Once it has been ascertained that neither of these conditions is present, begin treatment of the breasts with a hot compress. Make the compress of a thick towel and allow it to remain in place for from ten to fifteen minutes. Then, spreading the thumb and index finger wide, grip the base of the breast (Fig. 9) and, with a slight twisting motion, massage toward the nipple. Repeat this several times.

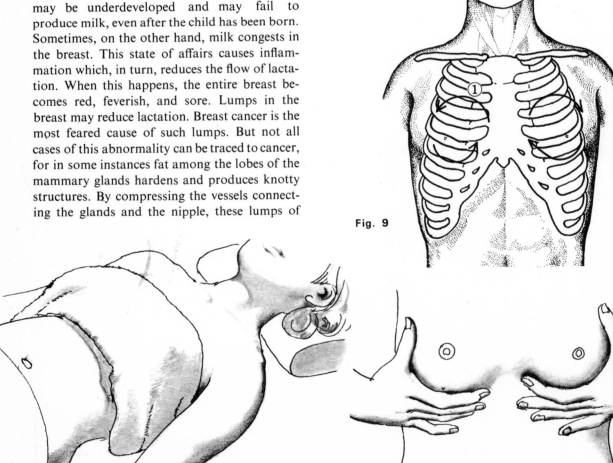

Fig. 9

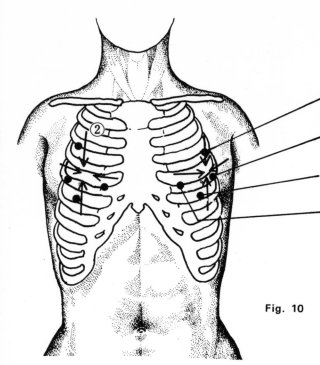

Fig. 10

1. ST-16 (膺窓, *Yin-chuang*)
On the line connecting the nipples; at the sternum at the third ribs.

2. SP-18 (天谿, *T'ien-hsi*)
Slightly above the fourth ribs two sun to the outer sides of ST-17.

3. ST-18 (乳根, *Ju-ken*)
About two fingers' width below ST-17; between the fifth and sixth ribs.

4. KI-23 (神封, *Shen-feng*)
Two sun to the right and left of the sternum slightly above the fourth ribs. Or points at the height of the nipples two sun to the right and left of a line from the base of the throat to the diaphragm.

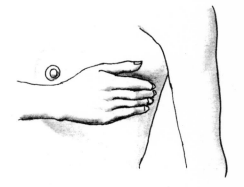

Then, gripping the breast, massage in the vicinities of the tsubo shown in Figs. 10 and 11. Massage toward the nipple. Next, carefully stroke the skin from the armpit to the nipple. Finally, gripping the breast at ST-17, pull and shake it lightly. Wipe the breast carefully with absorbent cotton dipped in hot water or in a 2-percent boric-acid solution. The entire treatment, including the hot pack, takes from twenty to thirty minutes; it must be repeated daily.

5. LU-1 (中府, *Chung-fu*)
Upper extremity of the exterior front chest wall at the second intercostal zone. Six sun on either side of the sternum.

6. ST-17 (乳中, *Ju-chung*)
The middles of the nipples.

Fig. 11

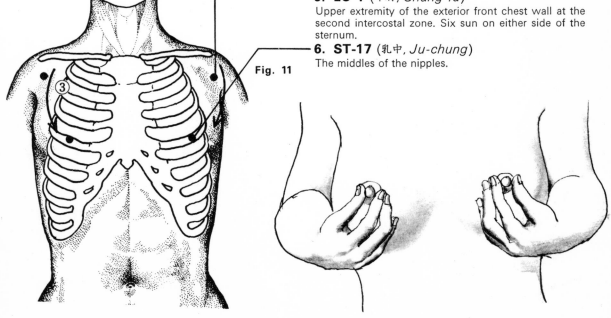

(4) Barrenness

When man and wife find it impossible to have children, the cause is on the male side in from 40 to 60 percent of all cases. If the woman is physiologically incapable of conceiving, she is usually the victim of one of the following three categories of disturbances: failure to ovulate, abnormality of the Fallopian tubes, abnormality of the uterus. In the first case, ovulation may take place; but it is rare, and the ova are abnormal. Furthermore, there is likely to be an irregularity in the production of the hormones regulating the functioning of the ovaries. In the second case, most frequently, there is an obstruction in the Fallopian tubes, through which the ova must pass to reach the uterus. Some of the main causes of cases of the third category include disturbance of the uterine membrane caused by invasion by tuberculosis bacilli, irregular development of the uterus, and uterine tumor. In addition to these factors, diabetes, Basedow's disease, malnutrition, and psychological stress can adversely influence female physiology and bring on barrenness. There is no tsubo on which treatment can immediately cure barrenness and enable a woman to bear children. The oriental therapeutic method is to strive to put the woman's body in excellent physical condition and, in this way, contribute to the cure of the problem.

First perform massage or shiatsu massage on KI-16, CV-6, and CV-3 (Fig. 12). Then treat SP-6 (Fig. 13) in the same way. Next massage or perform shiatsu on BL-23, GV-4, BL-33, and BL-48 (Fig. 14). If the cause of the barrenness is understood, medical or other treatment can be implemented. But when a married couple cannot have children for no ascertainable reason, patient and persevering oriental tsubo therapy may be the source of the help they need.

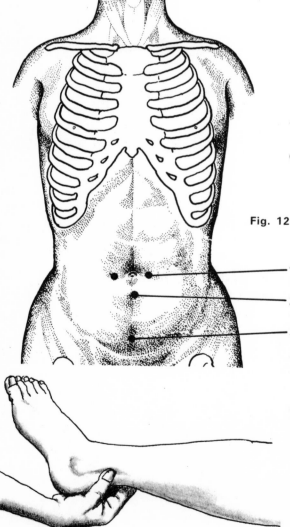

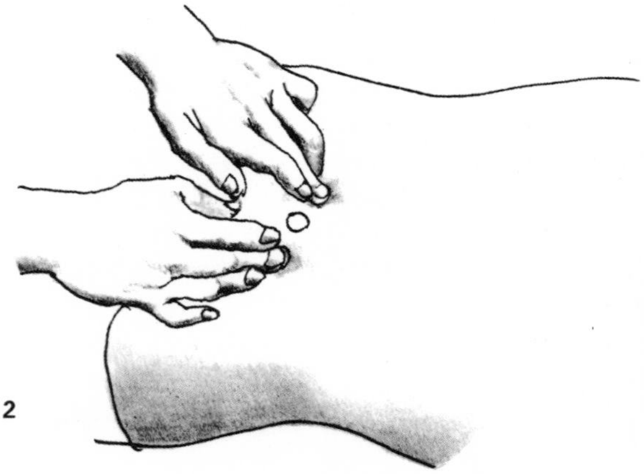

Fig. 12

1. KI-16 (肓兪, *Huang-yü*)
Points located five sun on either side of the navel.

2. CV-6 (気海, *Ch'i-hai*)
One sun and five bu below the navel.

3. CV-3 (中極, *Chung-chi*)
Four sun below the navel, or at points four-fifths of the way between the navel and the pubis.

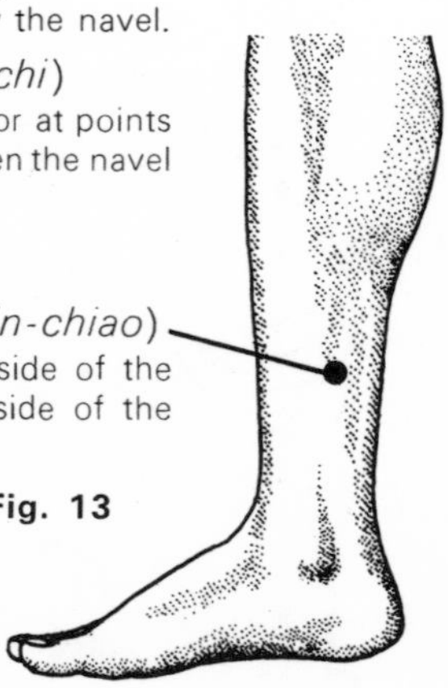

4. SP-6 (三陰交, *San-yin-chiao*)
Three sun upward on the side of the shin bone from the inner side of the ankle.

Fig. 13

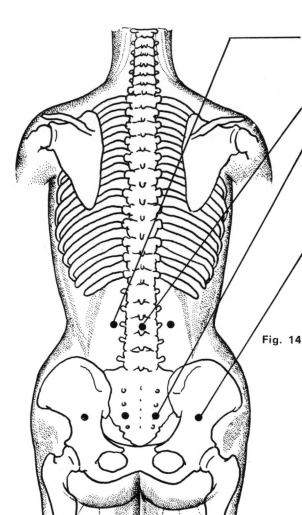

Fig. 14

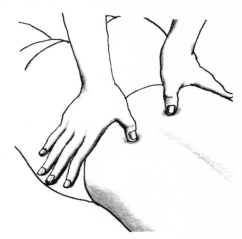

5. BL-23 (腎俞, *Shen-yü*)

One sun and five bu on either side of the spinal column at points below the spinal projections of the second lumbar vertebra, which is located at the height of the lowest ribs.

6. GV-4 (命門, *Ming-men*)

Between BL-23 and below the spinal projections of the second lumbar vertebra.

7. BL-33 (中髎, *Chung-liao*)

Five sacral vertebrae are fused to form a rear wall for the pelvic cavity. The four tsubo BL-31, BL-32, BL-33, and BL-34 are located beside the openings on either side of the projections of the top four of these vertebrae. The pair of tsubo designated BL-31 is on the level of the topmost of the sacral vertebrae, and the others proceed downward in ascending numerical order.

8. BL-48 (胞肓, *Pao-huang*)

Three sun on either side of the spinal column at points below the second sacral vertebra.

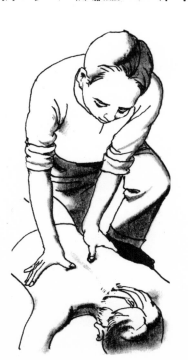

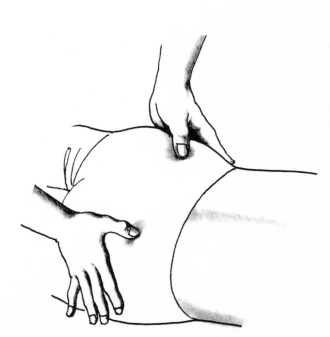

(5) Chilling

Because this kind of irregularity is not fatal or even extremely serious, little research has been done on it, and the exact causes have not been firmly established. In general, however, the explanation for chilling is as follows. The large cavities of the body—those housing the brain, the lungs, and the abdominal organs—must maintain a temperature of 36.5 degrees centigrade. The maintaining of this temperature is the function of the blood. During the summer, when surrounding temperatures are high, blood flows away from the body cavities to the surface, where internal temperatures are reduced as a consequence of the secretion and evaporation of sweat. In the winter, however, when surrounding temperatures are low, the blood flows from the extremities of the body to the cavities to warm them and to maintain the internal temperature required for normal functioning. The autonomic nervous system controls this regulation of the circulation system. And the operation of the autonomic nervous system is closely related to the secretion of various hormones by the different glands of the body. Consequently, irregularity in these glands causes the autonomic nervous system to fail to function as it ought to do and, in this way, affects the circulation of blood and

brings about either chilling or flushing. The temperatures of the cool parts of the body of a person subject to chilling will be found to be considerably lower than those of the other parts.

This condition is especially prevalent among thin women in menopause and thin girls at the age of puberty. Irregularities in the thyroid gland and the adrenal cortex can lower body temperatures and make it difficult for people to tolerate winter weather or even air-conditioned rooms in summer. When anemia is the cause, chilling is sometimes accompanied by palpitations and shortness of breath. The chilling generally manifests itself in the extremities and in the region of the hips because these places are less richly supplied with blood vessels than other zones. Some victims of chilling suffer from headaches, dizziness, and irritability as well.

To warm the feet, use hot packs, paraffin baths, or hot foot baths. For details on the first two treatments, see p. 56. For a hot foot bath, fill a bucket or other suitable container with water at a temperature of from 42 to 45 degrees centigrade. Submerge the feet in the hot water for from five to six minutes; repeat till the feet are thoroughly warmed. After this treatment, using either the thumbs or the four fingers of each hand, massage or perform shiatsu massage on the tsubo shown in Figs. 15 through 18. Acupuncture and moxa combustion too are effective on these tsubo. Do not expect the treatment to work suddenly and quickly. It takes time. Therapeutic effects will begin to be felt after about two or three weeks of regular treatment. Sometimes prolonged moxa therapy loses effect when the patient becomes accustomed to the stimulus of the heat. Should this happen, allow him to rest from moxa for a while and then resume treatment.

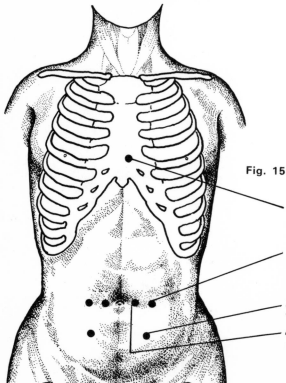

Fig. 15

1. CV-17 (膻中, *Shang-chung*)
Middle of the front of the sternum at the midpoint between the nipples.

2. ST-25 (天枢, *T'ien-shu*)
Two sun on either side of the navel. Easily found by lining the thumb and index and middle fingers on either side of the navel.

3. ST-27 (大巨, *Ta-chü*)
Two sun below ST-25.

4. KI-16 (肓俞, *Huang-yü*)
Points located five sun on either side of the navel.

5. BL-14 (厥陰兪, *Chüeh-yin-yü*)
One sun and five bu on either side of the spinal column at points below the spinal projections of the fourth thoracic vertebra.

6. BL-15 (心兪, *Hsin-yü*)
One sun and five bu on either side of the spinal column at points below the spinal projections of the fifth thoracic vertebra.

Fig. 16

7. BL-23 (腎兪, *Shen-yü*)
One sun and five bu on either side of the spinal column at points below the spinal projections of the second lumbar vertebra, which is located at the height of the lowest ribs.

8. BL-47 (志室, *Chih-shih*)
Three sun on either side of the spinal column at points below the spinal projections of the second lumbar vertebra; on the outer sides of BL-23.

9. BL-25 (大腸兪, *Ta-ch'ang-yü*)
One sun and five bu on either side of the spinal column at points below the spinal projections of the fourth lumbar vertebra.

10. BL-31 (上髎, *Shang-liao*)
11. BL-32 (次髎, *Tz'u-liao*)
12. BL-33 (中髎, *Chung-liao*)
13. BL-34 (下髎, *Hsia-liao*)
These four sets of tsubo are located adjacent to the sacral hiatuses of the four fused sacral vertebra.

14. KI-1 (湧泉, *Yung-ch'üan*)
In the center of the arch of the foot immediately behind the bulge of the big toe.

15. KI-9 (築賓, *Chu-pin*)
In the muscle that is the width of the index finger inward from the edge of the shin at a point five sun above the inner side of the ankle.

Fig. 17

Fig. 18

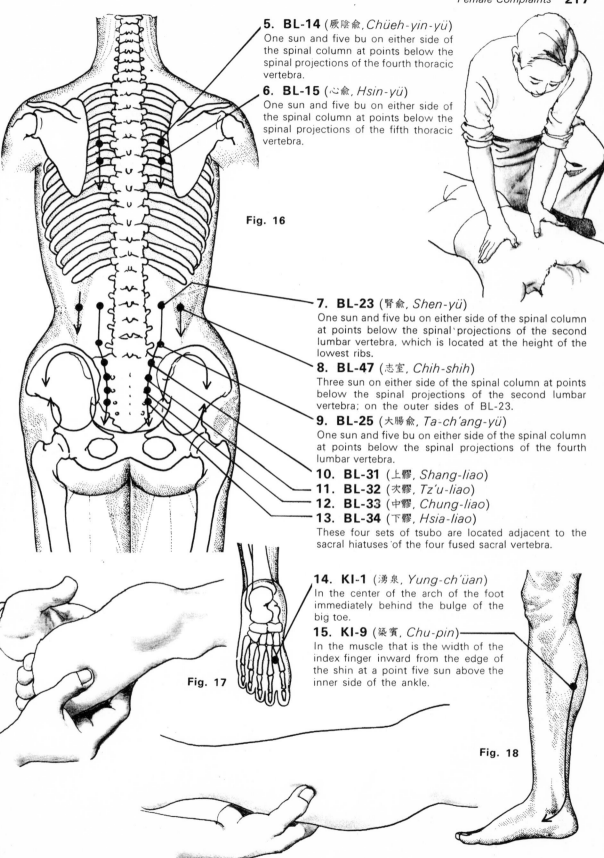

Recovery from Fatigue and Promotion of General Health

(1) Aching Back and Shoulders

The shoulders are called upon to play the very important role of supporting the arms and hands, among the most active parts of the whole body. It is not surprising that many people suffer from stiffness in the shoulders. This complaint can be classified according to the region it affects; but, in all cases, poor circulation and fatigue in the back, neck, shoulders, and shoulder blades are the cause. In older people, aging and consequent deformation of the back bone, neuralgia, rheumatism, sickness of the shoulder joints, high bood pressure, arteriosclerosis, neurosis, irregularities of the autonomic nervous system, irregularities in the digestive and respiratory systems, and female complaints bring on stiff shoulders.

The region in which the condition strikes most often is the area from the back of the head to the back of the neck and to the tips of the shoulders. Sometimes heaviness and discomfort arise in the head. At other times, the stiffness occurs from the back of the neck into the interscapular region and along both sides of the backbone. It may, however, begin below the shoulder blades and continue to the hips and the middle part of the back. Pain in the back of the neck and the tips of the shoulders affects people who bend forward or use their hands and fingers a great deal in their work. Pain along the sides of the backbone and in the interscapular region strikes people who are prone to coughs, palpitations, and shortness of breath. People with stomach and intestinal troubles and those who overwork are likely to suffer pain in the middle back.

Simple exercise is enough to cure light cases of aching back and stiff shoulders. The patient should bend forward and, holding it in both hands, lift a stick over his head and lower it several times. Lukewarm baths, too, are effective. While the patient is in the tub, he must massage his shoulders. Hot packs bring relief from this condition. The patient should place it under his back, wrap himself in a blanket, and lie still for about thirty minutes. It is sometimes believed that beating the shoulders is the best way to relieve stiffness. But sharp, prolonged tapping on this part of the body can physically upset people who are constitutionally weak.

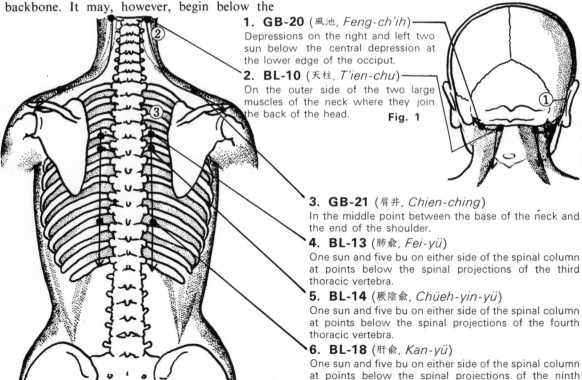

1. GB-20 (風池, *Feng-ch'ih*)
Depressions on the right and left two sun below the central depression at the lower edge of the occiput.

2. BL-10 (天柱, *T'ien-chu*)
On the outer side of the two large muscles of the neck where they join the back of the head.

Fig. 1

3. GB-21 (肩井, *Chien-ching*)
In the middle point between the base of the neck and the end of the shoulder.

4. BL-13 (肺兪, *Fei-yü*)
One sun and five bu on either side of the spinal column at points below the spinal projections of the third thoracic vertebra.

5. BL-14 (厥陰兪, *Chüeh-yin-yü*)
One sun and five bu on either side of the spinal column at points below the spinal projections of the fourth thoracic vertebra.

6. BL-18 (肝兪, *Kan-yü*)
One sun and five bu on either side of the spinal column at points below the spinal projections of the ninth thoracic vertebra.

Fig. 2

Overwork brings about a condition in which stiffness in the shoulders is accompanied by a heavy feeling in the head, tired eyes, general sluggishness, lack of spirit, poor appetite, sleepiness and yawning, and other similar symptoms. In such cases, massage in the direction of the arrow on the tsubos—especially meridians ①, ②, ③, ④, ⑤, ⑥, and ⑦—shown in Figs. 1 through 3. Follow the numerical order shown and use the thumbs.

7. SI-13 (曲垣, *Ch'ü-yüan*) —————
Inner side of the upper corner of the shoulder blade.

8. BL-37 (魄戸, *P'o-hu*) —————
On the right and left, three sun below the third thoracic vertebra.

9. BL-38 (膏肓, *Kao-huang*) —————
Three sun on either side of the spinal column at points below the fourth thoracic vertebra.

10. BL-39 (神堂, *Shen-t'ang*) —————
Three sun on either side of the spinal column at points below the fifth thoracic vertebra.

11. BL-25 (大腸兪, *Ta-ch'ang-yü*) —————
One sun and five bu on either side of the spinal column at points below the spinal projections of the fourth lumbar vertebra.

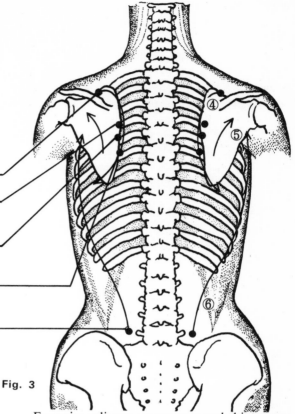

Fig. 3

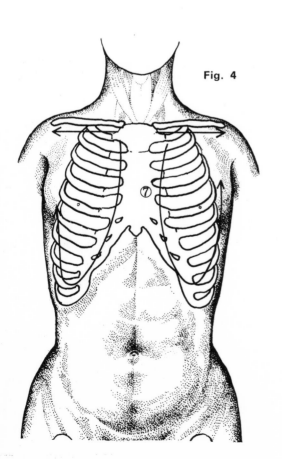

Fig. 4

Excessive reliance on massage and shiatsu can make the stiffness in the shoulders chronic. Should this happen, apply ice to GB-20, BL-10, GB-21, BL-37, and BL-39. Fill a small vessel —like a test tube—with crushed ice and salt. From one to three times a day, press the ice-filled vessel against the tsubo just listed. When each tsubo has turned red as a consequence of this treatment, move on to the next.

Some people complain of stiff shoulders that strike at the first sign of fatigue or whenever they do close work. For them, I suggest moxa combustion on the tsubo listed above. Should all therapy fail to relieve stiff shoulders, the patient is probably suffering from high blood pressure, arteriosclerosis, or a nervous ailment. All of these conditions require the attention of a specialist.

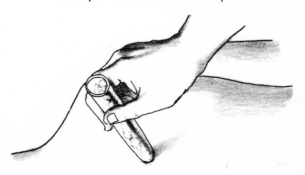

(2) Pain and Stiffness in Neck, Shoulders, and Arms

People approaching, or already in, their middle years frequently experience heaviness and numbness in the fingers, arms, neck and shoulders upon rising in the morning. These symptoms are signs of deformations or changes in the seven cervical vertebrae or in the intervertebral discs of the spinal column. Such deformations result in pressure on the bases of the nerves branching from the central spinal cord and traveling to the shoulders and arms.

The changes can be of a number of kinds. An intervertebral disc may have slipped from its proper place, and additional calcium may have deposited on it to form osteophytes. Congenital, riblike projections may be present on the cervical vertebrae. The *scalinus ventralis* muscles may be too tense. Overwork or aging may have caused obstructions in the circulation to the cervical vertebrae. The patient may be suffering from an external injury like the kind inflicted by the so-called whiplash syndrome (see p. 158). In cases involving the actual deformation of the bone or development of osteophytes, oriental therapy cannot effect a cure. Such conditions require the

attention of a specialist and may demand surgery. Oriental therapy is effective, however, in cases in which the cause is muscular or nervous.

In light instances, warm packs on the back of the neck are sufficient to limber the muscles and tendons in that part of the body and relieve pressure on the nerves. To find the best place to apply the hot pack, follow this procedure. First, press or tap the neck along the cervical vertebrae. When you reach a spot where pressure causes severe pain, you will have located the tsubo at which to place the hot pack. Leave it in place for about thirty minutes. Then stroke, press, or rub the vicinities of the following tsubo in the directions of the arrows: GB-20 and GB-21 (Fig. 5).

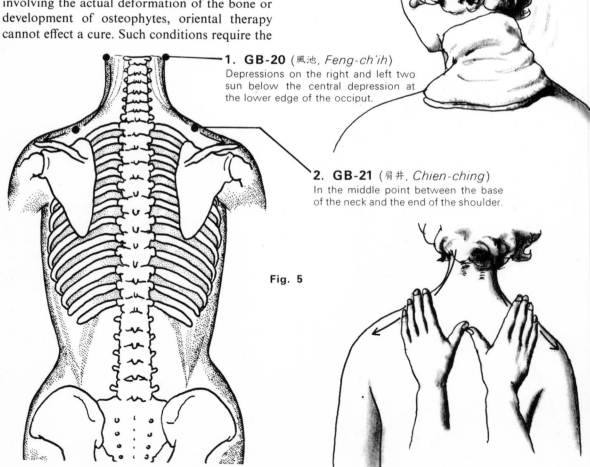

1. GB-20 (風池, *Feng-ch'ih*)
Depressions on the right and left two sun below the central depression at the lower edge of the occiput.

2. GB-21 (肩井, *Chien-ching*)
In the middle point between the base of the neck and the end of the shoulder.

Fig. 5

Next, thoroughly massage TH-16 and ST-11 (Fig. 6). Continue by massaging in the direction shown by the arrow in Fig. 7. The effect of treatment will be increased if you press each of these tsubo gently with the thumbs. Although people with stiff shoulders tend to minimize the movement of those joints and thus to overwork the joints of the arms and the hands, this is a bad thing to do. It is better to move the shoulder joints as much as possible.

Fig. 6

Fig. 7

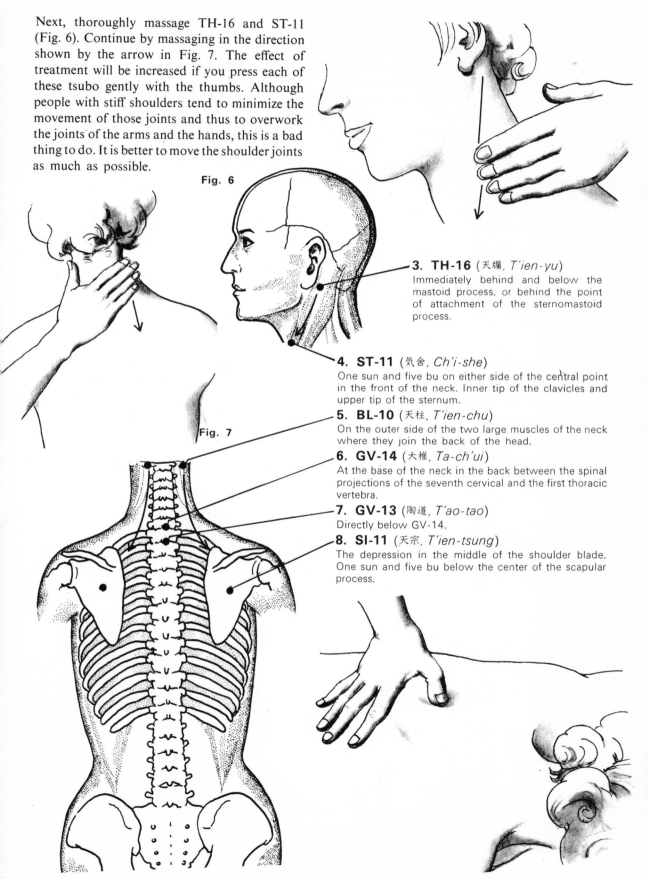

3. TH-16 (天牖, *T'ien-yu*)
Immediately behind and below the mastoid process, or behind the point of attachment of the sternomastoid process.

4. ST-11 (気舎, *Ch'i-she*)
One sun and five bu on either side of the central point in the front of the neck. Inner tip of the clavicles and upper tip of the sternum.

5. BL-10 (天柱, *T'ien-chu*)
On the outer side of the two large muscles of the neck where they join the back of the head.

6. GV-14 (大椎, *Ta-ch'ui*)
At the base of the neck in the back between the spinal projections of the seventh cervical and the first thoracic vertebra.

7. GV-13 (陶道, *T'ao-tao*)
Directly below GV-14.

8. SI-11 (天宗, *T'ien-tsung*)
The depression in the middle of the shoulder blade. One sun and five bu below the center of the scapular process.

(3) Sluggishness in Legs and Hips

Sluggishness and pain in the legs, the backs of the thighs and calves, and the lower parts of the back and hips are signs of the initial stages of sciatica. The legs, aside from their obvious importance in locomotion, cooperate with the hips and the lower regions of the back to protect and support the suprarenal glands, two of the most important hormone producers in the body. People who can work long hours without diminishing the strength and power of their legs are probably in good physical condition. But, when the legs begin to give way easily, it is symbolic of general debility. Furthermore, weariness in the legs affects the functioning of the suprarenal glands and, in this way, influences the health of the entire body. Perennial weariness and lack of strength in the legs and hips are a sign of age and the outcome of alterations and atrophy in the lumbar vertebrae and their intervertebral discs. Although this condition is sometimes congenital, it is more often brought on by alterations in the form of the bones; cold; chilling; and illness of the stomach, intestines, urinary tract, or sex organs. Long sitting or standing in the same position without exercise can bring on this condition because such immobility interferes with blood circulation. In addition, pregnancy and menstruation can cause pain in the legs, hips, and lower back.

To treat, follow this procedure. First, press KI-1 (Fig. 11) to determine whether this location is stiff. Stiffness in this tsubo traditionally indicates fever in the upper parts and chills in the lower parts of the body and means that treatment is required for fatigue, chilling, and stiffness in the legs. After applying a hot pack to the area from the lower back to the buttocks for from twenty to thirty minutes, massage meridian ①, with special attention given to BL-23, BL-47, and BL-25 (Fig. 8). Then lightly massage meridian ② from GB-29 to ST-36 (Fig. 9) with the palms of the hands. Next, employing light gripping motions with both hands, massage meridians ③, ④, and ⑤ in the direction of the arrow (Figs. 10 through 12). Although the tsubo given here are used in shiatsu, acupuncture and moxa combustion too are effective on them—especially on ST-36 and SP-6. Finally, apply gentle shiatsu to KI-1. In addition to this treatment, sitting in a chair and rolling a bottle over the floor with the insteps of the bare feet help bring relief to weary legs.

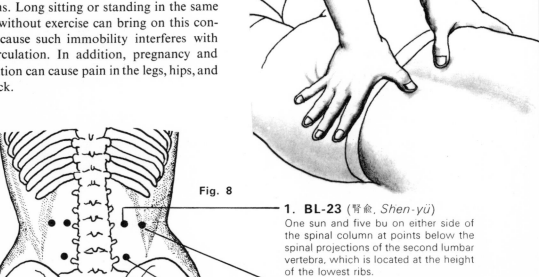

Fig. 8

1. BL-23 (腎俞, *Shen-yü*)
One sun and five bu on either side of the spinal column at points below the spinal projections of the second lumbar vertebra, which is located at the height of the lowest ribs.

2. BL-47 (志室, *Chih-shih*)
Three sun on either side of the spinal column at points below the spinal projections of the second lumbar vertebra; on the outer sides of BL-23.

3. BL-25 (大腸俞, *Ta-ch'ang-yü*)
One sun and five bu on either side of the spinal column at points below the spinal projections of the fourth lumbar vertebra.

4. GB-29 (居髎, *Chü-liao*)

Eight sun and three bu below the extremities of the eleventh ribs. Exactly in the middle, but somewhat to the rear, of the hucklebone.

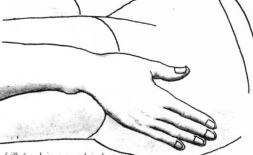

Fig. 9

5. ST-34 (梁丘, *Liang-chiu*)

Two sun above the upper edge of the kneecap. This can be easily located by fully extending the knee and finding the upper end of the groove formed on the outside of the kneecap. In other words, it is on the front of the thigh, two sun above the upper outer edge of the kneecap.

6. SP-10 (血海, *Hsüeh-hai*)

Two sun and five bu above the kneecap on the inner side of the thigh. The place where a depression is formed two sun and five bu above the knee when the leg is outstretched.

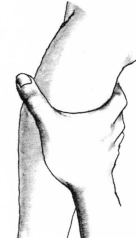

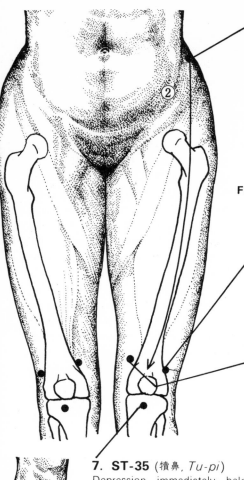

7. ST-35 (犢鼻, *Tu-pi*)

Depression immediately below the knee. The point in the exact middle of the zone between the kneecap and the shin bone.

8. ST-36 (足三里, *Tsu-san-li*)

On the outer side of the calf three sun below the knee. Outer edge of the shin bone.

9. ST-41 (解谿, *Chieh-hsi*)

Middle of the front part of the ankle.

10. BL-60 (崑崙, *K'un-lun*)

Immediately to the rear side of the outer ankle.

Fig. 10

13. SP-6 (三陰交, *San-yin-chiao*)

Three sun upward on the side of the shin bone from the inner side of the ankle.

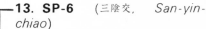
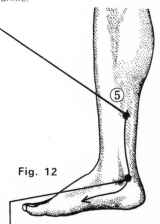

Fig. 12

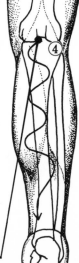

Fig. 11

11. BL-54 (委中, *Wei-chung*)

In the center of the groove formed behind the knee.

12. KI-1 (湧泉, *Yung-ch'üan*)

In the center of the arch of the foot immediately behind the bulge of the big toe.

14. KI-3 (太谿, *T'ai-hsi*)

Rear part of the inside of the ankle.

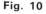

(4) Increasing Potency

Of course, I am speaking of sexual potency; but, since sexual vigor depends on the total strength and vitality of the body, oriental therapy strives to promote the former by maintaining the latter. As has been mentioned elsewhere, it is the oriental belief that the human body can call on two kinds of energy: the energy imparted to it before birth and the energy received by it after birth. If both kinds of energy are used in harmony and to the maximum, the body remains vigorous; and, as a consequence, sexual powers do not fail as rapidly as they might.

Peak operation of the hormones of the human body occurs during the twenties. After this age, hormone activity declines gradually. This means that masculine sexual powers begin slowly to fail. Total bodily power and sexual power follow a descending curve after the beginning of middle age, though sexual strength is the more enduring of the two. Massage, shiatsu, acupuncture, and moxa combustion on the tsubo can enable the body to use its innate and its later-acquired energies to the full and, in this way, increase sexual potency in middle age and after. The main tsubo to treat to achieve this effect are as follows: BL-18, BL-22, BL-23, GV-4 (Fig. 13), CV-17, CV-12, KI-16, ST-27, CV-4, LV-11 (Fig. 14), KI-10, LV-7, KI-1 (Fig. 15), KI-9, KI-3 (Fig. 16), and TH-4 (Fig. 17).

Before beginning this treatment, always press KI-16, on the sides of the navel, and KI-1, in the center of the instep. If there is stiffness or pain at these tsubo, the person's sexual powers are probably in a declining state. First, massage in the area of KI-1, then massage or perform shiatsu massage on the tsubo listed above. Moxa combustion is an effective home treatment on these tsubo; and, if you can call on the services of a professional, acupuncture has a highly therapeutic effect in cases of this kind. In massaging, pay special attention to places where the muscles are stiff and tense.

Fig. 13

1. BL-18 (肝兪, *Kan-yü*)
One sun and five bu on either side of the spinal column at points below the spinal projections of the ninth thoracic vertebra.

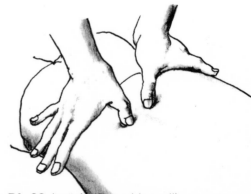

2. BL-22 (三焦兪, *San-chiao-yü*)
One sun and five bu on either side of the spinal column at points below the first lumbar vertebra.

3. BL-23 (腎兪, *Shen-yü*)
One sun and five bu on either side of the spinal column at points below the spinal projections of the second lumbar vertebra, which is located at the height of the lowest ribs.

4. GV-4 (命門, *Ming-men*)
Below the spinal projections of the second lumbar vertebra and between the tsubo designated BL-23.

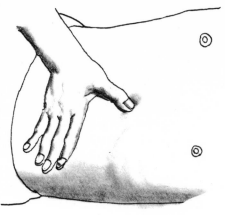

Fig. 14

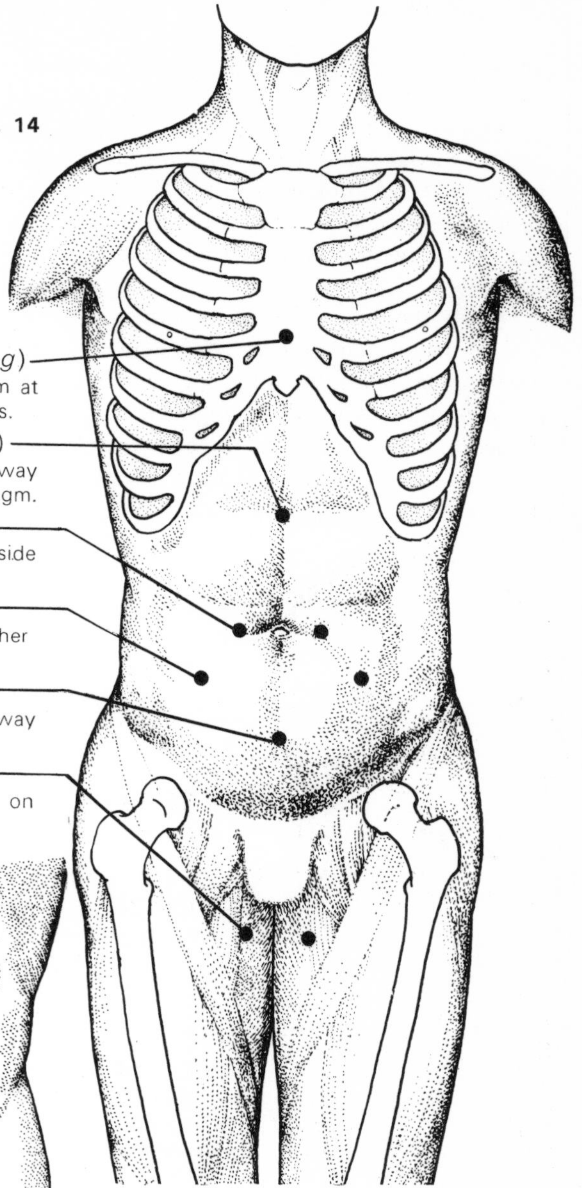

5. CV-17 (膻中, *Shang-chung*)
Middle of the front of the sternum at the midpoint between the nipples.

6. CV-12 (中脘, *Chung-wan*)
Four sun above the navel; midway between the navel and the diaphragm.

7. KI-16 (肓俞, *Huang-yü*)
Points located five sun on either side of the navel.

8. ST-27 (大巨, *Ta-chü*)
Two sun below poins two sun on either side of the navel.

9. CV-4 (関元, *Kuan-yüan*)
Three sun below the navel, or midway between the navel and the pubis.

10. LV-11 (陰廉, *Yin-lien*)
About two sun below the crotch on the inner side of the thigh.

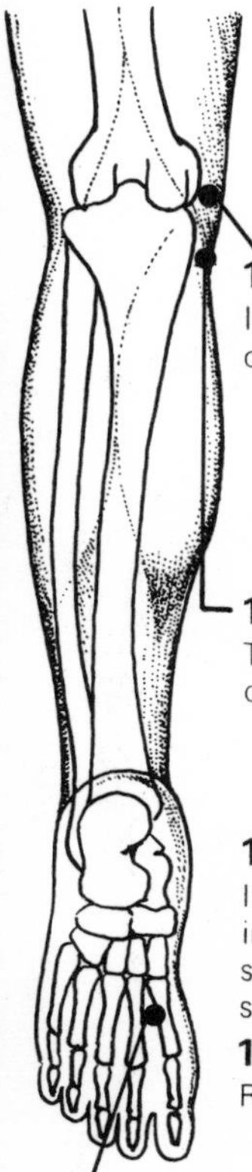

11. KI-10 (陰谷, *Yin-ku*)
In the crease behind the knee on the outer side at the top of the calf.

Fig. 15

12. LV-7 (膝関, *Hsi-kuan*)
Two sun below the bend of the knee on the inner side.

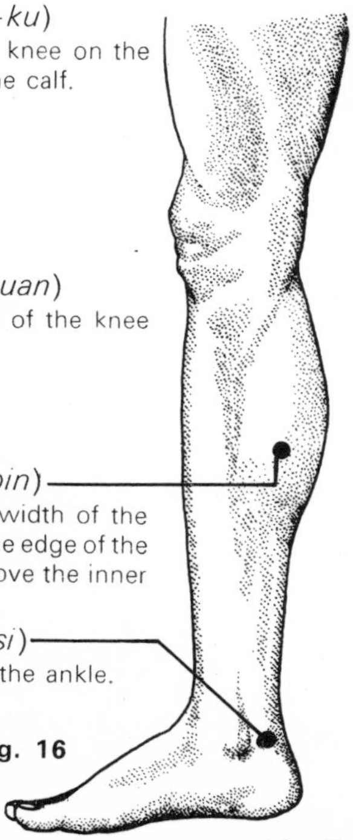

13. KI-9 (築賓, *Chu-pin*)
In the muscle that is the width of the index finger inward from the edge of the shin at a point five sun above the inner side of the ankle.

14. KI-3 (太谿, *T'ai-hsi*)
Rear part of the inside of the ankle.

Fig. 16

Fig. 17

15. KI-1 (湧泉, *Yung-ch'üan*)
In the center of the arch of the foot immediately behind the bulge of the big toe.

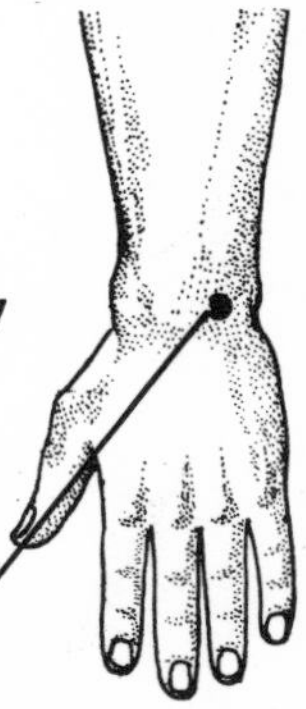

16. TH-4 (陽池, *Yang-ch'ih*)
When the palm is outstretched, on the back of the hand at the back of the wrist a hard, thick muscles becomes apparent. This tsubo is on the little-finger side of that muscle; that is, it is slightly to the little-finger side of the middle of the wrist.

(5) Dispelling Sleepiness

Long period of monotonous work inevitably make a person drowsy. Often overwork and increasing fatigue make people sluggish and sleepy throughout the entire morning, thus impairing their abilities to work efficiently. Accumulated fatigue creating obstructions in the autonomic nervous system is the cause of this condition.

During the daytime, the sympathetic subdivision of the autonomic nervous system keeps the involuntary operations of the body and its organs proceeding as required. At night, the parasympathetic subdivision of the same nervous system takes control. In order to make it possible for a person to wake bright and clear in the morning,

it is necessary to enable him to effect a quick changeover from the control of the parasympathetic to the control of the sympathetic nervous system. This cannot be done consciously, of course; but it can be facilitated by massaging the tsubo that activate the autonomic nervous system. Incidentally, the massage and the tsubo outlined below are very helpful for students and other people who find that they must remain alert for study or work late into the night.

First, thoroughly massage GV-20, BL-10, GB-20, CV-14, LV-14, CV-12, and KI-16 (Figs. 18 and 19) in the shiatsu fashion. Proceed to perform shiatsu massage on GV-14, BL-13, BL-17, BL-18, and BL-23 (Fig. 20). Finally, firmly press LI-10, ST-36, SP-6, and KI-3 (Figs. 21 through 23). The person who wishes to clear his head of drowsiness in the morning may perform this shiatsu massage on his own body for five or six minutes before rising.

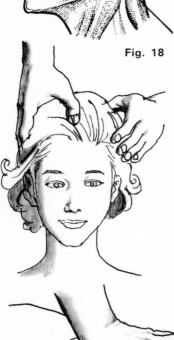

1. GV-20 (百会, *Pai-hui*)
At the point where a line directly upward from ear to ear crossing the top of the head and a line straight upward from the midpoint of the area between the shoulders to the top of the head intersect.

2. BL-10 (天柱, *T'ien-chu*)
On the outer side of the two large muscles of the neck where they join the back of the head.

3. GB-20 (風池, *Feng-ch'ih*)
Depressions on the right and left two sun below the central depression at the lower edge of the occiput.

Fig. 18

4. CV-14 (巨闕, *Chü-ch'üeh*)
Immediately below the diaphragm; two sun below the lower extremity of the sternum.

5. LV-14 (期門, *Ch'i-men*)
Extermities of the ninth ribs. Or a place located at the boundary between the rib and the abdomen directly below the nipple of the breast. The zone between the edge of the rib and the diaphragm.

6. CV-12 (中脘, *Chung-wan*)
Four sun above the navel; midway between the navel and the pubis.

7. KI-16 (肓兪, *Huang-yü*)
Points located five sun on either side of the navel.

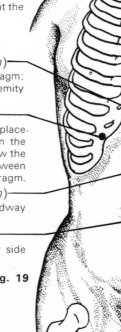

Fig. 19

8. GV-14 (大椎, *Ta-ch'ui*)
At the base of the neck in the back between the spinal projections of the seventh cervical and the first thoracic vertebra.

9. BL-13 (肺俞, *Fei-yü*)
One sun and five bu on either side of the spinal column at points below the spinal projections of the third thoracic vertebra.

10. BL-17 (膈俞, *Ke-yü*)
One sun and five bu on either side of the spinal column at points below the spinal projections of the seventh thoracic vertebra.

11. BL-18 (肝俞, *Kan-yü*)
One sun and five bu on either side of the spinal column at points below the spinal projections of the ninth thoracic vertebra.

12. BL-23 (腎俞, *Shen-yü*)
One sun and five bu on either side of the spinal column at points below the spinal projections of the second lumbar vertebra, which is located at the height of the lowest ribs.

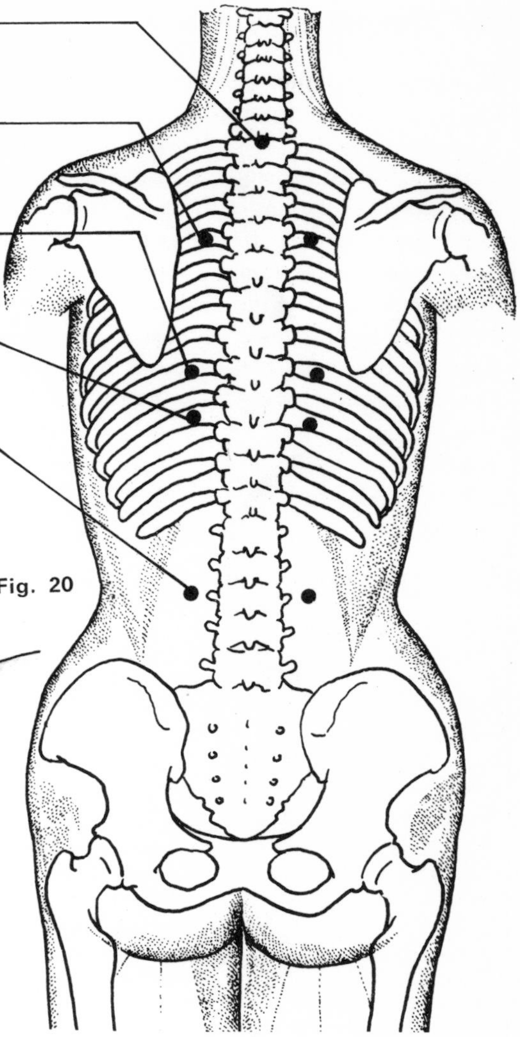

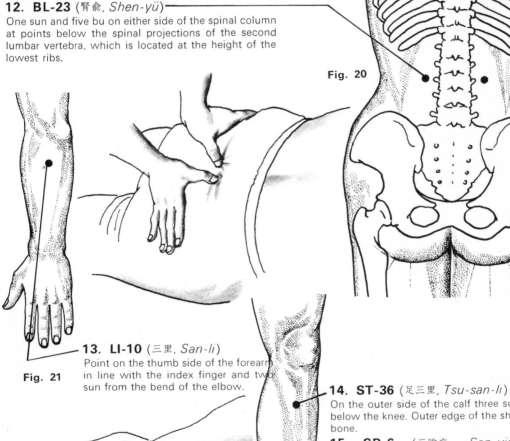

Fig. 20

Fig. 21

13. LI-10 (三里, *San-li*)
Point on the thumb side of the forearm in line with the index finger and two sun from the bend of the elbow.

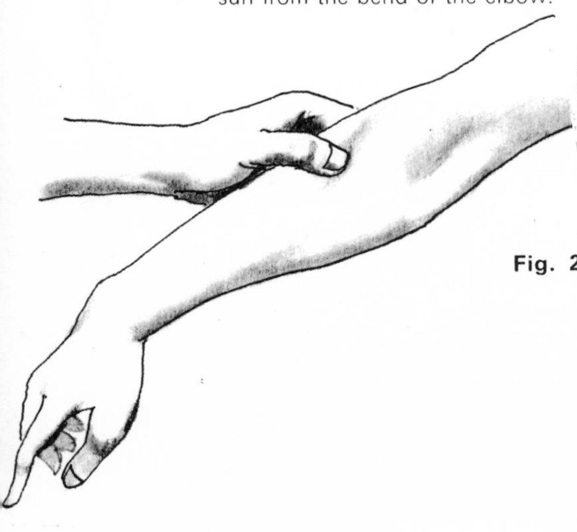

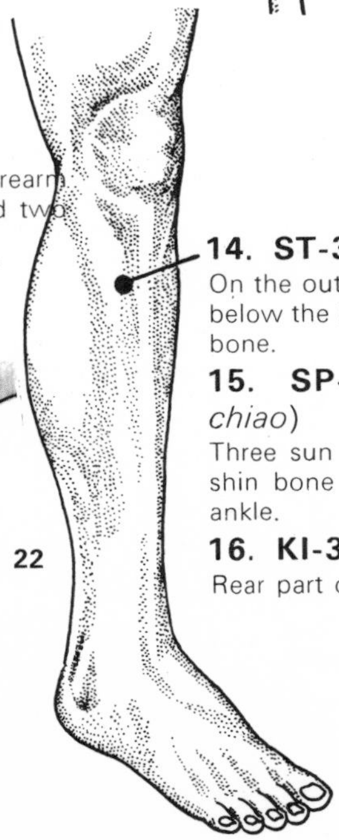

Fig. 22

14. ST-36 (足三里, *Tsu-san-li*)
On the outer side of the calf three sun below the knee. Outer edge of the shin bone.

15. SP-6 (三陰交, *San-yin-chiao*)
Three sun upward on the side of the shin bone from the inner side of the ankle.

16. KI-3 (太谿, *T'ai-hsi*)
Rear part of the inside of the ankle.

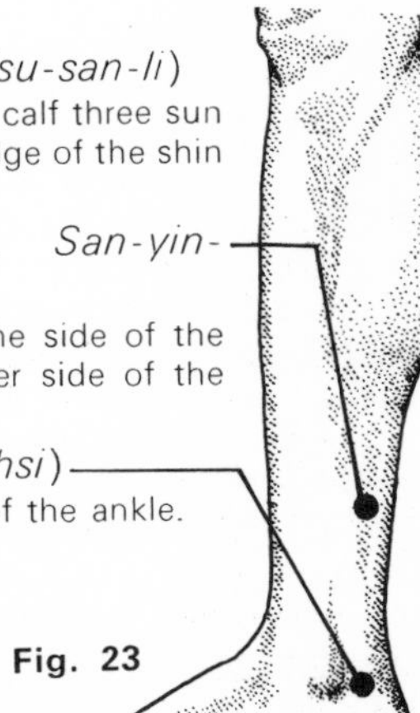

Fig. 23

(6) Preventing Aging

Accompanying the conveniences of modern living—rapid transportation, electrical home appliances, and so on—is a pervasive lack of exercise that tends to accelerate the aging process. It is thought that aging in the human body begins during the twenties. If this is true, aside from those people who remain active in sports for many years, most of the readers of this book are already in the process whereby bones will alter their shapes and the tendons and muscles supporting and moving those bones will harden

and lose tone and resilience. The first thing to do to slow down the aging process is to restore tone to the muscles on both sides of the neck and spinal column. Following this, it is essential to use oriental tsubo therapy on the muscles of the hips, abdomen, arms, palms, fronts of thighs, buttocks, calves, and insteps.

First, using the four fingers of each hand for massage and the thumbs for shiatsu, massage GB-20, BL-10, GV-14, LI-15, GB-21, SI-13, BL-13, BL-17, BL-21, BL-22, and BL-25 (Figs. 24 and 25) in the direction of the arrows. Next, similarly, massage or perform shiatsu massage on the following: CV-12, KI-16, CV-4, ST-25, GB-29, ST-32, ST-34 (Fig. 26), LU-5, LU-9, HC-7, HT-7 (Fig. 27), LI-14, TH-10, and TH-4 (Fig. 28), BL-50, BL-51, BL-54, BL-57, KI-1 (Fig. 29). Treatment on ST-41 and BL-60 too is effective in retarding aging. It is advisable to combine this regimen with simple warmup exercises.

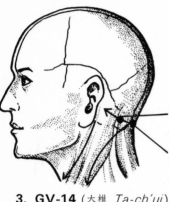

Fig. 24

1. GB-20 (風池, *Feng-ch'ih*)
Depressions in the lower edge of the occiput two sun on either side of BL-10.

2. BL-10 (天柱, *T'ien-chu*)
On the outer side of the two large muscles of the neck where they join the back of the head.

3. GV-14 (大椎, *Ta-ch'ui*)
At the base of the neck in the back between the spinal projections of the seventh cervical and the first thoracic vertebra.

4. LI-15 (肩髃, *Chien-yü*)
At the depression between the tip of the shoulder and the triceps muscle when the arm is held outstretched in a horizontal position. Thumb side of the upper arm at the tip of the acromion process.

5. GB-21 (肩井, *Chien-ching*)
In the middle point between the base of the neck and the end of the shoulder.

6. SI-13 (曲垣, *Ch'ü-yüan*)
Inner side of the upper corner of the shoulder blade.

7. BL-13 (肺兪, *Fei-yü*)
One sun and five bu on either side of the spinal column at points below the spinal projections of the third thoracic vertebra.

8. BL-17 (膈兪, *Ke-yü*)
One sun and five bu on either side of the spinal column at points below the seventh thoracic vertebra.

9. BL-21 (胃兪, *Wei-yü*)
One sun and five bu on either side of the spinal column at points below the spinal projections of the twelfth thoracic vertebra.

10. BL-22 (三焦兪, *San-chiao-yü*)
One sun and five bu on either side of the spinal column at points below the first lumbar vertebra.

11. BL-25 (大腸兪, *Ta-ch'ang-yü*)
One sun and five bu on either side of the spinal column at points below the spinal projections of the fourth lumbar vertebra.

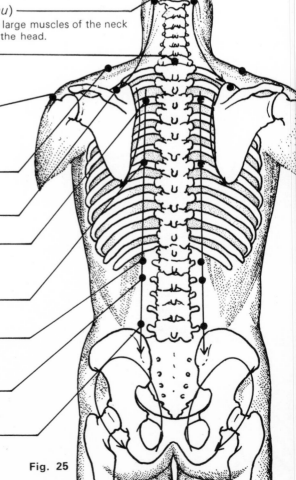

Fig. 25

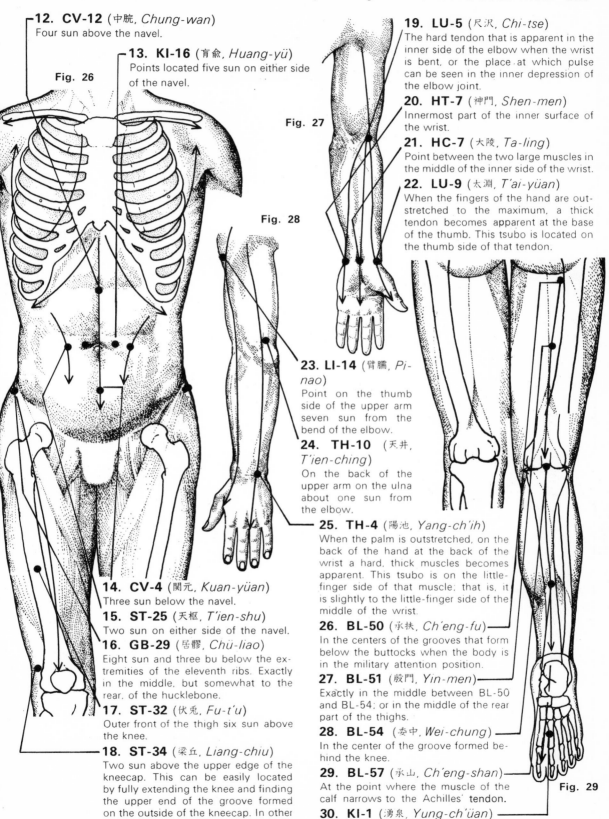

12. CV-12 (中脘, *Chung-wan*)
Four sun above the navel.

13. KI-16 (肓俞, *Huang-yü*)
Points located five sun on either side of the navel.

Fig. 26

Fig. 27

Fig. 28

19. LU-5 (尺沢, *Chi-tse*)
The hard tendon that is apparent in the inner side of the elbow when the wrist is bent, or the place at which pulse can be seen in the inner depression of the elbow joint.

20. HT-7 (神門, *Shen-men*)
Innermost part of the inner surface of the wrist.

21. HC-7 (大陵, *Ta-ling*)
Point between the two large muscles in the middle of the inner side of the wrist.

22. LU-9 (太淵, *T'ai-yüan*)
When the fingers of the hand are outstretched to the maximum, a thick tendon becomes apparent at the base of the thumb. This tsubo is located on the thumb side of that tendon.

23. LI-14 (臂臑, *Pi-nao*)
Point on the thumb side of the upper arm seven sun from the bend of the elbow.

24. TH-10 (天井, *T'ien-ching*)
On the back of the upper arm on the ulna about one sun from the elbow.

25. TH-4 (陽池, *Yang-ch'ih*)
When the palm is outstretched, on the back of the hand at the back of the wrist a hard, thick muscles becomes apparent. This tsubo is on the little-finger side of that muscle; that is, it is slightly to the little-finger side of the middle of the wrist.

26. BL-50 (承扶, *Ch'eng-fu*)
In the centers of the grooves that form below the buttocks when the body is in the military attention position.

27. BL-51 (殷門, *Yin-men*)
Exactly in the middle between BL-50 and BL-54; or in the middle of the rear part of the thighs.

28. BL-54 (委中, *Wei-chung*)
In the center of the groove formed behind the knee.

29. BL-57 (承山, *Ch'eng-shan*)
At the point where the muscle of the calf narrows to the Achilles' tendon.

30. KI-1 (湧泉, *Yung-ch'üan*)
In the center of the arch of the foot immediately behind the bulge of the big toe.

14. CV-4 (関元, *Kuan-yüan*)
Three sun below the navel.

15. ST-25 (天枢, *T'ien-shu*)
Two sun on either side of the navel.

16. GB-29 (居髎, *Chü-liao*)
Eight sun and three bu below the extremities of the eleventh ribs. Exactly in the middle, but somewhat to the rear, of the hucklebone.

17. ST-32 (伏兎, *Fu-t'u*)
Outer front of the thigh six sun above the knee.

18. ST-34 (梁丘, *Liang-chiu*)
Two sun above the upper edge of the kneecap. This can be easily located by fully extending the knee and finding the upper end of the groove formed on the outside of the kneecap. In other words, it is on the front of the thigh, two sun above the upper edge of the kneecap.

Fig. 29

(7) **Retarding Muscular Atrophy**

In recent years, a massage system called connective-fiber massage has gained wide popularity in America and Europe. This method involves massaging the ankles and wrists—places where there are few muscles and blood vessels—to retard muscular atrophy. This approach is in complete accord with the principles of oriental therapy because the tsubo are often located, not on the full parts of muscles, but at their points of origin and attachment. In other words, the tsubo are frequently in such places as the ankles and wrists. The origins and attachment points of muscles are the places where treatment increases muscular strength. For the further prevention of atrophy, it is good to massage thoroughly the area around ST-9 (Fig. 30) on the sternomastoid muscle, which is in the location of important blood vessels leading to the head and the heart. Perform the massage in the direction of the arrow. Massage or shiatsu on the trepezius muscle, too, is vitally important, since this muscle must support the head, which in some individuals weighs as much as four kilograms.

It is unnecessary to massage all of the tsubo shown in the chart all of the time. But for the sake of retarding atrophy, select the tsubo related to the muscle that seems to be weakening. This kind of treatment has the additional effect of relieving stiff shoulders and other muscular irregularities. Consequently, for health and for prolonged youthfulness and vigor, massage the tsubo and the meridians shown in Figs. 30 through 37.

Since the insteps are called upon to bear the weight of the body, special attention must be paid to massaging KI-1. Rolling a bottle over the floor with the bare insteps is an excellent way to massage these tsubo. Therapy of this kind is essential since, if fatigue builds up in the insteps, the tendency is to overwork the knees and hips, thus destroying the muscular balance of the entire body.

Fig. 30

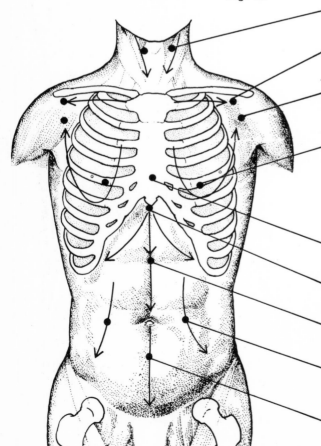

1. ST-9 (人迎, *Jen-ying*)
Points one sun and five bu on either side of the Adam's apple. The pulse is felt strongly in these places.

2. LU-2 (雲門, *Yun-men*)
Middle of the depression at the underside of the external extremity of the clavicle. One sun above LU-1.

3. LU-1 (中府, *Chung-fu*)
Upper extremity of the exterior front chest wall at the second intercostal zone. Six sun on either side of the sternum.

4. KI-23 (神封, *Shen-feng*)
Two sun to the right and left of the sternum slightly below the fourth ribs. Or points at the height of the nipples two sun to the right and left of a line from the base of the throat to the diaphragm.

5. CV-17 (膻中, *Shang-chung*)
Middle of the front of the sternum at the midpoint between the nipples.

6. CV-15 (鳩尾, *Chiu-wei*)
On the diaphragm or one sun below the lower extremity of the sternum.

7. CV-12 (中脘, *Chung-wan*)
Four sun above the navel; midway between the navel and the diaphragm.

8. ST-25 (天枢, *T'ien-shu*)
Two sun on either side of the navel. Easily found by lining the thumb and index and middle fingers on the side of the navel.

9. CV-4 (関元, *Kuan-yüan*)
Three sun below the navel, or midway between the navel and the pubis.

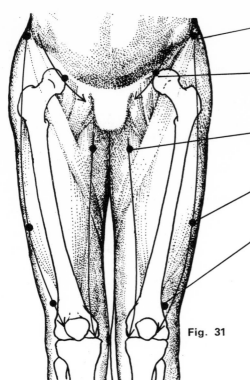

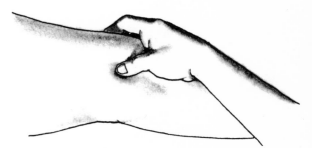

10. GB-29 (居髎, *Chü-liao*)

Eight sun and three bu below the extremities of the eleventh ribs. Exactly in the middle, but somewhat to the rear, of the hucklebone.

11. SP-12 (衝門, *Ch'ung-men*)

Five sun below the points four sun to the right and left of the navel. These points are at the bases of the pelvic joints.

12. LV-11 (陰廉, *Yin-lien*)

About two sun below the crotch on the inner side of the thigh.

13. GB-32 (中瀆, *Chung-tu*)

In the depressions located five sun above the knee on the outsides of the thighs.

14. ST-34 (梁丘, *Liang-chiu*)

On the front of the thigh two sun above the upper outer edge of the patella.

Fig. 31

15. TH-10 (天井, *T'ien-ching*)

On the back of the upper arm on the ulna about one sun from the elbow.

16. TH-4 (陽池, *Yang-ch'ih*)

When the palm is outstretched, on the back of the hand at the back of the wrist a hard, thick muscle becomes apparent. This tsubo is on the little-finger side of that muscle; that is, it is slightly to the little-finger side of the middle of the wrist.

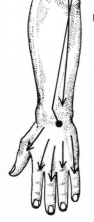

Fig. 32

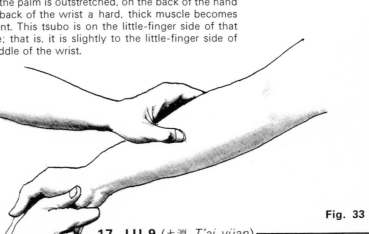

17. LU-9 (太淵, *T'ai-yüan*)

When the fingers of the hand are outstretched to the maximum, a thick tendon becomes apparent at the base of the thumb, This tsubo is located on the thumb side of that tendon.

18. HT-7 (神門, *Shen-men*)

Innermost part of the inner surface of the wrist.

Fig. 33

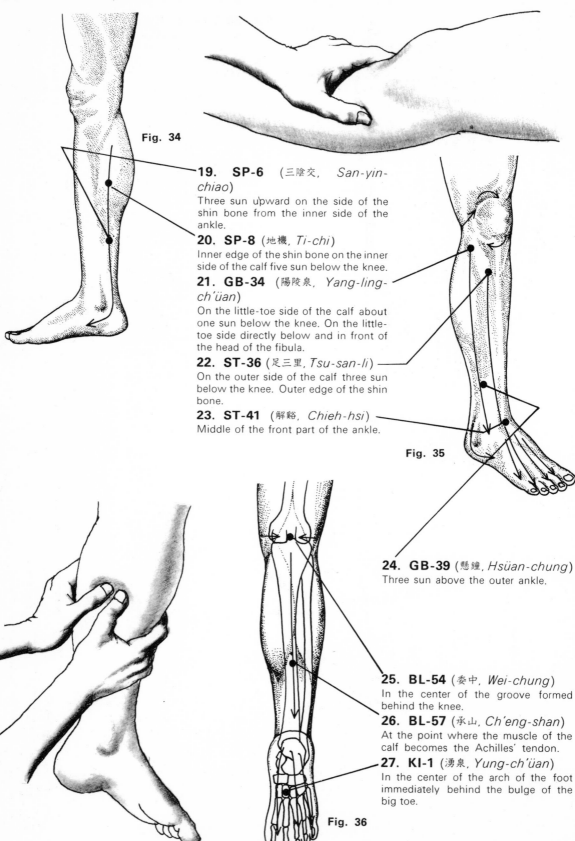

Fig. 34

19. SP-6 (三陰交, *San-yin-chiao*)
Three sun upward on the side of the shin bone from the inner side of the ankle.

20. SP-8 (地機, *Ti-chi*)
Inner edge of the shin bone on the inner side of the calf five sun below the knee.

21. GB-34 (陽陵泉, *Yang-ling-ch'üan*)
On the little-toe side of the calf about one sun below the knee. On the little-toe side directly below and in front of the head of the fibula.

22. ST-36 (足三里, *Tsu-san-li*)
On the outer side of the calf three sun below the knee. Outer edge of the shin bone.

23. ST-41 (解谿, *Chieh-hsi*)
Middle of the front part of the ankle.

Fig. 35

24. GB-39 (懸鐘, *Hsüan-chung*)
Three sun above the outer ankle.

25. BL-54 (委中, *Wei-chung*)
In the center of the groove formed behind the knee.

26. BL-57 (承山, *Ch'eng-shan*)
At the point where the muscle of the calf becomes the Achilles' tendon.

27. KI-1 (湧泉, *Yung-ch'üan*)
In the center of the arch of the foot immediately behind the bulge of the big toe.

Fig. 36

28. BL-10 (天柱, *T'ien-chu*)

On the outer side of the two large muscles of the neck where they join the back of the head.

29. GV-14 (大椎, *Ta-ch'ui*)

At the base of the neck in the back between the spinal projections of the seventh cervical and the first thoracic vertebra.

30. GB-21 (肩井, *Chien-ching*)

In the middle point between the base of the neck and the end of the shoulder.

31. TH-14 (肩髎, *Chien-liao*)

Depression at the under edge of the external tip of the acromion process.

32. BL-38 (膏肓, *Kao-huang*)

Three sun on either side of the spinal column at points below the fourth thoracic vertebra.

33. BL-17 (膈俞, *Ke-yü*)

One sun and five bu on either side of the spinal column at points below the seventh thoracic vertebra.

34. BL-18 (肝俞, *Kan-yü*)

One sun and five bu on either side of the spinal column at points below the spinal projections of the ninth thoracic vertebra.

35. BL-23 (腎俞, *Shen-yü*)

One sun and five bu on either side of the spinal column at points below the spinal projections of the second lumbar vertebra, which is located at the height of the lowest ribs.

36. BL-25 (大腸俞, *Ta-ch'ang-yü*)

One sun and five bu on either side of the spinal column at points below the spinal projections of the fourth lumbar vertebra

37. BL-50 (承扶, *Ch'eng-fu*)

In the centers of the grooves that form below the buttocks when the body is in the military attention position.

Fig. 37

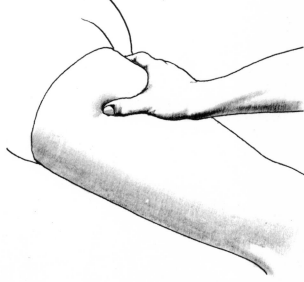

(8) Restoring Vitality

Vitality is that special drive that makes people seek to fulfill their wishes, to pursue what is pleasing, and to avoid what is displeasing. Vitality is the active phase of life; emotional reactions are often passive. Sometimes, however, people lose vitality and become generally listless. Stress often causes this condition, which, in the past, was frequently considered under the catch-all heading of neuroses. Medical science now recognizes slight contractions of many different kinds of diseases as major causes of total listlessness. If the sickness giving rise to the condition is definitely known, by all means provide the therapy that is effective in combatting it. When the illness has been cured, vitality will be restored. Allowed to go untreated, loss of vitality can lead to a serious melancholic depression, a state in which the patient finds all movement distressing and loses power to make decisions or even to think normally.

In these instances, oriental tsubo therapy performed regularly and for an extended period can be of great help. Perform shiatsu massage on GV-20, BL-10, and GB-20 (Fig. 38). Then, having the patient lie on his back, massage LU-1, CV-17, CV-12, CV-6, and ST-27 (Fig. 39). Then treat GV-14, BL-13, BL-18, GV-8, BL-23, BL-47, GV-4, BL-26 (Fig. 40), LI-11, LI-4 (Fig. 41), ST-36, LV-3 (Fig. 42), KI-9, and KI-3 (Fig. 43).

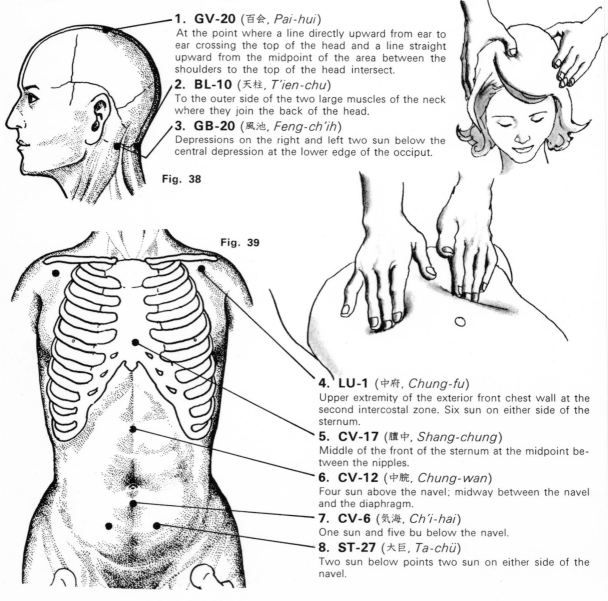

1. GV-20 (百会, *Pai-hui*)
At the point where a line directly upward from ear to ear crossing the top of the head and a line straight upward from the midpoint of the area between the shoulders to the top of the head intersect.

2. BL-10 (天柱, *T'ien-chu*)
To the outer side of the two large muscles of the neck where they join the back of the head.

3. GB-20 (風池, *Feng-ch'ih*)
Depressions on the right and left two sun below the central depression at the lower edge of the occiput.

Fig. 38

Fig. 39

4. LU-1 (中府, *Chung-fu*)
Upper extremity of the exterior front chest wall at the second intercostal zone. Six sun on either side of the sternum.

5. CV-17 (膻中, *Shang-chung*)
Middle of the front of the sternum at the midpoint between the nipples.

6. CV-12 (中脘, *Chung-wan*)
Four sun above the navel; midway between the navel and the diaphragm.

7. CV-6 (気海, *Ch'i-hai*)
One sun and five bu below the navel.

8. ST-27 (大巨, *Ta-chü*)
Two sun below points two sun on either side of the navel.

---

9. GV-14 (大椎, *Ta-ch'ui*)

At the base of the neck in the back between the spinal projections of the seventh cervical and the first thoracic vertebra.

10. BL-13 (肺俞, *Fei-yü*)

One sun and five bu on either side of the spinal column at points below the third thoracic vertebra.

11. BL-18 (肝俞, *Kan-yü*)

One sun and five bu on either side of the spinal column at points below the spinal projections of the ninth thoracic vertebra.

12. GV-8 (筋縮, *Chin-so*)

Below the spinal projections of the ninth thoracic vertebra; between BL-18.

13. BL-23 (腎俞, *Shen-yü*)

One sun and five bu on either side of the spinal column at points below the spinal projections of the second lumbar vertebra, which is located at the height of the lowest ribs.

14. GV-4 (命門, *Ming-men*)

Below the spinal projections of the second lumbar vertebra; between BL-23.

15. BL-47 (志室, *Chih-shih*)

Three sun on either side of the spinal column at points below the spinal projections of the second lumbar vertebra; on the outer sides of BL-23.

16. BL-26 (関元俞, *Kuan-yüan-yü*)

One sun and five bu on either side of the spinal column at points below the spinal projections of the fifth lumbar vertebra.

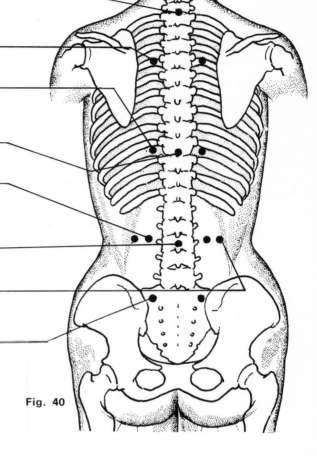

Fig. 40

17. LI-11 (曲池, *Ch'ü-ch'ih*)

Thumb side of the bend of the elbow.

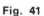

Fig. 41

18. LI-4 (合谷, *Ho-ku*)

The point exactly between the thumb and index finger on the back side of the hand.

19. ST-36 (足三里, *Tsu-san-li*)

On the outer side of the calf three sun below the knee. Outer edge of the shin bone.

20. LV-3 (太衝, *T'ai-ch'ung*)

Two sun upward on the instep from the crotch between the first and second toes.

Fig. 42

21. KI-9 (築賓, *Chu-pin*)

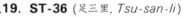

In the muscle that is the width of the index finger inward from the edge of the shin at a point five sun above the inner side of the ankle.

22. KI-3 (太谿, *T'ai-hsi*)

Rear part of the inside of the ankle.

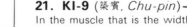

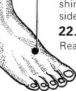

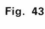

Fig. 43

(9) Increasing Powers of Concentration

Stimuli delivered to the nervous system by the sensory organs become material for memory. The human brain matures more quickly than some of the other organs. Consequently, it must be put to active use early if it is to fulfill its potential. The powers to concentrate and to remember depend on the brain, but they can be greatly influenced by external stimuli of all kinds. For instances, illness can sharply diminish an individual's powers of concentration. This is especially true when a sickness that has not yet been diagnosed preys on a patient's mind, making him fear that he is sicker than he is. In such instances, of course, the thing to do is to have a physician discover the cause of the trouble and set the patient's mind at rest by telling him the scientific truth.

Although it is impossible to increase the powers of a developed brain, ability to concentrate and remember can be strengthened by making maximum use of the brains' potential. This is best accomplished by providing as much intellectual, emotional, and rational stimulation as possible.

Sometimes illness—tuberculosis, gastritis, colitis, hepatitis, diabetes, disturbances of the thyroid glands, high blood pressure, alcoholism, brain tumor, whiplash syndrome, empyema, and so on—reduce powers of concentration. If the sickness is one that medical methods can treat, consult a physician and accelerate recovery by removing as many aggravations as possible from the patient's daily life. This will relieve irritability, enable the patient to sleep, eliminate headaches, and prevent him from feeling persecuted and depressed. When all of this has been done, the patient will once again be able to concentrate and will find that he is able to lead a well-ordered life. Oriental therapy on the tsubo shown in Figs. 44 through 50 facilitates the achievement of these aims.

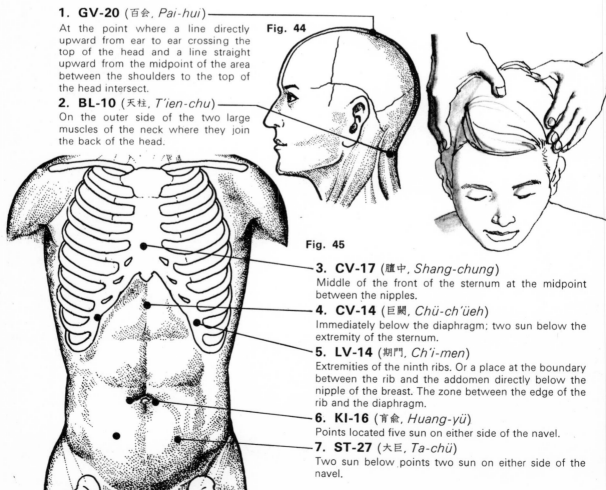

1. GV-20 (百会, *Pai-hui*)

At the point where a line directly upward from ear to ear crossing the top of the head and a line straight upward from the midpoint of the area between the shoulders to the top of the head intersect.

2. BL-10 (天柱, *T'ien-chu*)

On the outer side of the two large muscles of the neck where they join the back of the head.

Fig. 44

Fig. 45

3. CV-17 (膻中, *Shang-chung*)

Middle of the front of the sternum at the midpoint between the nipples.

4. CV-14 (巨闕, *Chü-ch'üeh*)

Immediately below the diaphragm; two sun below the extremity of the sternum.

5. LV-14 (期門, *Ch'i-men*)

Extremities of the ninth ribs. Or a place at the boundary between the rib and the addomen directly below the nipple of the breast. The zone between the edge of the rib and the diaphragm.

6. KI-16 (肓兪, *Huang-yü*)

Points located five sun on either side of the navel.

7. ST-27 (大巨, *Ta-chü*)

Two sun below points two sun on either side of the navel.

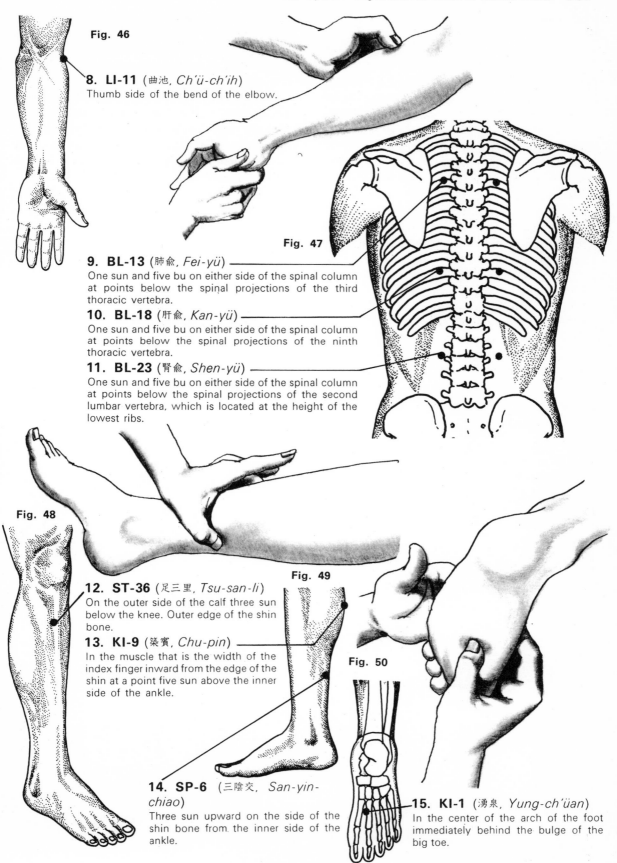

Fig. 46

8. LI-11 (曲池, *Ch'ü-ch'ih*)
Thumb side of the bend of the elbow.

Fig. 47

9. BL-13 (肺俞, *Fei-yü*)
One sun and five bu on either side of the spinal column at points below the spinal projections of the third thoracic vertebra.

10. BL-18 (肝俞, *Kan-yü*)
One sun and five bu on either side of the spinal column at points below the spinal projections of the ninth thoracic vertebra.

11. BL-23 (腎俞, *Shen-yü*)
One sun and five bu on either side of the spinal column at points below the spinal projections of the second lumbar vertebra, which is located at the height of the lowest ribs.

Fig. 48

Fig. 49

12. ST-36 (足三里, *Tsu-san-li*)
On the outer side of the calf three sun below the knee. Outer edge of the shin bone.

13. KI-9 (築賓, *Chu-pin*)
In the muscle that is the width of the index finger inward from the edge of the shin at a point five sun above the inner side of the ankle.

Fig. 50

14. SP-6 (三陰交, *San-yin-chiao*)
Three sun upward on the side of the shin bone from the inner side of the ankle.

15. KI-1 (湧泉, *Yung-ch'üan*)
In the center of the arch of the foot immediately behind the bulge of the big toe.

Cosmetic Treatments

(1) Eliminating Facial Wrinkles

The tissues of the muscles and skin in the face are closely interwoven, instead of being entirely separate, as they are in the other parts of the body. This means that highly active parts of the face—the ends of the eyes, the forehead, and the area from the chin to the neck—wrinkle easily in persons of more than thirty years of age unless extremely good care is taken to prevent this phenomenon. The facial skin wrinkles more noticeably in people whose skin is thin. Thick skin preserves nutrients and oils; thin skin, because it cannot do this, is often dry and wrinkled. The following treatment helps prevent wrinkling in the face. It must be performed regularly and over the entire area of facial skin; that is, from the hairline to the base of the neck.

Perform shiatsu massage on BL-2, TH-23, GB-1, and BL-1 (Fig. 1). At the same time, using the thumbs and index fingers, massage the upper and lower edges of the eye sockets from the inside in an outward, radial pattern from ST-2 (Fig. 2). The most important tsubo for removing wrinkles from the forehead is GB-14 (Fig. 3), located slightly above the middle of the eyebrow. Massage and stroke with the fingertips from this tsubo in the direction of the arrows; that is, right and left toward the temples from the center of the forehead and to the hairline. Continue the therapy by massaging in the areas of ST-8 and GB-7 and from the hairline to the ears (Fig. 4). Next massage at the right and left corners of the mouth (Fig. 5). To massage the neck, spread the thumbs and fingers fully, raise the chin as high as possible, and massage the tsubo on the neck. The massage must extend to the base of the neck. If there is no one to assist you, use your left hand in massaging the right of the neck and your right hand in massaging the left. Conclude the treatment by standing in front of a mirror and making many faces in order to exercise the facial muscles.

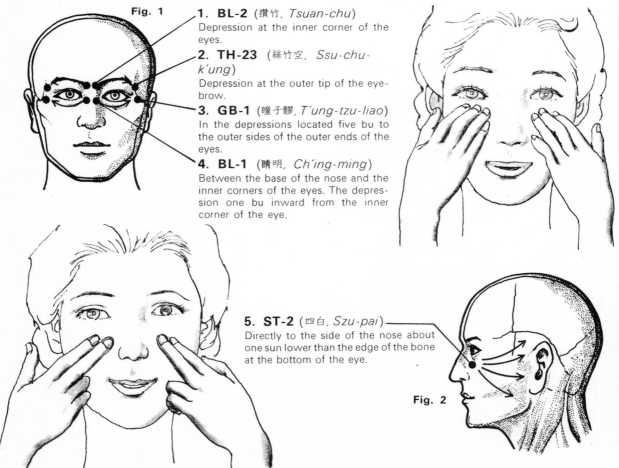

Fig. 1

1. BL-2 (攅竹, *Tsuan-chu*)
Depression at the inner corner of the eyes.

2. TH-23 (絲竹空, *Ssu-chu-k'ung*)
Depression at the outer tip of the eyebrow.

3. GB-1 (瞳子髎, *T'ung-tzu-liao*)
In the depressions located five bu to the outer sides of the outer ends of the eyes.

4. BL-1 (睛明, *Ch'ing-ming*)
Between the base of the nose and the inner corners of the eyes. The depression one bu inward from the inner corner of the eye.

5. ST-2 (四白, *Szu-pai*)
Directly to the side of the nose about one sun lower than the edge of the bone at the bottom of the eye.

Fig. 2

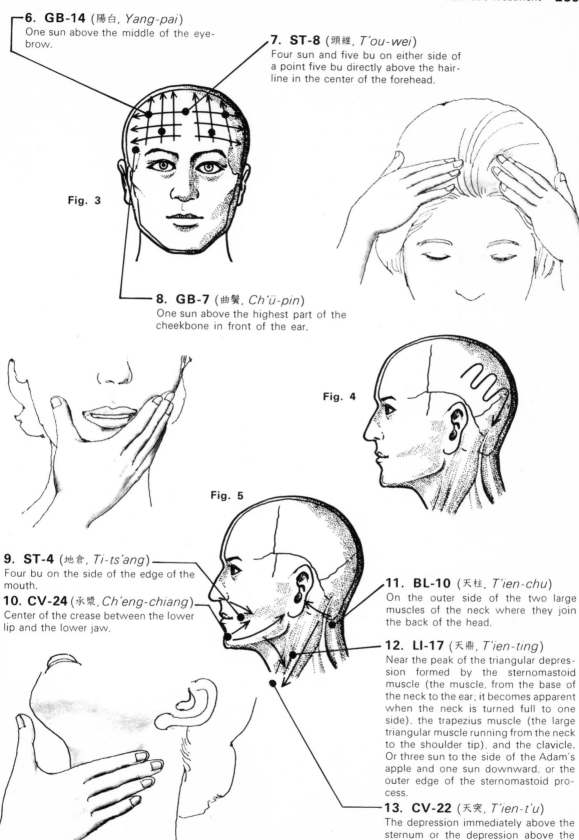

6. GB-14 (陽白, *Yang-pai*)
One sun above the middle of the eyebrow.

7. ST-8 (頭維, *T'ou-wei*)
Four sun and five bu on either side of a point five bu directly above the hairline in the center of the forehead.

Fig. 3

8. GB-7 (曲鬢, *Ch'ü-pin*)
One sun above the highest part of the cheekbone in front of the ear.

Fig. 4

Fig. 5

9. ST-4 (地倉, *Ti-ts'ang*)
Four bu on the side of the edge of the mouth.

10. CV-24 (承漿, *Ch'eng-chiang*)
Center of the crease between the lower lip and the lower jaw.

11. BL-10 (天柱, *T'ien-chu*)
On the outer side of the two large muscles of the neck where they join the back of the head.

12. LI-17 (天鼎, *T'ien-ting*)
Near the peak of the triangular depression formed by the sternomastoid muscle (the muscle, from the base of the neck to the ear; it becomes apparent when the neck is turned full to one side), the trapezius muscle (the large triangular muscle running from the neck to the shoulder tip), and the clavicle. Or three sun to the side of the Adam's apple and one sun downward, or the outer edge of the sternomastoid process.

13. CV-22 (天突, *T'ien-t'u*)
The depression immediately above the sternum or the depression above the midpoint between the clavicles.

(2) Treating Pimples

Almost all young people go through a phase in which their faces break out in pimples. These unsightly spots are a cause of embarrassment and suffering to the young person and an unpleasant spectacle for people around him. The causes of the condition are highly complicated. Pimples may be the result of irregularities in hormone secretions, upset of vitamin balance, disorders in the digestive or autonomic nervous systems, excessively oily skin, or sometimes bacterial infection. At first, red bumps develop on the face, arms, and back. Later, as the young person undergoes the physiological changes accompanying sexual maturity, the pimples appear and disappear with relative regularity. In very serious cases, the pimples fester and sometimes leave ugly reddish-blackish stains on, or even pits in, the skin. Festering pimples are painful. Frequently, people must consult a physician to treat stubborn cases of pimples; but, in most instances, when puberty has passed, the condition clears up by itself.

Oriental tsubo therapy strives to relieve the emotional and physical discomfort of pimples by putting the entire physical organism in good condition. When the body is functioning normally, pimples are less likely to occur. The most important tsubo for this kind of treatment are GV-4 and BL-23 (Fig. 6). Perform thorough shiatsu massage on these two, both of which are related to restoring to the body the vigor and strength that is innate to it. To stimulate the functioning of the digestive system, massage BL-22 and CV-12 (Fig. 7). Shiatsu on BL-13, BL-18, and BL-20 invigorates the skin and muscles. Thorough shiatsu on LU-1, LV-14, and KI-16 (Fig. 7) is excellent for the skin and muscles

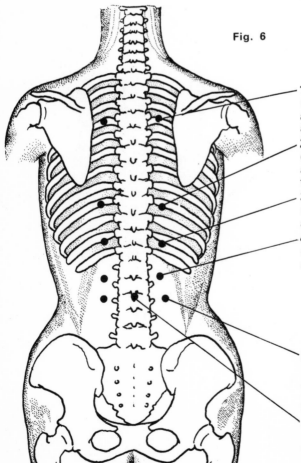

Fig. 6

1. BL-13 (肺兪, *Fei-yü*)
One sun and five bu on either side of the spinal column at points below the spinal projections of the third thoracic vertebra.

2. BL-18 (肝兪, *Kan-yü*)
One sun and five bu on either side of the spinal column at points below the spinal projections of the ninth thoracic vertebra.

3. BL-20 (脾兪, *P'i-yü*)
One sun and five bu on either side of the spinal column at points below the eleventh thoracic vertebra.

4. BL-22 (三焦兪, *San-chiao-yü*)
One sun and five bu on either side of the spinal column at points below the first lumbar vertebra.

5. BL-23 (腎兪, *Shen-yü*)
One sun and five bu on either side of the spinal column at points below the spinal projections of the second lumbar vertebra, which is located at the height of the lowest ribs.

6. GV-4 (命門, *Ming-men*)
Between BL-23 and below the spinal projections of the second lumbar vertebra.

since these tsubo are related to the liver and spleen, which, according to ancient oriental thought, control the condition of the muscles and skin.

Moxa combustion is effective in situations of this kind; but, since it can disfigure the skin, it is not recommended for women. People who are constipated are subject to attacks of pimples. Take care to guard against constipation and to treat for it should it occur (see p. 108). Shiatsu on SI-6 (Fig. 8) is effective against carbuncles.

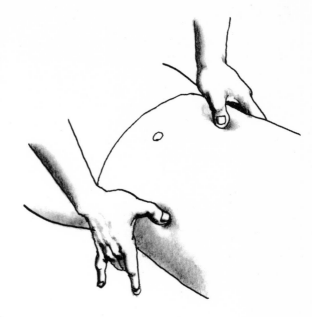

Fig. 7

7. LU-1 (中府, *Chung-fu*)
Upper extremity of the exterior front chest wall at the second intercostal zone. Six sun on either side of the sternum.

8. LV-14 (期門, *Ch'i-men*)
Extremities of the ninth ribs. Or a place located at the boundary between the rib and the abdomen directly below the nipple of the breast. The zone between the edge of the rib and the diaphragm.

9. CV-12 (中脘, *Chung-wan*)
Four sun above the navel; midway between the navel and the diaphragm.

10. KI-16 (肓兪, *Huang-yü*)
Points located five sun on either side of the navel.

11. SI-6 (養老, *Yang-lao*)
Depression in the upper surface of the wrist.

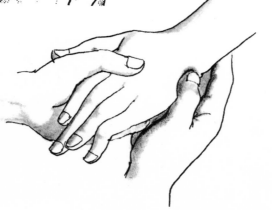

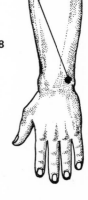

Fig. 8

(3) Discolorations and Freckles

Women who are very much concerned about their appearance are often distressed by such discolorations of the facial skin as birthmarks, moles, and freckles. A wide range of elements may contribute to the development of these marks. Direct sunlight, overwork, menstruation, ovulation, uterine illnesses, upsets in the suprarenal cortex, liver troubles, emotional disturbances, and so on can be the causes of, or can intensify, these spots. When a definite cause is known, the advice and treatment of a specialist are required. It is not unusual, however, for discolorations and freckles to arise for no apparent reason. In such instances, the person must avoid direct sunlight —which often brings on or darkens freckles— must get plently of rest, and must not overwork. In some people with pale skin, freckles are hereditary. They become more numerous in the summer when the skin is exposed to direct sunlight.

Oriental tsubo therapy cannot suddenly make skin discolorations disappear. It can, however, minimize the manifestations of such discolorations by promoting total and general good physical condition. To this end, shiatsu and massage on the following tsubo are effective: BL-22, BL-23, GV-4 (Fig. 9), CV-17, CV-12 ,CV-7 (Fig. 10), TH-4 (Fig. 11), and KI-3 (Fig. 12).

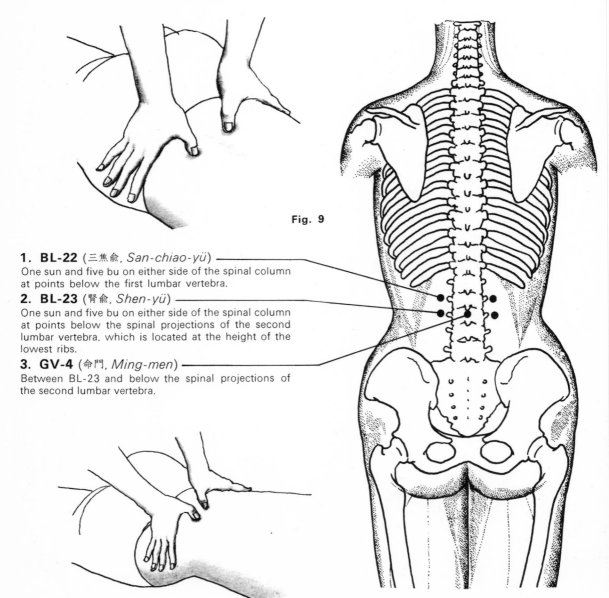

Fig. 9

1. BL-22 (三焦兪, *San-chiao-yü*) ——————
One sun and five bu on either side of the spinal column at points below the first lumbar vertebra.

2. BL-23 (腎兪, *Shen-yü*) ——————
One sun and five bu on either side of the spinal column at points below the spinal projections of the second lumbar vertebra, which is located at the height of the lowest ribs.

3. GV-4 (命門, *Ming-men*) ——————
Between BL-23 and below the spinal projections of the second lumbar vertebra.

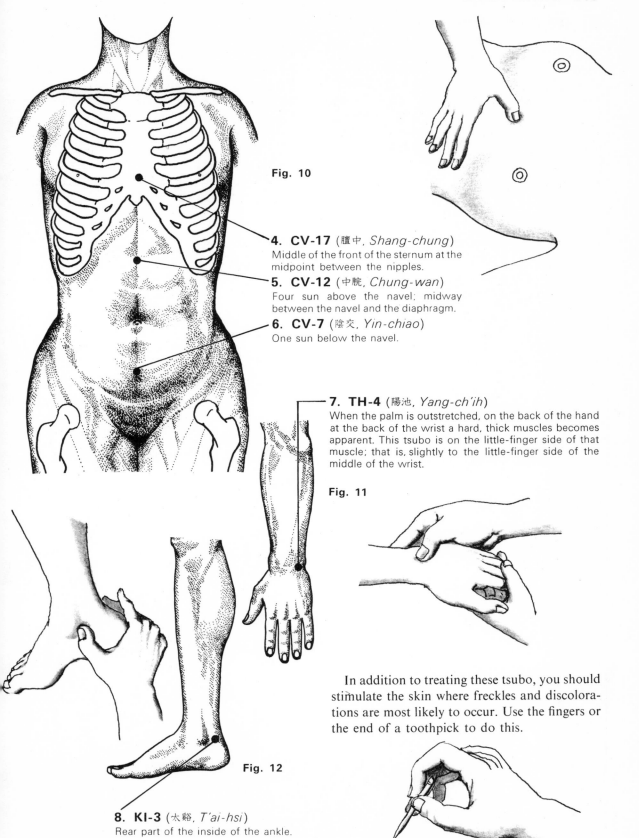

Fig. 10

4. CV-17 (膻中, *Shang-chung*)
Middle of the front of the sternum at the midpoint between the nipples.

5. CV-12 (中脘, *Chung-wan*)
Four sun above the navel; midway between the navel and the diaphragm.

6. CV-7 (陰交, *Yin-chiao*)
One sun below the navel.

7. TH-4 (陽池, *Yang-ch'ih*)
When the palm is outstretched, on the back of the hand at the back of the wrist a hard, thick muscles becomes apparent. This tsubo is on the little-finger side of that muscle; that is, slightly to the little-finger side of the middle of the wrist.

Fig. 11

In addition to treating these tsubo, you should stimulate the skin where freckles and discolorations are most likely to occur. Use the fingers or the end of a toothpick to do this.

Fig. 12

8. KI-3 (太谿, *T'ai-hsi*)
Rear part of the inside of the ankle.

(4) Adding Luster to the Hair

When the hair is lusterless and tends to fall out or break easily, the cause may be either internal or external. Fevers and other sicknesses sometimes cause falling or unhealthy hair. Bacteria—for instance, trichophytons—attack from the outside and ruin the condition of hair. In instances of such sickness, consult a specialist at once. But the way to keep hair healthy is to ensure adequate nourishment to the roots and to regulate the functioning of the autonomic nervous system. Treatment on the tsubo listed below can assist in doing these things.

BL-22 and BL-23 (Fig. 13) are especially important in this connection because they help control the use of the energy the body receives before and after birth. Although shiatsu, massage, and acupuncture are good too, moxa combustion is most effective. Other tsubo that provide excellent places for therapy designed to improve body strength and condition and thus to add luster and beauty to the hair are these: CV-17, CV-12, CV-7, CV-4 (Fig. 15), TH-4, (Fig. 16), and KI-3 (Fig. 17). And, using both hands and exerting a fairly great degree of pressure, massage the tsubo in Fig. 14.

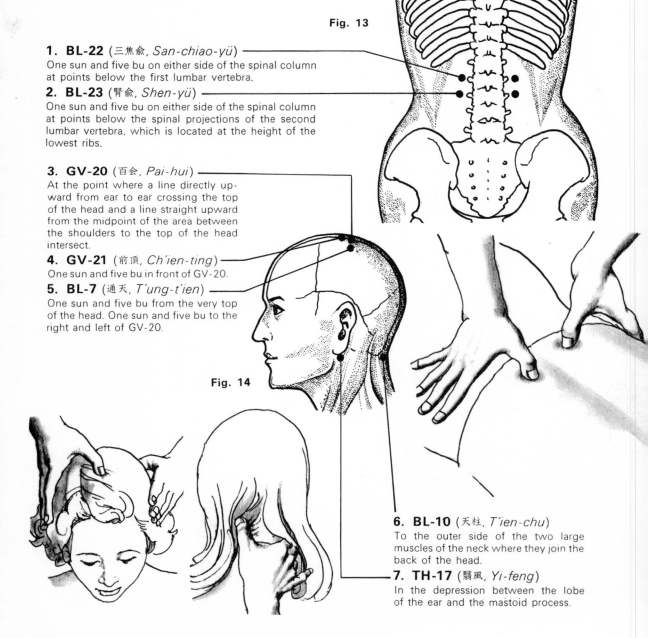

Fig. 13

1. BL-22 (三焦兪, *San-chiao-yü*)
One sun and five bu on either side of the spinal column at points below the first lumbar vertebra.

2. BL-23 (腎兪, *Shen-yü*)
One sun and five bu on either side of the spinal column at points below the spinal projections of the second lumbar vertebra, which is located at the height of the lowest ribs.

3. GV-20 (百会, *Pai-hui*)
At the point where a line directly upward from ear to ear crossing the top of the head and a line straight upward from the midpoint of the area between the shoulders to the top of the head intersect.

4. GV-21 (前頂, *Ch'ien-ting*)
One sun and five bu in front of GV-20.

5. BL-7 (通天, *T'ung-t'ien*)
One sun and five bu from the very top of the head. One sun and five bu to the right and left of GV-20.

Fig. 14

6. BL-10 (天柱, *T'ien-chu*)
To the outer side of the two large muscles of the neck where they join the back of the head.

7. TH-17 (翳風, *Yi-feng*)
In the depression between the lobe of the ear and the mastoid process.

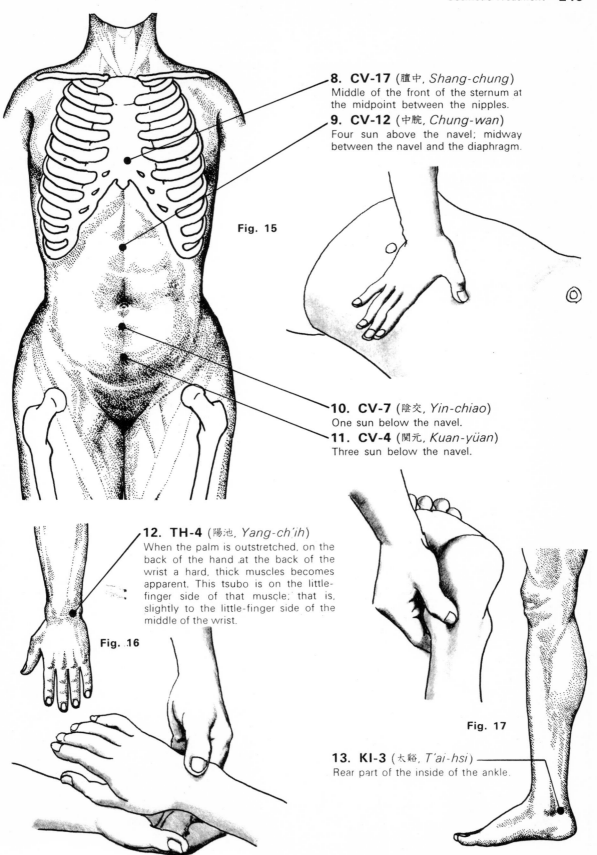

8. CV-17 (膻中, *Shang-chung*)
Middle of the front of the sternum at the midpoint between the nipples.

9. CV-12 (中脘, *Chung-wan*)
Four sun above the navel; midway between the navel and the diaphragm.

Fig. 15

10. CV-7 (陰交, *Yin-chiao*)
One sun below the navel.

11. CV-4 (関元, *Kuan-yüan*)
Three sun below the navel.

12. TH-4 (陽池, *Yang-ch'ih*)
When the palm is outstretched, on the back of the hand at the back of the wrist a hard, thick muscles becomes apparent. This tsubo is on the little-finger side of that muscle; that is, slightly to the little-finger side of the middle of the wrist.

Fig. 16

Fig. 17

13. KI-3 (太谿, *T'ai-hsi*)
Rear part of the inside of the ankle.

(5) Developing the Breasts

Size, proportions, texture, and shape are all important aspects of the beauty of the female breasts. To improve the loveliness of the bust, it is important to improve the conditions of the chest muscles. Since the chest, shoulders, and arms are closely related to each other, exercising the latter two does much to exercise—consequently to beautify—the chest and the breasts. To round out an ideal regimen for the beautification of the bust, it is good to combine such exercise with massage or shiatsu on the tsubo listed below. This total system is not magical. It cannot ensure swelling bustlines in short times. The beautiful body is one that is healthy, that curves outward where it should, and that is slender and graceful elsewhere. The tsubo that can assist in developing this kind of body are as follows: GV-12, BL-15, and BL-17 (Fig. 19). Therapy on these tsubo cures round shoulders and, by doing no more than this, greatly improves the lines of these tsubo cures round shoulders and, by doing no more than this, greatly improves the lines of the bust. Stroking massage on LU-1, GB-23, SP-18, KI-23, CV-17 (Fig. 18), and GB-22 (Fig. 19) helps supply nourishment to the breasts. Finally, regulate the action of the stomach, relieve constipation and help make menstruation normal by massaging in the area of CV-14, CV-12, ST-25, and CV-4 (Fig. 20). This too helps develop both the muscles and the skin of the breasts.

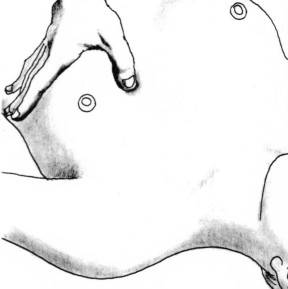

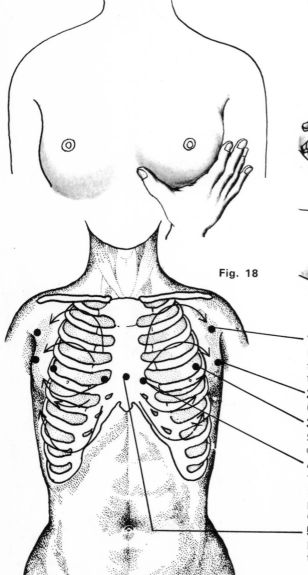

Fig. 18

1. LU-1 (中府, *Chung-fu*)
Upper extremity of the exterior front chest wall at the second intercostal zone. Six sun on either side of the sternum.

2. GB-23 (輙筋, *Ch'e-chin*)
One sun behind SP-18; one sun in front of GB-22.

3. SP-18 (天谿, *T'ien-hsi*)
Slightly below the fourth ribs two sun to the outer sides of the nipples.

4. KI-23 (神封, *Shen-feng*)
Two sun to the right and left of the sternum slightly below the fourth ribs. Or points at the height of the nipples two sun to the right and left of a line from the base of the throat to the diaphragm.

5. CV-17 (膻中, *Shang-chung*)
Middle of the front of the sternum at the midpoint between the nipples.

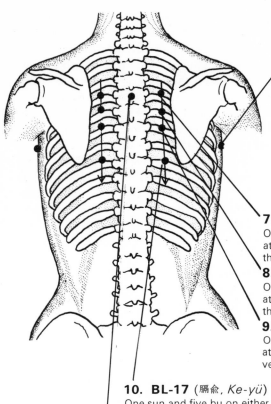

6. GB-22 (淵腋, *Yüan-yeh*)
In the armpit between the fourth and fifth ribs. Behind LU-1.

Fig. 19

7. BL-13 (肺俞, *Fei-yü*)
One sun and five bu on either side of the spinal column at points below the spinal projections of the third thoracic vertebra.

8. BL-14 (厥陰俞, *Chüeh-yin-yü*)
One sun and five bu on either side of the spinal column at points below the spinal projections of the fourth thoracic vertebra.

9. BL-15 (心俞, *Hsin-yü*)
One sun and five bu on either side of the spinal column at points below the spinal projections of the fifth thoracic vertebra.

10. BL-17 (膈俞, *Ke-yü*)
One sun and five bu on either side of the spinal column at points below the seventh thoracic vertebra.

11. GV-12 (身柱, *Shen-chu*)
Below the spinal projections of the third thoracic vertebra.

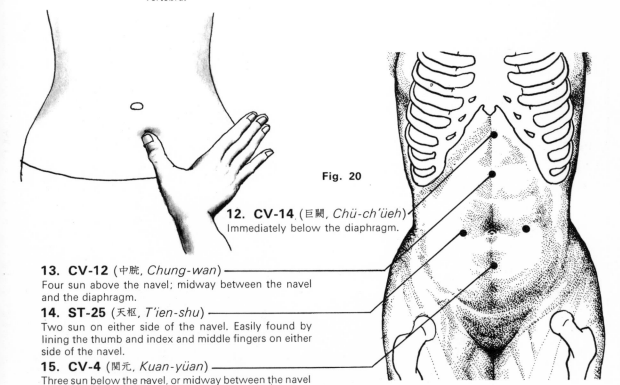

Fig. 20

12. CV-14 (巨闕, *Chü-ch'üeh*)
Immediately below the diaphragm.

13. CV-12 (中脘, *Chung-wan*)
Four sun above the navel; midway between the navel and the diaphragm.

14. ST-25 (天枢, *T'ien-shu*)
Two sun on either side of the navel. Easily found by lining the thumb and index and middle fingers on either side of the navel.

15. CV-4 (関元, *Kuan-yüan*)
Three sun below the navel, or midway between the navel and the pubis.

(6) Beautifying the Skin

Women tend to have less oily skins than men. Indeed, bright oily skin occurs only in young girls. In women of greater age, the skin is likely to be dry and therefore susceptible to wrinkles, cracks, and other disfigurements, most of which are more prevalent among people whose skin is thin. Diets low in fats reduce the oil in women's skin still further. To beautify the skin, it is necessary to take full advantage of the natural strength of the body. Massage on BL-23 (Fig. 22) helps do this. Treatment on BL-22, ST-9 (Fig. 21), CV-12 (Fig. 23), TH-4 (Fig. 24), and KI-3 (Fig. 25) are important in allowing the body to make use of the foods that it takes in for the sake of energy. For this reason, it is important for the preservation of a beautiful skin, which depends on sound nourishment. Because it causes gas and other wastes to accumulate, constipation is especially bad for the skin. Guard against it and treat for it as explained on p. 108 should it occur.

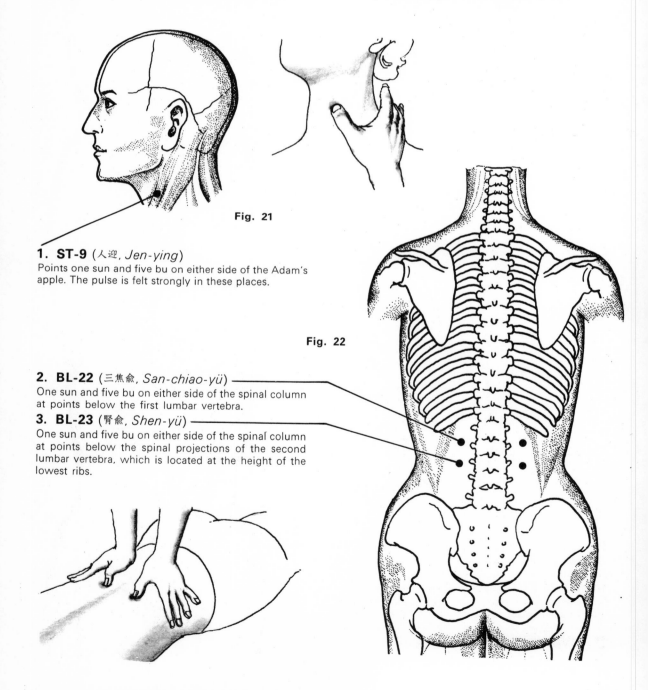

Fig. 21

1. ST-9 (人迎, *Jen-ying*)
Points one sun and five bu on either side of the Adam's apple. The pulse is felt strongly in these places.

Fig. 22

2. BL-22 (三焦兪, *San-chiao-yü*)
One sun and five bu on either side of the spinal column at points below the first lumbar vertebra.

3. BL-23 (腎兪, *Shen-yü*)
One sun and five bu on either side of the spinal column at points below the spinal projections of the second lumbar vertebra, which is located at the height of the lowest ribs.

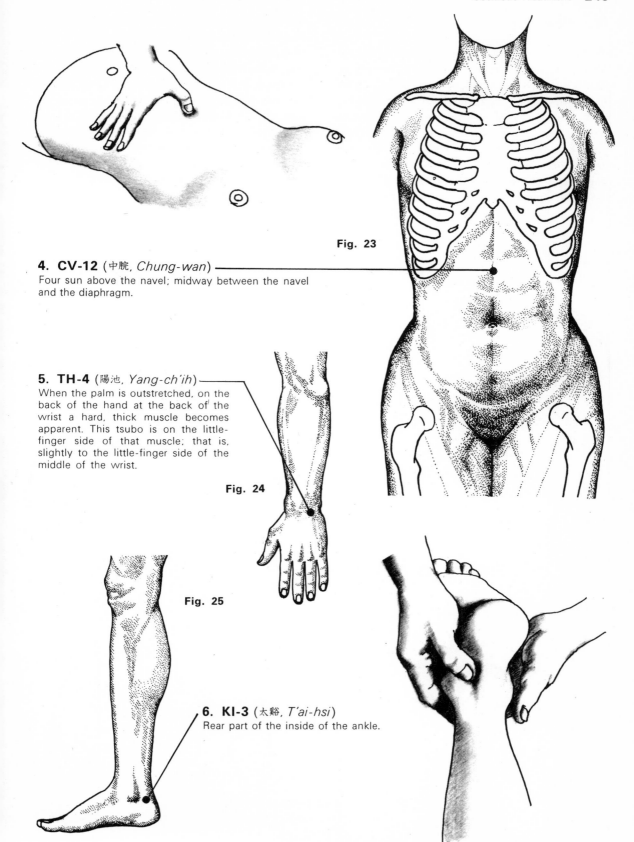

Fig. 23

4. CV-12 (中脘, *Chung-wan*)
Four sun above the navel; midway between the navel
and the diaphragm.

5. TH-4 (陽池, *Yang-ch'ih*)
When the palm is outstretched, on the
back of the hand at the back of the
wrist a hard, thick muscle becomes
apparent. This tsubo is on the little-
finger side of that muscle; that is,
slightly to the little-finger side of the
middle of the wrist.

Fig. 24

Fig. 25

6. KI-3 (太谿, *T'ai-hsi*)
Rear part of the inside of the ankle.

(7) **Reducing**

In some cases, overweight is the result of assignable pathological upsets in the endocrine system. When this is true, the patient must consult a physician. In this section, I am talking about the kind of overweight, generally brought on by excess caloric consumption, that is more a cosmetic than a health problem. The places on the female body where fat is most likely to accumulate are the lines from the chin along both sides of the body to the breasts, the zones around the abdomen and hips at the level immediately below the navel, the thighs, the areas behind the knees, and the ankles. Help prevent fat from accumulating in these places by means of regular oriental massage on the following tsubo: BL-22, BL-23, BL-50 (Fig. 26), BL-60 (Fig. 27), LU-1, CV-12, GB-29, CV-4, SP-10, ST-34 (Fig. 28), BL-54, BL-57, KI-1 (Fig. 29), SP-8, and KI-3 (Fig. 30). Using either the palms of the hands or the four fingers of each hand, massage in these areas, paying special attention to the soft zones between muscles.

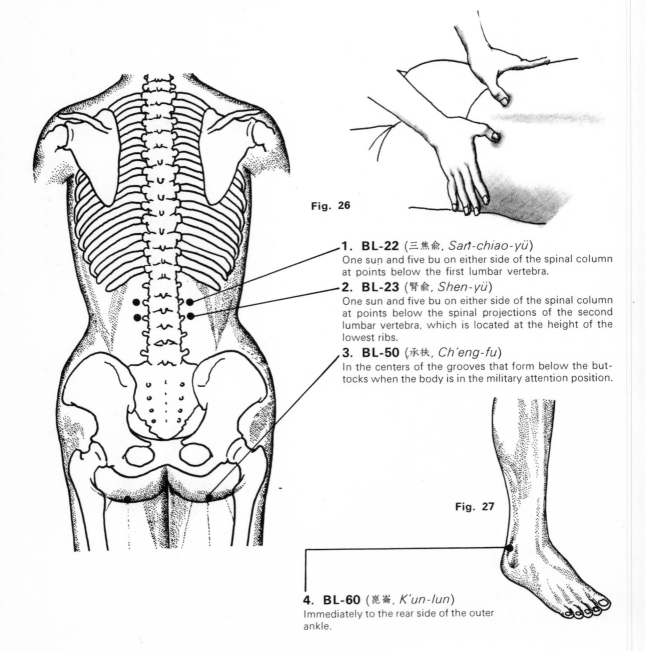

Fig. 26

1. BL-22 (三焦兪, *Sań-chiao-yü*)
One sun and five bu on either side of the spinal column at points below the first lumbar vertebra.

2. BL-23 (腎兪, *Shen-yü*)
One sun and five bu on either side of the spinal column at points below the spinal projections of the second lumbar vertebra, which is located at the height of the lowest ribs.

3. BL-50 (承扶, *Ch'eng-fu*)
In the centers of the grooves that form below the buttocks when the body is in the military attention position.

Fig. 27

4. BL-60 (崑崙, *K'un-lun*)
Immediately to the rear side of the outer ankle.

5. LU-1 (中府, *Chung-fu*)
Upper extremity of the exterior front chest wall at the second intercostal zone. Six sun on either side of the sternum.

Fig. 28

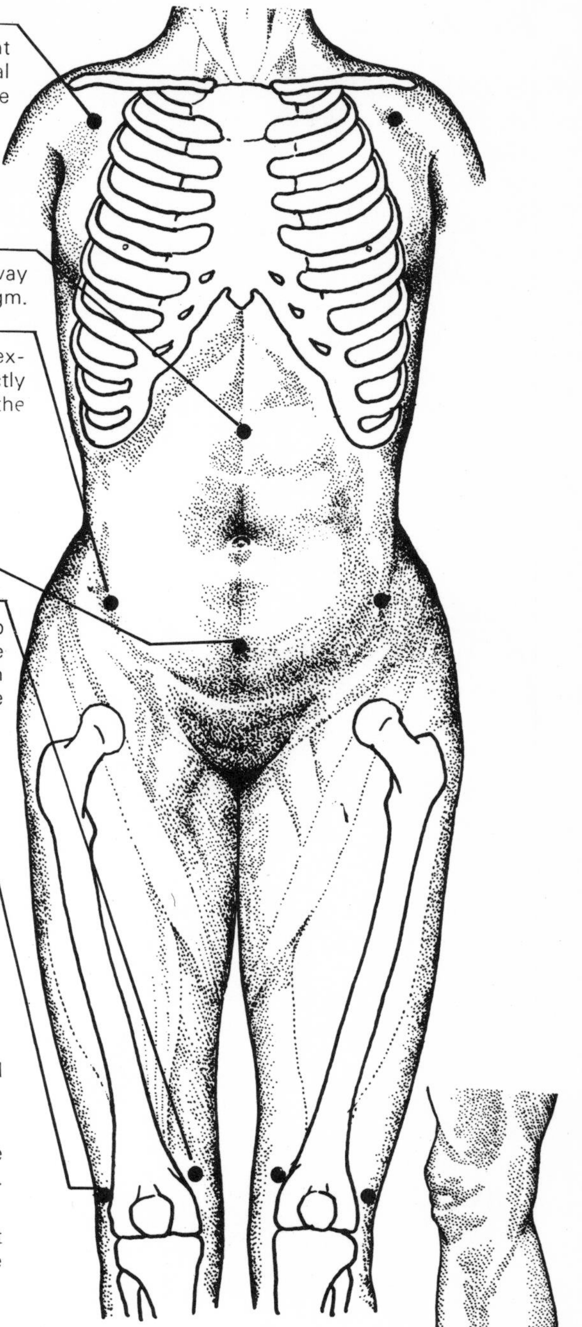

6. CV-12 (中脘, *Chung-wan*)
Four sun above the navel; midway between the navel and the diaphragm.

7. GB-29 (居髎, *Chü-liao*)
Eight sun and three bu below the extremities of the eleventh ribs. Exactly in the middle, but somewhat to the rear, of the hucklebone.

8. CV-4 (関元, *Kuan-yüan*)
Three sun below the navel.

9. SP-10 (血海, *Hsüeh-hai*)
Two sun and five bu above the kneecap on the inner side of the thigh. The place where a depression is formed two sun and five bu above the knee when the leg is outstretched.

10. ST-34 (梁丘, *Liang-chiu*)
Two sun above the upper edge of the kneecap. This can be easily located by fully extending the knee and finding the upper end of the groove formed on the outside of the kneecap. In other words, it is on the front of the thigh, two sun above the upper outer edge of the kneecap.

Fig. 29

11. BL-54 (委中, *Wei-ch'ung*)
In the center of the groove formed behind the knee.

12. BL-57 (承山, *Cheng-shan*)
At the point where the muscle of the calf narrows to the Achilles' tendon.

13. KI-1 (湧泉, *Yung-ch'üan*)
In the center of the arch of the foot immediately behind the bulge of the big toe.

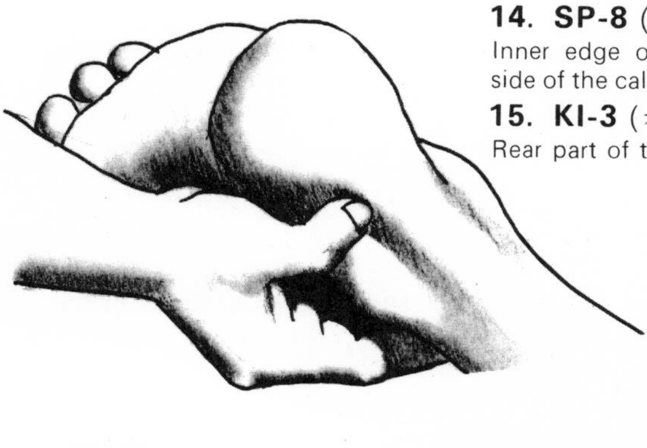

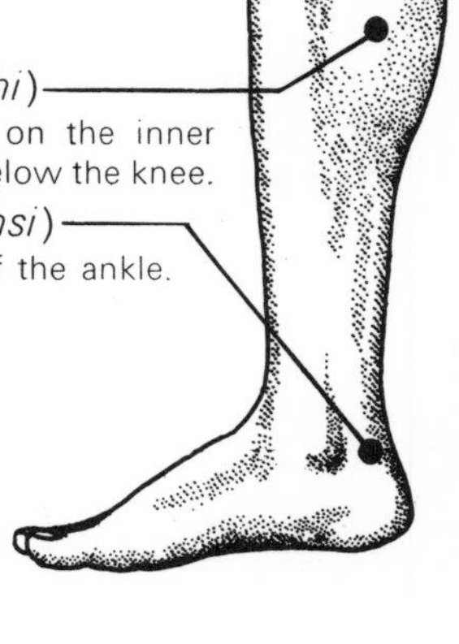

14. SP-8 (地機, *Ti-chi*)
Inner edge of the tibia on the inner side of the calf five sun below the knee.

15. KI-3 (太谿, *T'ai-hsi*)
Rear part of the inside of the ankle.

Fig. 30

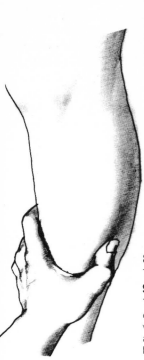
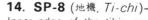

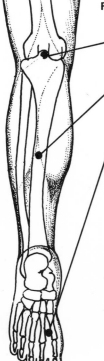

Index of Tsubo, Ailments, and Minor Complaints